The Live-it Lifestyle

Dropping Die-its Forever!

Ronnie Landis

INFINITY
PUBLISHING

ISBN 978-0-7414-7300-4

Printed in the United States of America

Published January 2013

Disclaimer: This book is being sold for informational purposes only and is not designed in any way to substitute a professionally licensed physician. This book is not intended as medical advice and should not be construed as such. The author, the publisher, nor the distributor of this material will be held responsible for the use, misuse, or the lack there of relating to this information. The author does not prescribe anything contained in this book as a treatment or cure for any illness and suggests the advice from a medical professional when reviewing health information. The author does not advocate the use of cooked, processed, denatured, and demineralized food in order to alleviate health crises.

INFINITY PUBLISHING
1094 New DeHaven Street, Suite 100
West Conshohocken, PA 19428-2713
Toll-free (877) BUY BOOK
Local Phone (610) 941-9999
Fax (610) 941-9959
Info@buybooksontheweb.com
www.buybooksontheweb.com

Ronnie Landis is the newest generation of superhero magical inspiration come to life. This is a man who not only humbly walks his talk, but also lives, breathes, and eats it! With bold eloquence, "The Live It Lifestyle: Dropping Diets Forever!" simply speaks the truth as would a grand master martial artist. This book is destined to become the Magna Carta of diet abolishment.

Sacred Steve Adler- Raw Chocolate Pioneer & Founder of Sacred Chocolate

Ronnie Landis shares his powerful message of health with such passion that you just know he is going to positively influence our world. He is bringing forth information that will no doubt awaken people on a grand scale, and delivering it in a way that those new to this uncompromising approach will want to grab hold of, and those who are within our community will make greater strides. There is really something to be said for a young man that exudes such charisma, deep knowledge, and ambition. I expect Ronnie's book will shake things up for the better as he undeniably speaks the truth.

Bethanne Wanamaker-Founder, EdibleGoddess.com, Co-Author, Superfood Beauty Elixirs & Co-Author, Thank God I: Stories of Inspiration for Every Situation, vol 3.

Ronnie is an amazing raw educator. His background in sports, nutrition, raw foods and super foods has given him some valuable information to share with many others.

Chef BeLive- Raw Food Cuisine Pioneer & Co-Author of 'Going Going Gone Raw'

Ronnie Landis is truly one of the finest examples of a New Breed of "Superhero" emerging today! Wise beyond his years, Ronnie is driven with an unbridled passion and determination to make his mark in the world by sharing his years of knowledge, research, and intuitive knowing in the field of Wellness Education. In this amazing book he is taking us on a journey into areas of Nutrition and Superfoods where few have gone before; a journey where truth, freedom, and optimal health can be discovered, and easily applied in each and every one of our lives. This is a "must read", and after doing so, you will become part of the Ripple Effect of "The Live It Lifestyle"!!!

Debra Cornell (alias Deb"Raw") -Certified Health Coach, Certified Raw Foods Chef and Instructor, Nutrition Educator, and Motivational Speaker, CHC, AADP

'As someone who knows first hand when things go wrong with your health, and how bad it can get, I encourage everyone to heed Ronnie Landis' words of wisdom shared in the LIVE IT LIFESTYLE. Whether you're seeking physical healing or are looking to optimize your health and/or lifestyle, there are valuable tools in this book that should not be missed.'

Carolyn Marie Solton- HHC, AADP, Owner/Director www.HealingNRG.org, Certified Raw Food Nutritionist, Author of DYING TO BE WELL

I first met Ronnie when he approached me about a book he was writing. He was incredibly excited about Raw Foods and the book he envisioned writing. I had seen so much of this enthusiasm in people, here one day and then gone in the next moment. However this was not the case with Ronnie. Just a few years before when I hit 50 years of age, I suffered from extreme obesity weighing in at 430 lbs. I also had Cancer, kidney problems, Diabetes, Acid Reflux Disease, High Blood Pressure and survived a heart Attack and Stroke. I was living on a DEAD FOOD DIET for my entire life from the time I was born. I was a bottle-fed baby. What I discovered at the age of 50 is something that Ronnie has discovered and latched onto at such an incredibly young age. This young man has completely changed his LIFE. He now lives a lifestyle that millions of others only dream of. Come and partake in LIFE ITSELF as you enter into a new dimension of life, reality, health and happiness that is yours for the taking !!!!! Thank you Ronnie for having the courage to help others...I say to people who read this:

Here is a sample of the next Generations Super Hero...Ronnie Landis.

Dave Conrardy, "The Raw Food Trucker"- Raw Food & Motivational Speaker

Ronnie Landis is a fresh and powerful new voice on the raw food scene. His passion and clarity make it obvious that he will succeed at his mission of bringing great light and health to the world.

~ Laura Chiraya Fox, Founder, Best of Raw and the Raw Living Expo

Dedications

To my mother who showed me what hard work and incredible resilience looks like. Even though we did not always see eye to eye, you never gave up on me or neglected me. You always supported my interests and worked over time to help me find my way. I love you!

To my grandmother who fought with me in the adolescent years. You knew how I felt deep down inside and did your very best to help guide me along. You encouraged me through this entire process. I understand who you are and how much you sacrificed so our family could have a better life.

To my grandfather who took the role of the father figure in my life. You showed me how to be self reliant and never stop striving for personal improvement. Your spirit lives deep inside of me and I hope my life is a adequate reflection of the invaluable lessons you left with me.

To Cher Till who entered my life for a brief period and left me with the confidence that I may utilize on this path. You whispered words of encouragement as I began this undertaking and your example will live on through me. Your work in the raw food community has blessed so many!

To Hoi Sauce who's uncompromising attention to detail has help to tranform this book into a work of art. Your editing has successfully allowed me to convey my message to all those who are introduced to this labor of love!

Foreword

Many seekers of higher health will scan and skim their way through the nutrition section of their local bookstore where they will soon find books on the latest gimmick diet programs to be pervasive throughout the shelves. It is my sincerest hope that they be lucky enough to find this particular book as it has the potential to serve as the primer in sparking your greater curiosity in this subject.

There are so many great books on this particular subject yet there are no books available on this particular subject all at the same time, as you the reader will soon discover. As you immerse yourself within the pages of this book, you will realize that this book is not limited to the subject as suggested by the category this book falls under. This book is the summation of Ronnie Landis' tireless efforts to collectively compile, condense, and compress years upon years of knowledge from the greatest minds to grace recorded history, sharing a broad range information from the most powerful success literature, philosophies, and comprehensive research that he decisively selected to be included in this work and to be applied into the concept of the "live it".

When I was initially approached to be the editor of this book I accepted this responsibility with great reluctance (despite being enticed by some of the most delicious homemade raw chocolates ever created) as I knew the task ahead of me would be to inspect, review, and polish four years worth of content. I must admit that I was intimidated by the thought of accepting such a task ahead me because I had no idea what I was getting myself into. I must say that I was accurate in my assessment; I really had no idea what I was getting myself into. However, do not be mistaken by my tone because I say this in a positive light!

As the pages turned in editing this work, I became deeply absorbed into the material, inspired by what Ronnie had diligently put into words. I hope you, the reader, will find it as obvious as I have that each chapter, section, page, and detail in this book was intimately constructed to provide you with the tools and knowledge to expand the boundaries of your beliefs and imagination on what is possible for your life and for your health. Drawing from the greatest minds, Ronnie has assembled a piece of literature that explores all facets that pertain to empowering you, which is ultimately the purpose of this book. In reviewing this book, I now consider all other books on health and nutrition that I have personally read to be one-dimensional in comparison. There really are no other works like this that have come before it as this book introduces you to pioneering concepts that would take several generations before any brick and mortar educational institutions to catch up to (if ever). The concepts presented within this book are so universal yet flexible enough that it will withstand the changing of the times, and will continue solidifying its validity as more people reach breakthroughs in their own health as they traverse the pages within. The database of knowledge in the 2nd Edition of The Live It Lifestyle has undergone a maturation process that I, the editor, have personally witnessed the author undergo in his own personal health quest. The author has subjected himself to the potential perils of this health quest so that you may see the rewards of embarking on this journey, and perhaps you will reap these same rewards as well. If you feel called to realize your own potential then read on.

Hoi Sauce 1/7/2013

Table of Contents

Introduction

"We can't know anything except our own experience.
Everything else is programming"
EL Ron Hubbard

This book is designed for those who want to know the truth behind nutrition, health, and a conscious approach to life style. This book is both practical and far reaching, it is an open invitation to expand ones mind with action steps presented along the way. This is a gift for those who are no longer entertained with the confusion and contradictions that have been delivered by the diet and health industries. Those who wish to activate true genius in every area of their lives, this book was written specifically for you. This is not a structured dietary program that promises short term gain at the expense of long term results. This is a deeply researched compilation of information infused with practical wisdom guaranteed to produce tangible results. You are the captain of your own ship, therefore this book acts as a manual which you may use to design your own unique lifestyle in any way you choose. This book is for the individual who identifies with their own greatness and values their life. This can be read by a complete beginner into nutrition, the intermediate student, and those who are advanced. All the information sealed within these pages is intended to plant the seeds of transformation. Some seeds sprout immediately, some take a bit longer to produce fruit. The goal is not to master this information right away, it is to allow a single idea to take ahold of you and see where it may take you. This is a journey, not only into your health, but into new and undiscovered possibilities for the rest of your life. I suggest you read this from beginning to end the first time through and revisit this material frequently as you may find new insights take shape.

For the student of health, nutrition, and wellness this book will serve as a powerful tool to expand your understanding of these subjects. We are exploring the long upheld theories of diet, raw food philosophy, the nature of disease, and the unquestioned scientific basis for these concepts. The information laid out here is direct and applicable yet it is also wrapped in a riddle that the reader must step by step solve in order to pull out deep insights for their own advancement. By applying this information I know you will not only reach for higher levels of health but you may notice the level of your intellect greatly improve. The sophistication of obstacles in our world call for us to activate a greater degree of sophistication towards their solutions. The over-simplification in the mainstream diet and medical model have actually dampened our abilities and reduced our consciousness. It is time to take back the noble ideal of self-accountability and venture into unexplored territory. That is what this book offers. You will produce great and even life transforming results if you dedicate yourself. Find key aspects of this book that speak to you and work them out as you would a muscle. Eventually it becomes second nature and what seemed impossible and far out of reach one day becomes a part of your unique lifestyle.

The Live-it Lifestyle

Life is a magnificent exploration that may never be adequately communicated or articulated with mere words, no matter how eloquently those words are delivered. Each breath is to be appreciated as if it were our last, to be held with great intention, and a released expression of all possibilities. The light we all have inside must be shown to the world; even if barely flickering, it can be reignited into a flurry of fireworks in likes the world has never seen but desperately is yearning to witness.

The live-it lifestyle is the idea that all of our thoughts, words, habits, choices, and associations can literally take us to any destination we choose. For endless generations, people have been inundated with the idea of struggling their way to the top of the mountain while pushing a boulder, in hopes of finally one day being rewarded for such a task. The results of such actions never seem to match the effort, yet people repeat these patterns haphazardly exhausting time, money, resources, health and relationships.

You are the creator of the masterpiece you call your life. You are a radiant beacon of potential untapped until this very moment. Within you is all the knowledge, wisdom, possibility, and skill sets of all of your ancestors, whether you know it or not. Whether you believe it or not, this energy is residing deep inside a reservoir of hope that what you are reading is accurate, and that you do have what it takes to eventually blaze a trail that will be followed by countless others who are inspired to march to the beat of their own drums. Just as Van Gogh, Leonardo Da Vinci, and William Shakespeare gifted the world works of art that can never be duplicated by human hands, you have the very same opportunity to explore the depths of your heart and uncover diamonds that may be deposited into the history books for all time. We can recall the great masters that have solidified their place in our memory because the work of these individuals is just as relevant now as it was in their own time. Each and everyone of us has the potential to be remembered for the work we leave behind, and it is our choice how we choose to be remembered that leads to life transformation!

The live-it lifestyle is a process of doing away with the problem orientation in our society that has plagued us with confusion, conflict, indirect communication, inner turmoil, dis-ease, and completely replacing it with solution-based mantras such as love, prosperity, responsibility, positive language, and a sense of well being that never seems to cease. The primary focus of this idea is centered in and around our food choices because the most common way we interface with our world is through eating. The planet we live on is tremendously impacted in many ways by what we eat, and because of this, we must consider the implications it may cause, depending on the direction we are choosing to go.

True living is all about passion, enthusiasm, joy, and an infectious engagement for each day. Since these qualities resemble the true nature of life, we focus primarily on living foods to bring this kind of vibrant energy out of each of us. Living foods are foods that are kept in their raw natural energetic state, filled with the touch of love from the dedicated farmer, and contain the vitality of the sun and earth.

All life transforms from seed to sprout under the sun, which is why someone who thrives from a lifestyle of primarily raw plant-based foods could be called a sun foodist. The sun is the contributor of all life, increasing feelings of wellness and ease to all who bask in its presence. The nourishment of the sun reaches far beyond our rational understanding, and taps deep into the center of healing the more one aligns with its energy. The lifestyle of a sun foodist is based on integrity with one's own values, authenticity of character, conscious awareness of actions, respect for all living creatures, and deeper connection to our planet.

I truly believe, as inhabitants on this earth, we have a real responsibility not only to our own well being, but to the whole of life that surrounds our every breath. The connection of all living organisms is so intricate that it literally flows through our veins, giving us a deeper sense of our own purpose so long as we choose to live with awareness, compassion, and reverence for this magnificent body. The choice to remove oneself from the painful patterns of a negative lifestyle can be likened to finding a light switch in a dark room. It may involve some bumps, some fumbling, and some confusion, but as soon as you flick the switch the darkness clears away and clarity begins.

The breaking point for all limited beliefs and behaviors is when someone heals from a condition that is conventionally considered to be irreversible. To witness a seemingly insurmountable obstacle remove itself from your life with ease, one that was previously attacked with invasive strategies, is not only incredible but it is very probable. We remove the die-it from the equation, thus leaving out the struggle and the strife to better concentrate on the healing power of a focused life. The limited attitude of the past is left in the past because we must live in the flow of continued vitality that never slows down, much like the fluidity of the river that only knows the path of least resistance.

We exist in the most amazing universe that always responds to our most residually focused thoughts and emotions. Our thoughts create actions that lead to results that either promote our dreams or detour them. Eating closest to the earth will literally transform your thoughts from scarcity to abundance. Your actions may have once been all about sustaining your own self interests before, but after following the living-foods lifestyle, you will become a great promoter of global sustainability projects that open doors for massive positivity where endless generations may walk through.

The beauty of our times lies within the incredible choices we all have to choose and act upon, and all information that has been made widely available through reliable media. I would caution the use of free information because anyone can go online and write any article without any references or factual basis. I recommend that you do your own due diligence before taking anyone's word to heart, especially mine as you read this. All goal-achieving individuals know how to saturate their minds with valuable information, and they also learn how to discern between the useful and the useless. I suggest you polish these skills as well while being on your way to achieving all of your goals.

This book, the **Live It Lifestyle: Dropping the Die it Forever**, was inspired by a conversation with a good friend that took place on the way back from a raw food health seminar. Everyone reading this, I'm sure, has tried the ever revolving door of try this, try that, don't do this, but do that in the die-it world. The idea that you need to suffer your way to excellent abundant health is not only incorrect, it is absolutely absurd because it completely goes against the natural laws of the universe. You can only attract what you align with, and if you want more vitality and exuberance for life, you must align with what produces this energy. In my experience, what produces this energy is living plant-based foods.

We live in a health food culture full of propaganda, misinformation, extreme belief systems, and what would appear to be religious agendas. Fascism and absolutism are thought processes that have ignited every major dispute, war, and break down of constructive relationships we know of today. Those that are sincerely searching for answers to help upgrade their life, and remove the unnecessary stresses, should be aware of proponents of the infamous one-way-is-the-only-way approach to diet and lifestyle. In most cases, these ideas are merely distractions and illusions that we must apply critical thinking towards. Otherwise, we may get wrapped up in a cult-like mentality that holds no foundation and no viable future.

A foundational lifestyle formed around natural eating habits, comprised of foods from the sun and earth, have an effect on the human nervous system, brain chemistry, bone health, metabolism, heart health, muscular efficiency, response time, hormonal balance, mental acuity, depth of creative imagination, heartfelt relationships, and abundance of life force energy unlike anything else known in modern civilization.

It is my hope that you will use this book as a consistent reference to help guide you on your path to the massive transformation of your mind, body, spirit, and eventually your overall environment. It is a firm belief of mine that in order to get to where you want to be, it is critical that you find, research, and model someone that has already been there first. The world is full of the blind leading the blind into impenetrable walls of sorrow and desperation. We are doing away with the old model of do-what-I say-but - not-what-I-do. Instead, we are embarking on a crash course in human ingenuity that can only lead to the expansive and always pleasurable expression of your greatest excellence. You are a gifted creator with untapped abilities the world is eagerly waiting for. Do not wait any longer to become the architect of your future. Lay down all excuses that lead nowhere now, and reroute the course of your life in the direction of your heart's desires.

This book was put together for the reader to use in any way they see fit as a resource for informational purposes. Throughout this work, we will visit and revisit common subject matters in order to not only reinforce, but also display how our food and lifestyle choices are affecting every aspect of our lives, and the world around us. I encourage you to become a health detective; someone who is always investigating the mysteries, intrigue, and unknowns of what health could be like when we remove the chains of doubt and distress from our lives.

Remember, you cannot achieve life from death. You cannot develop a mind set of wealth from poverty, and you cannot attract what you want from focusing on that which you don't want. Let's focus all of our collective and individual efforts on creating the world we all want through removing the problem and fully embracing the solution!

Enjoy the process!

Begin Where You Are

"Vitality shows in not only the ability to persist but the ability to start over."
F. Scott Fitzgerald

"The secret to a rich life is to have more beginnings than endings."
David Weinbaum

"He who chooses the beginning of the road chooses the place it leads to. It is the means that determines the end."
Harry Emerson Fosdick

The most important thing to remember when making any transformative changes in your life, and often the most neglected piece of it, is to begin exactly where you are at right now. All too many times we get wrapped up in the ideas, strategies, and long-term results we need to achieve, and we forget that we must gauge our readiness to take that first step into new and exciting possibilities.

A mass combination of emotions and thoughts could be entering your mind as you embark on this journey into deeper levels of self discovery from the inside out. It is important to understand that this is completely normal. Whenever anyone makes a concrete decision to change their habitual routine of living their life, a multitude of interferences will seemingly bombard you in an effort to keep you in your comfort zone. Do not let this throw you off track. Work with this energy, and learn to redirect it in your favor as you progress in your newly-chosen path of growth.

In the late 1600's, the famous mathematician, Sir Isaac Newton, presented to the world what is known as Newton's Three Laws of Motion. The first law states, *"an object that is at rest will stay at rest unless an unbalanced force acts upon it"*. This means unless a force outside of us acts upon us, we may never move our feet; we become comfortable with stagnation. The other half of this law states, *"an object that is in motion will not change its velocity unless an unbalanced force acts upon it"*. This means if we begin to move our feet in a certain direction, we will build up momentum. By virtue of this law, we generate more speed the more we move our feet, and while resisting the temptation of stagnant behavior.

You are bigger than any challenge. You have more light inside you than the deepest and darkest shadows of the world could ever hope to extinguish. By this information showing up in your life, you are exactly where you need to be, and need not burden yourself with ideas about the contrary. The first step is the hardest because you know deep inside that if you make the move, you will make another. Eventually the more steps you take, the harder it is to go back to old way of doing things.

It is easy to overwhelm ourselves at first, but remember small actions taken repeatedly will lead to great achievements eventually. Anyone who ever did anything in their lives had to step out on faith at some point. It wasn't always comfortable or always pleasurable, but if you asked those same people today, I am willing to bet they would say it was definitely worth it. The fulfillment of your heart's desire is always worth the process of finding the right bridge to cross.

Regardless of what pursuit you begin in life, you will be met with opposition from peers and family, especially when you make powerful changes in your eating and lifestyle choices. Most individuals who grew up in the world of microwaves and instant results are accustomed to doing things the way society dictates. When these individuals step outside of that mold, it makes other people uncomfortable. When you begin to glow more and smile more, due to the cleaning up of your body, others might criticize you out of their own insecurities at first, but eventually even they will grow tired of their own stagnation, and inquire about what you're doing. It's human nature to resist anything they do not understand at first. However, just like all major trends we have today, they begin with ridicule, followed by violent opposition, then finally followed by obvious acceptance, as if they never had a disagreement in the first place.

"If one advances confidently in the direction of one's dreams, and endeavors to live the life which one has imagined, one will meet with a success unexpected in common hours."
Henry David Thoreau

We must take complete responsibility for our lives every step of the way if we are to transform ourselves into the people we truly aspire to be. It can become easy to fall back on our laurels when we achieve a certain level of results, and start telling everyone else what to do, much like the old boss at the assembly line enforcing rules to the workers below him. That old model is long gone, and we are not interested in going backwards. We are living and breathing examples of our most noble thoughts, aspirations, and progressive qualities.

With each step you take, you will transform yourself into a new being. You may take periodic breaks if you wish but there is no avoiding the positive addiction of personal growth once the process has begun. After all, it was Brian Tracy who said that the great thing about personal development is once you get in it, you can't get out. Be certain that you want to step into the future of becoming all that you can be because it will take from you all that you have to give. But once that light inside has been sparked, it will happily give back to you in return.

Test your Limits

In the accepted model of society, we are constantly told to limit our scope of what is possible. The consciousness of a sun food superhero does not exist in a cage of restrictions. The world is completely open to your wildest dreams, expanding as far as you give it permission to do so. When exploring the world of living foods, I encourage you to test the limits of your digestive powers for it is through the stomach that the mind can reach new heights. In the beginning, you may need to start slow on certain things, but as you move forward, you should add in as much raw plant food as possible. As you progress, you will educate yourself, you will meet new people that have the knowledge you are looking for, and you will learn as you follow this path out. So do not fear road blocks because they are going to arise either way. You might as well deal with them as soon as possible, and be done with it.

If you have strong desires to eat a lot, then embrace this urge by making the best choices to cater to it. You do not have to deprive yourself in order to transform yourself. You just have to understand the situation, and select the best option available at the time. If you over eat, do not feel ashamed because when you over eat raw foods, you do not suffer the same consequences as dense cooked foods. Your body will recover much faster if flooded with raw foods that contain dense nutrients than with cooked foods that contain bulk calories and little nutrition, if any. When the food contains nutrients that the body can recognize, it will be utilized quickly and the excesses will be released. This is the intelligence of moving towards a living foods lifestyle, and you will get ahold of yourself in a much shorter amount of time. There is a philosophy I have begun to live by, which is, at every moment possible, stack the odds in your favor. If you feel the periodic urge to lay out in front of the television, feel free to do so, but have this book sitting next to you each time. The lessons contained in these pages will slowly speak to you as long as you remain open to the possibility that one day, in the near future, your ears will hear the message.

Upgrade the Operating System

An idea I would encourage you to play with is looking at your physical body as an operating system that is fully functional, and capable of performing tasks in relation to the different types of fuel we feed it. The food we take in is different depending on what we require at the time. We need food for the body, food for the mind, food for the soul, and food for relationships as well. What I have noticed in my own journey, and after speaking with many long-term raw foodists, is that the food is merely a key to unlock a realm of larger possibilities. This topic of adding in raw foods, super foods, herbs, and higher-quality water, and sharing these topics with others is really a call for humanity to upgrade their life in every way possible, which is completely available by making intelligent choices moment to moment.

We have all been brought up in a system that educates only within the confines of outdated modalities. It would be advantageous to understand that our current school system was designed during the industrial revolution in order to train future workers. The way we have been instructed to live our lives is not in accordance with the laws of nature. For this reason alone, we need to be given a new set of instructions, a few of which are "you are what you eat", "you become what you think about", and "you are who you associate with". If we begin to assimilate these phrases into our consciousness each day, the world will deliver options, events, people, and circumstances that will further enhance your health, your brain transmissions, and your immune system to a point where the idea of getting sick will no longer be entertained. You can upgrade your nervous system to a level where you are responding to multiple things instantly without even thinking about it. You can reach a space in time where you literally fall into your heart, and where the old model of blocked-off possibilities no longer exists.

As we proceed to upgrade our lifestyle choices the advice I commonly recommend is we begin adjusting the habits we already have. It is very difficult to completely revamp your entire life over night, we need to take incremental steps towards ours goals and health pursuits. Most people fail not because of a lack of effort, but more commonly because of the now or never syndrome that grips our health food culture. In extreme cases of health crisis, it may be imperative that someone makes rapid lifestyle shifts, but in the case of the average individual short term goals with smaller actions steps can prove more beneficial in the long term. For example, if someone is a long term habitual cigarette smoker the chances of them dropping this habit automatically is slim. I would recommend that person looks into upgrading what they are already doing by purchasing organically-grown-chemical-free-open-tobacco-leafs with a non-fiber glass containing cotton filter(or no filter), and 100% hemp paper to roll it in. This simple change in behavior can yield greater results without adding on additional stress in our already stress filled world. If someone is into drinking alcohol regularly I suggest moving into organically-produced-bio-dynamic-wine. Done in appropriate fashion these upgrades can produce much more attractive results, done in excess they can create similarly negative results as their much more artificial counter parts.

Asking the Right Questions

"Life will pay whatever price you ask of it"
Anthony Robbins

"A man may fulfill the object of his existence by asking a question he cannot answer, and attempting a task he cannot achieve."
Oliver Wendell Holmes

"Asking is the beginning of receiving. Make sure you don't go to the ocean with a teaspoon. At least take a bucket so the kids won't laugh at you."
Jim Rohn

If you had to ask me what was the one thing I could do right now to immediately change the direction of my thoughts, feelings, and actions, it would be to start asking yourself the right questions. The most powerful skill anyone can cultivate is the ability to ask themselves more accurate and honest questions about any situation. Asking sets the stage of future events in the movie of your life, and you may ask questions that lead into any direction of your choosing.

The quality of your questions will become the quality of your life. This should be sealed in the hearts and minds of every aspiring individual because when you put a question out to the universe, the answer is coming. It may not happen on your time table, but you can rest assured that it will respond like a boomerang. I have a theory that when inspired ideas drop into our lap seemingly out of nowhere, they are actually just the answers to questions we have asked in the past. Sometimes it takes a while for the answers to reach us because we must mature a bit in order to be fully receptive to them. The higher quality of the question we ask, the higher quality person we must become in order to take action on the answers we are given.

"Asking the right questions takes as much skill as giving the right answers."
Robert Half

Many times people will say I can't seem to find any solutions to my problems. But if you look carefully, you will find that the answers are always there, and you may not have realized how general your questions are. If all you say is "I want to make more money", and someone gives you a quarter, that is all you deserve because you failed to ask the right question. If you say "I want to be healthy", and you are coasting along just enough to not get sick, you are also getting exactly what you asked for. The ability to ask selectively focused questions, ones that are fueled with strong emotion, is what separates those that have the best time with their lives and those that are riding the emotional roller coaster.

I know that if I am in full alignment with my goals, then the answers to all of my questions from the past and the present will flow naturally to me, and with no conscious effort; it is more dependent on vibrational effort. Start asking yourself questions like "how can I find myself in the most pleasurable circumstances having the best day possible", or "how can I enjoy the best health possible while enjoying all my favorite foods and drinks in a way that feels amazing". When you start gearing your personal language in this kind of manner, the doors of opportunity open in all directions.

We all know of the iconic story of Aladdin and the magic lamp. Aladdin trails out of a snow storm into a cave to find a magic lamp on the ground. He rubs the magic lamp on accident and a genie comes out to grant him three wishes. Without knowing the power he had received, he makes unthought-out wishes and then realizes he blew it. The moral is, of course, be careful what you wish for because it will most certainly come true!

"Asking and being open to receive is one of the first steps required to receive some of the gifts of the quantum field. Taking control via our lifestyle to tune to specific channels within the universal field is a basic and easy art to learn."

Jasmuheen

If the brain is the receiver for electrical conduction of the body, then the heart is the magnetic generator that produces a field of energy which attracts all things in our life. The Law of Attraction is used through our finely-tuned heart chakra; it is not from analytical calculations that attempt to interpret the flux of reality from which we create our greatest results. It is in our hearts that the God force energy is cultivated and expanded into the world; wrapping around the globe more than a million miles an hour and reaching everyone within a similar thought frame. Our thoughts only create the display we wish to see, and that display represents a state of feeling where our true power is. The questions we ask should be rooted within our power. If we can make this a habit, what we receive may far exceed the display we create in the linear mind. If we are reaching others in the world, and they are reaching us unconsciously, then perhaps the questions we are asking are being answered somewhere across the globe, and those answers are making their way to us so long as we remain connected but not attached. Most people get so attached to the answers they want that they end up overlooking the answers that they are given.

Ask questions that radiate from your core; your heart and soul must be lined up for the power of the mind to take form. The right nutrition will help you conduct perfect tuning with the ideal radio station, and at the same time, lower the resistance to your heart which has been built up over time from living in concrete cities that are isolated from nature's ease and perfection.

(Recommended Books: Ask and its Given: Esther Hicks)

You are your Associations

"A man only learns in two ways, one by reading, and the other by association with smarter people."
Will Rogers

"Always be yourself, have faith in yourself, do not go out and look for a successful personality and duplicate it"
Bruce Lee

Beware of the company you keep because we as human beings are easily influenced by our surroundings at the subconscious level. The thoughts, ideas, words and energies coming from those around us will do one of two things: help propel us in the direction of our goals and dreams, or knock us off track from what we are aiming to accomplish. It is not only a good idea to limit the time spent with negative people, but it is imperative if your goals are of a higher quality than the goals of those around you.

It is important to keep yourself in the right group setting that is in accordance with your highest values. You don't have to completely alienate yourself from those you love, people who may not be ready right now to meet you where you are at, but that does not mean they never will be, so keep an open mind to all things because you can still benefit from everyone. You just have to develop certain skills for filtering out negativity that we will all face in our journey. Remember, if you want to help bring others along, you must be a fully fledged example of excellence in all that you do.

The truth of the matter is that everyone has an inherent desire for personal growth and expressing their gifts through a creative outlet, but they just don't know how to do it. They have never been given a proper manual for using their tools. It is important to focus on yourself for awhile. People just need examples to look to because, in the matrix of everyday living, there is mass confusion and chaos. I have found in my own experience that by being a person of disciplined action and empathy for all people, friends of mine who I counted out long ago have come back around because they finally reached their breaking point; the point where they were sick and tired of being sick and tired. I learned long ago that people are good at the core, and we all want the same things in our lives, but most just don't know what that looks like. You can be that bright light that is so clear that it will one day become obvious, and others will wonder why it took them so long to come your way.

Solitude

Solitude from the outside world can be a precious thing when the disruptive energies take their toll. All of us on the path of profound health in all areas of our lives will go through these times. It can be a very frustrating experience to be around others who seem to have not a care in the world for their health, the environment, and for contributing to others. These are exactly the type of people you should separate yourself from as much as you're willing too.

When you become more of a naturalist(living naturally), meaning you begin gravitating towards a eating protocol dominant in plant based foods, it has a way of completely opening you up to higher levels of awareness, mental clarity, and emotional and physical toxic release. You will develop a completely new outlook on life and the way you view the beauty of nature. I would highly suggest everyone to spend as much time being inspired and captivated by the subtle energies that are all around us; from the weeds growing in your front yard to the magnificent forests most of us all have instant access to. This can have dramatic effects on your temporarily unbalanced emotions since nature has a way of delivering calm and tranquil vibrations to your mind and spirit. Get barefoot on the grass, bring your favorite book, and just let all the troubles of the world fall away with ease.

Master Mind Principle

The importance of partnerships is one that is overlooked in mainstream society. There is so much going on that many people forget the benefits of forming genuine relationships with like-minded individuals. Ideas that you would never have grasped are now available for your usage. Actions towards your goals can be taken by those in your camp in order to double the results you seek. It is important to remember that nobody goes it alone in life; we are always being helped along every day, whether we know it or not.

The success philosopher Napoleon Hill focused much of his work on this key idea. In his success principles, it is necessary to form a collective master mind alliance. This is a group of two or more people that have a like and sound mind, and are in agreement on their definiteness of purpose and willingness to work together in its ultimate completion. The ability to leverage the ideas, resources, talents, and energy of those around you is a key ingredient for accomplishing more in a shorter amount of time. This is why it is always a good idea to surround yourself with those more skilled and outgoing than yourself. Those that have more experience in the field of health, nutrition, personal development, ethical business practice, and fitness. Whatever you're looking to improve on, find the leaders to aid you in your pursuits.

Start getting people together for living food potlucks; introduce this idea to the community and watch how fast it will expand. By actively engaging in other people's lives, you will be amazed at how fast you can get into contact with all of their friends, and build huge networks of positively powerful relationships where people you didn't even know are now a part of your core group. If you can promote your passion for better health, inner and outer growth, sustainable and ethical food growing operations, and better choices for all, then the right people to help your ideas take off will appear; it is the law of attraction responding to your convictions.

Hope

"Everyone who has ever built anywhere a "new heaven" first found the power thereto in his own hell"
Fredrick Nietzsche

"When you get to the end of your rope, tie a knot and hang on"
Anonymous

"The human body experiences a powerful gravitational pull in the direction of hope. That is why the patient's hopes are the physician's secret weapon. They are the hidden ingredients in any prescription"
Norman Cousins

Those who strive with all their might will be blessed with a power unforeseen to them in waking hours, but will be revealed in times of great struggle when they need it most. This power flows through all living things naturally, and if channeled correctly, it can flow with ease. The ability for a flower to grow vigorously through the cracks of concrete, making its way to the sun, depends on its ability to endure the process. The process of maturity is something we all must endure as it brings its own set of growing pains, and when we find ourselves in these transitions of life, we would do well to develop our sense of indisputable hope.

No matter what challenges you may find yourself in, there is hope. You may be severely overweight, a binge eater due to emotional disturbances or physiological cravings, and surrounded by the clutter of a life out of balance, but you know what, I still believe in you. The ability you have to rise above the obstacles you face is greater than any stumbling block that could ever come your way. Never forget that you are a being of life-force energy, and you run the show of your own life; you are the director, the producer, the funding agency, and most importantly, the lead role in the life you have yet to showcase for the world.

We harbor the feelings of hope in all layers of life deep inside all of us. We hope to be successful, we hope to find our soul mate, and we hope to be accepted. So the idea of hope is very familiar but, unfortunately, it is often only applied out of comfort for many. I believe this is due to the idea that we are living in an instant result-orientated society. If we are not granted the result of our desire immediately or shown evidence that it is possible, we dismiss it and choose a side of life that will not require all that we have to give, and that is why many people feel hopeless in their lives. This feeling of hopelessness can be instantly overcome by taking a new direction in your life. You must decide on what it is you really want and then take action.

"A real decision is measured by the fact that you've taken a new action. If there's no action, you haven't truly decided"
Anthony Robbins

Action

The ability to take action on your hopes and dreams is what will inevitably lead you from bread crumb to bread crumb to finding your ultimate destiny. Those that remain in a state of self doubt and worry are those that have developed a strong habit of inaction. The capacity for how much inaction you allow into your life will ultimately determine how much self defeating opportunities you give yourself, and how far you're willing to dig yourself into a deeper hole that has no end. You are always exactly where you're at right now based on the thoughts you think, the people you associate with, and the actions you take or don't take.

When I was pursuing a career as a professional athlete I was committed to a lifestyle of massive action. I remember all my friends would be glued to the television during sports games and they would sometimes ask me if I saw the latest game. My response was always the same: "no I didn't see the game I was too busy playing it". I was never satisfied watching other people live out their dreams unless I was right alongside of them. This is an important key to your success in any field. Those who work hard when the lights are turned off will be rewarded when the lights are turned on. Develop a habit of action at all times whenever possible.

If you are committed to losing the weight that has been holding you back, then take steps towards your goal. Make some small changes in your eating habits, go out and get a decent juicer, get some carrots, celery, cucumbers, and cilantro(all organic preferably), and get accustomed to doing this once a day. If you are committed to reducing artificial sugar cravings, then begin by replacing bad habits for good habits. Trade in that junky candy bar for a fresh apple, a small bag of grapes(with seeds), a slice of juicy watermelon, or a delicious mango. The steps you take do not have to be huge at first because the most important thing is to begin taking steps.

Expectation

The thoughts we have about ourselves mold the looking glass for possible future events. The reality we perceive is being scripted step by step in our own thought process. What you expect you will always project. So what are you expecting for yourself right now? Do you expect to have a great day when you wake up? Do you expect to have a clean, healthy body that is clear of toxins and negative energy? Do you expect to attract people, events, circumstances, and a mass amount of synchronicity that is beyond your own common understanding? Your expectations are a direct result of your own belief system about life, and if you believe you are a success, then it will eventually become a reality; starting from the core and working its way to the surface.

The super successful individuals in the world have all had one thing in common: they expected to be where they are at right now. Donald Trump, who is renowned for his skills in business, has faced massive defeats of losing entire billion-dollar fortunes. However, in a matter of a few years, not only did he regain what was lost, but also achieved much more. Lance Armstrong had been stricken with testicular cancer at the peak in his cycling career. When facing such a life threatening obstacle, no one expected him to get back on the bike. However, it made no difference what anyone else thought as long as his expectation was on point. He ended up going through brain and lung treatments along with massive chemotherapy before he made a complete recovery, and went on to win the Tour de France 6 times. That is an amazing display of powerful forces of human will and being on purpose.

"I am not in this world to live up to other people's expectations, nor do I feel that the world must live up to mine."
Fritz Perls

To be in full alignment with your expectation is to be backed by faith. If you are struggling with weight loss, then it takes a lot of faith to affirm your goals everyday in the midst of temptation. If you are overcoming a chronic injury or a so called incurable dis-ease, then it takes the kind of hope that's generated from a place deep down inside; a place where your rational thoughts of doubt cannot infiltrate. To be the kind of person you were designed to be by the creator, it takes faith to see yourself as that person every day. You have to expect to walk in those shoes every day, and persist even when you sometimes fall short and can't resist. Your expectations of yourself in the end will determine the outcome of your life, and since you are going to be thinking anyways, you might as well think about what you want.

Expect the best for yourself; don't accept any less than what you deserve. When you make a firm resolve, the universe will conspire to shape the perfect path for you to walk in order to achieve it. In *Napoleon Hill*'s classic book, **Think & Grow Rich**, he instills the power of taking possession of your mind, determining a definiteness of purpose, and directing your attention onto that purpose each day, fueled by the passion that comes from knowing its presence is soon to arise.

I heard a personal development speaker talk about the effect Napoleon Hill's work had on his life. He said the book is called think and GROW rich, not think and work really hard and get rich. This is very important in understanding the difference between those who are just working hard to make a living and those who are working smart and growing in order to create a lifestyle. There is a saying: "don't tell me to reach for the stars when there is clearly footprints on the moon".

Planting Seeds of Hope in Children

"If theres no hope for the youth then theres no hope for the future"
Tupac Shakur

There has been many different points of view on the direction we must take in order to ensure the survival of our species. I find many of the opinions from politicians and corporate appointed officials to be drastically out of alignment with the most obvious starting point. Flaring like wild fire, arguments about the environment, animal welfare, economic and social equality are critical issues. But before we can address those issues, we must first kneel down and touch the heart of a child. There is a saying I once heard which goes something like: children grow so tiresome of always teaching grown ups lessons they have forgotten along the way. Children are unburdened by the restrictive factors modern living tends to impose. Their lights have not been blown out. For this reason, the children of the future are our only hope for a positive outcome.

There is a special place in my heart for the youth, especially the kids that are less fortunate than others, yet somehow still manages to create magic in their lives. When I was teaching Tae Kwon Do, I had the great pleasure of interacting with and leading hundreds of children through the years. I believe this experience was the seed that was planted in my heart to do the work that I do now. I got to know a variety of personalities, from the most outgoing to the most shy and hesitant. One thing they all had in common was the innate ability to excel with the encouragement of those they followed. I was raised to respond to threats and fear, but as a teacher, I had learned it was much more effective to instruct from passion and hope.

The truth is, everything a child learns begins at home. As products of our environment, we absorb information relevant to our surroundings at the unconscious level. Kids will always take on the behavioral patterns of their parents. I know this from my own experience, although it took me years to actually admit that fact. If parents use foul language, then so will the child. If the parent smokes or drinks alcohol, then chances are, so will the child. If a single mom or dad disrespects the opposite sex, then this attitude will pass through the generational barrier. No single celebrity, athlete, model, teacher, musician, or marketing tool has more power of influence than the lead players in the household. With this said, I suggest every parent take strict attention to the food selections that are allowed to enter into their household. Over the years of working with parents, I have seen them sincerely attempt to correct their children's behavioral problems through discipline with little to no thought as to what they were feeding their children. According to the CDC(Centers for Disease Control and Prevention), childhood obesity has tripled in the past 30 years. In 2008 alone, more than one third of children and adolescents alike were considered overweight or obese. These are very unsettling statistics. It is very difficult to instill hope for our world when the recipients of it are predicted to die before their parents do.

These facts may seem very frightening for many people, and I know it can seem hopeless at certain low points in our lives, but if you are that parent, you must muster up all the strength in your soul to hold the wheel tight. This book, and many others like it, was written for you. The first thing you can do is educate yourself, which is what you are doing here. Now is the time to implement this information. In the immortal words of Bruce Lee, *"It is never enough to know, we must do"*. If you are willing to create a space for change in your life, then you may be surprised how effortlessly your children follow your lead. I advise you to study the following chapters in close detail: **Symptoms of Society: Diabetes Type 1, The Raw Naked Truth, Asking the Right Questions, & Begin Where Your Are.**

I understand it can be a challenge to reverse negative nutrition habits of kids these days. The over exposure to addictive processed, sugary, cooked, and animal-based foods has created opposition, but not an impenetrable wall. I am not suggesting you take away your kids favorite snack, and attempting to replace it with a stalk of celery or head of lettuce. The best thing you can do is to meet them where they are at. By this, I mean substituting what they already eat with a better form of it. The chart below is a simple and easy to understand way to get started with implementing changes that your children will actually enjoy following! (You may look into the vast library of raw food cuisine recipe books for more ideas)

Current Food Choice	**New Food Choice**
Peanut Butter W/Bread	Raw Almond Butter W/Celery
Soda, Sugary Drinks	Kombucha, Celery-Apple-Ginger Juice
Assorted Processed/Sugary Snacks	Goji Berries, Cashews, Cacao Nibs, Fruit
Glass of Milk	Almond, Hemp, Brazil Nut Milk
Butter & Toast	Raw Honey spread over Ezekiel Bread
Meat Sandwich	Avocado W/ Chia or Flax Crackers
Cheese	Nut Butters (Cashew, Almond, Tahini, ect)
Spagetti	Zucchini Strips W/ Home Made Sauce
Processed Chocolate Bars	Raw Organic Chocolate (Cacao) Bars
Sports Drinks	Coconut Water (From Coconut if possible)
Milk Ice Cream	Raw Coconut Cashew Ice Cream (Dairy Free)
No matter what have at all times-	A Bowl of "Fresh" Juicy Fruit on the Table!

Vision

"It is a terrible thing to see and have no vision."
Helen Keller

"It takes someone with a vision of the possibilities to attain new levels of experience. Someone with the courage to live his dreams."
Les Brown

"Wisdom is obtained by reading the mind of god"
Wallace Wattles

Achievements of all stature, from small to large, started as an idea, a thought, and a vision put into creation. The most powerful asset we possess as human beings is our ability to create the world around us as we see fit. It is said that the outer manifestations of your reality are in direct proportion to that of the inner visions you harbor. Nothing comes into the world without it starting as the seed of an idea, growing inside the garden of one's mind, and fertilized by powerful emotions that will fuel a positive or negative outcome.

The vision you hold inside is entirely yours to create. You are the artist holding the brush, and you control the strokes of genius that have yet to be discovered. In knowing this important wisdom, do not give your power away to another who may manipulate your path. Although many may seem to have good intentions, ultimately, most people are coming from a place of self interest due to the vision they have created. No one has any way of knowing the portrait you have inside your heart, so therefore you must protect it.

If your vision is hazy at times or undeveloped, all this means is now is the time you can begin piecing together the illustration of your life. Start to tell the story of the life you wish to live from moment to moment, and from this day forward, no longer entertain the life you don't wish to live, even if that is the life currently in front of you. By taking positively focused action on your dreams daily, you can dramatically alter the results you are receiving. You have the power to interrupt the pattern of mediocrity that most lock themselves in until the end of their days. You do not have to fall into this group. You are meant for more, you are meant to explore your greatness despite all evidence of the contrary.

Do you want to be merely healthy or do you want unshakable vitality that never ceases or weakens? Do you want a moderate level of energy or do you want a never ending flow of electrically concentrated energy? The truth is, your wish is your command, and it begins from the constructs of your own mind in partnership with the willingness of an open heart. Consider the wise words of *Florence Scovel-Shinn* in her classic work, **The Game of Life**: *"If one asks for success and prepares for failure, he will get the situation he has prepared for.* I have found in my own life that it is always better to be prepared for an opportunity, and not have it, then to be given an opportunity that you are unable to pursue. Read Florence's next words closely and imprint them onto the forefront of your mind, *"man must prepare for the thing he has asked for, when there isn't the slightest sign of it".*

Begin changing the thoughts you think by changing the food you eat. Fresh food that carries the energy of the sun with all of its nutrient profile fully intact can have tremendous effects on ones overall sense of well being. When you feel better, you will think better. When you think better, your actions will be better. Positive results follow positive action; positive people follow positive people, like attracts like and life attracts life.

If you want to explore your creativity, explore the colorful rainbow of fresh organic fruits and berries mother nature has to offer. Start playing with a wide collection of amazing choices ranging from blueberries, raspberries, blackberries, strawberries, goji berries, raisins, honey dew melons, juicy watermelon, apples and peaches ripe from the tree, savory coconut water with a side of grapes, and a smile. The options are endless, and the more you play around in the cornucopia of nature's offerings, the more your creative imagination will flourish into realms of artistic potential you didn't even know was available. It has been said in ancient shamanistic wisdom that if you want to see better eat more colors.

Explore the Unexplored

"The only way to discover the limits of the possible is to go beyond them into the impossible"
Arthur C. Clarke

We live in a world of unparalleled possibility that has yet to be realized or even grasped by the human mind. The tools for achievements of all sizes are at our finger tips. All we must do is recognize the opportunity, and move towards its realization. Sounds easier said than done, right? If we consistently listen to the influx of negative voices that surround us, then I completely agree. It is easier to say something positive than to live it. Our world has suppressed the idea of limitless exploration to the point where you might as well be a cult leader if you are a confident and positive leader. It is so much easier to just go with the flow of mediocrity and lead a life of mild expectations, asking very little from the grand designer of the universe, or is it?

I know for myself, if I played life safe on a regular basis, then the internal conflict would have become much more unbearable than the initial struggles of pursuing my greater plans for life. The vision we have grafted on the screen of our mental projector is presented to inform us of the growing possibilities. At no time is any idea out of our reach. We are given all that is required to climb the rungs of a ladder we build either out of solid oak or flimsy plastic. The foundation for what we create in life is solidified in the melting pot of our imagination and formed with the hands of the higher powers; at no point do we ever go it alone.

The greater part of the population tend to gauge their expectations somewhere between what they have done themselves and what they have witnessed others do. Everything we believe about what is possible is merely assumptions created in the mind, based upon beliefs that can be dramatically shifted at any time we choose. People all throughout history have shown us that limited ways of thinking are just the tipping point, and our social expectations are being stretched all the time. In 1954 a man named Roger Bannister had done something where at the time was considered out of reach even by the most talented athlete. Bannister broke the four-minute mile barrier as a runner. It did not happen overnight; he had to refine his stride over years of practice and making mistakes. Luckily, for every runner following Bannister, he did not believe it was too far out of reach. What is interesting about his example is after he showed it was possible, other runners started breaking this record also. This type of phenomena seems to be a trend in our world: when a new idea that challenges our current limits is introduced, we resist it until we see evidence of it, and only then it becomes a completely normal idea.

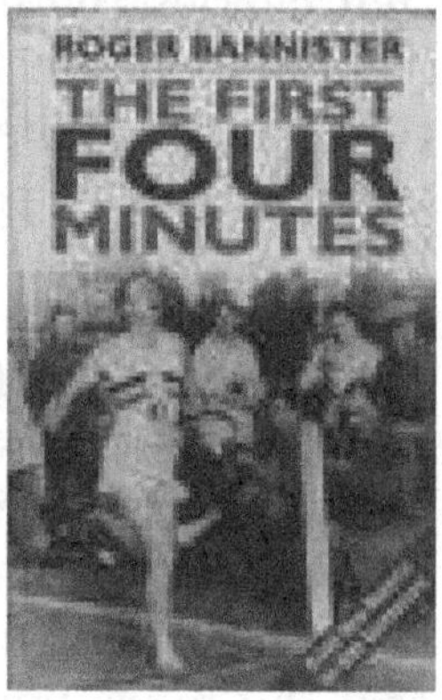

The concept of what is realistic is one I have always thought to be a little silly. Seeing as how individuals with big dreams that create new innovations have existed all throughout time, we can now take advantage of letting go of barriers. I am sure most people are thankful that in 1903 the two Wright Brothers, Orville and Wilbur, put together the very first operational flying machine. The idea of even doing such a thing at that time, with absolutely no evidence before, was met with extreme criticism and disbelief to say the least. Those that criticize others' ideas are also those that measure themselves entirely to others instead of the divine spark of creativity that exists in all. When your embarking on your raw journey, you will undoubtably be met with opposition from those who do not understand. Within every segregated community in health, there are unfamiliar ideas, such as the ones I present in this book. In the conventional theories of health, the idea of vegetarianism or veganism is highly uncomfortable for many. Even in the vegan community, the idea of a completely raw food lifestyle can seem totally absurd. Interestingly enough, in the general raw food community, many of the ideas on plant-based super foods, herbalism, and natural supplements seem out of reason. Human skepticism does not seem to escape any field of interest. This is an important thing to remember as you pursue your innermost inspirations. Do not be led astray by conflicting voices; be your own internal guidance vehicle moving you closer to your ultimate vision!

The original idea of our planet was that the earth was flat, and all ideas of the contrary were considered ridiculous. All throughout history, brave men and women have opposed the paradigms set up by short-term thinkers. Although we have over 150 years of accessible raw food knowledge, it is still very much a conscious shift many are hesitant to explore. I have been so empowered by the single choice I made to embody this lifestyle that I believe it is a part of my purpose to be a major voice for the greatest message of the twentieth century. This message is exposing one of the greatest mysteries in the field of nutrition: it is entirely possible to sustain ones most vital life force mostly or entirely on raw plant foods. I truly wish to explore the depths of health, nutrition, and endless abundance from this beautiful way of life.

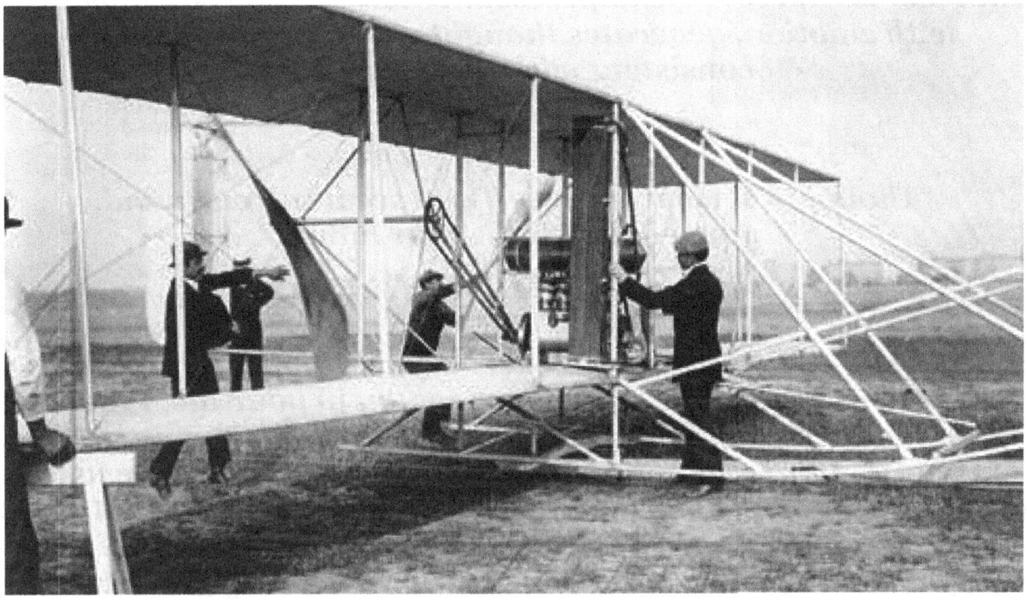

The Wright Brothers constructing the worlds first airplane

"You are not here merely to make a living. You are here in order to enable the world to live more amply, with greater vision, with a finer spirit of hope and achievement. You are here to enrich the world, and you impoverish yourself if you forget the errand."

Woodrow Wilson

The Thinking Stuff

"Whatever is expressed is impressed. Whatever you say to yourself, with emotion, generates thoughts, ideas and behaviors consistent with those words."
Brian Tracy

"Thoughts become things. If you see it in your mind, you will hold it in your hand."
Bob Proctor

"I believe that you're great, that there's something magnificent about you. Regardless of what has happened to you in your life, regardless of how young or how old you think you might be, the moment you begin to think properly, this something that is within you, this power within you that's greater than the world, it will begin to emerge. It will take over your life. It will feed you, it will clothe you, it will guide you, protect you, direct you, sustain your very existence. If you let it! Now that is what I know, for sure."
Michael Bernard Beckwith

There is a natural order set up in the universe that is in complete balance with all living things. There is a catalytic power that thrusts intention into the unseen perils of space and time. This intangible yet vibrant power is directing our every move, our every word, our every action, and our every result. This is the power of our thoughts.

You are the magnificent orchestrator of your own destiny; you have the power to direct all circumstances and get into alignment with the perfect events that could shape everything you have ever wanted into your life. I could say this to you all day long, but unless you believe it and reinforce it from within more than you deflect it, you will never know this truth.

As rational people, we constantly down play the magnitude that we may influence any single aspect of our lives simply by redirecting the route that our thinking is taking us. If you're in a ship that's heading for a big iceberg, you don't just keep pushing forward. You're going to grip the edge of the wheel and pull that ship in the opposite direction. Life is exactly the same, yet so many people see the iceberg coming and they continue in the same direction until it's too late. This is why they build guard rails on freeways, so that you know you're heading for trouble if you are hitting it.

It's interesting after studying psychology for years, and observing people, including myself over my own life, I have come to a profound insight. The majority of the thoughts we think are not actually our own. We are so bombarded throughout our lives with other people enforcing their own opinions, judgments, insecurities, and prejudices that we barely have enough time to form our own opinions from our unique and individual perspective of the world. As we go through our adult life, the voices in our head from parents, pastors, teachers, spouses, and so on follow us everywhere we go. In *Shad Helmstetter's* book, **What to say when you talk to yourself**, he effectively points out that many of the pitfalls of our subconscious mind in terms of learning information, retaining it, and making long-term changes. The fact that most of our internal language is negatively driven plays a major part in the outer results we are witnessing.

Beliefs:

Our belief about ourselves is the dominant factor in all of our efforts to make any changes, to take any positive action, and to incorporate healthier choices of food into our daily routine. A great question to ask yourself is: "what is my most underlying belief about myself, and is it serving me or disempowering me?" Most people's thoughts and beliefs about themselves are destructive, disempowering, and will ultimately lead them into a place of constant denial, pessimism, fear, shame, and guilt. If you have all of that going on in your life, any kind of positive change will feel like carrying a backpack of stones up a mountain top without a compass.

Regardless of what our beliefs are, we are being affected by them. Whether they are correct or not, all you need to do is look around and discern as to how your life looks, and decide if you like what you see or if something's got to give. The fact is, it is never what we say that proves our belief; it is always what we do that shows what we truly believe in. The story we tell ourselves about our life is usually just another form of comfort food we stuff our face with to distract us from making a choice. Little do we realize that in not making a choice we are still making a choice.

Vince Lombardi, who was coach of the Green Bay Packers NFL team in the 1960's, and wrote the great book **What it takes to be #1**, had a core belief about his approach to football that translated into life. He believed that there is no point in playing to lose. If you are going to play the game, you might as well play to win and go full out. This was his core belief, and because it was so strong, it rubbed off on all the players he ever coached. His conviction led him to achieve a legacy of greatness in his field, all because of a simple belief.

The truth is, every single person on earth has the capability to be, do, and have the greatest of all worlds as long as they are willing to adopt a more powerful belief system. How different would your life be if you believed you deserved the most abundant health ever. What if you woke up every morning believing without a quiver of a doubt that you were tapped in, tuned in, and turned on at all times, regardless of the possible chaos going on around you. How about believing you were worth the extra investment of going completely organic, or rearranging your schedule to make sure you were at every farmers market, or knowing you had such a depth of greatness waiting to burst out of you that you began going to health seminars, personal development and success mastery workshops. I wonder how different life would look for you then when you have developed that kind of belief about yourself.

Beautify your Garden:

In the classic book by *James Allen,* **As a man Thinkth,** he brilliantly likens the mind to that of a garden. We are the masters and gate keepers of our gardens, we decide what kind of fertilizer we use, we decide the quality of seeds we plant in the soil, and we decide that the final product is that of our own making. You have complete control and responsibility for your own garden, and if you do not diligently tend to the weeds that will periodically show up, you will become overrun and poisoned by your own passive negligence to the details of your own life. Success information pioneer Earl Nightingale said it this way: *"We're comparing the human mind with the land because the mind, like the land, doesnt care what you plant in it. It will return what you plant, but it doesn't care what you plant".*

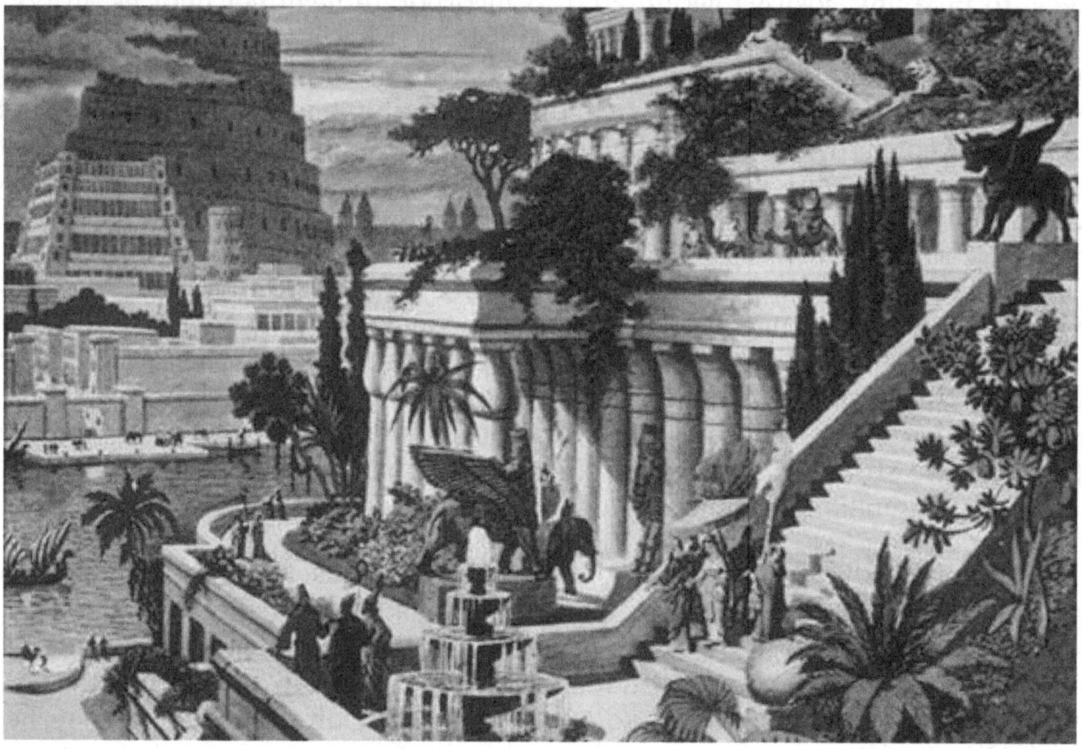

Ancient Babylonian Garden, The garden of our mind can look like this!

Every day we are planting the seeds of our future, regardless of whether we are conscious of this fact or not. Every time we think a certain type of thought, we are creating neuron connections that attach themselves in our brain to thoughts of a like kind. The more we think negative thoughts, the more we are likely to be connected to more thoughts of the same nature, and the more powerful the emotion behind it become, the deeper rooted those connections become. This is called the neuron network of the brain. The human brain according to *Dr. Joe Dispenza* receives around 400 billion bits of information a second but we are only consciously aware of about 2,000 bits per second. In the amount we are aware of, it is mostly of our environment, our interactions, and things we are responding to moment by moment. That leaves out a considerable amount of data that is roaming around somewhere in our mental store house. Since we are unaware of this data, we have no way of knowing the effects it may have on our lives subconsciously.

(Recommended book: Evolve your Brain: The Science of Changing your Mind, Dr. Joe Dispenza)

The beautiful thing about taking responsibility for the thoughts you are thinking is that no matter how many neuron networks you have formed in a self-destructive manner, you can always pattern interrupt those connections, and rewire the network receptors by thinking a more positively-charged thought. The brain is constantly reassembling this process in response to the different experiences, emotions, and thoughts we are being exposed to on an immediate basis. If you become self-directed and aware of your thoughts as you are thinking them, then you can alter negative thinking and replace it with more self-assured, noble, prosperous, and exciting thoughts even when your conscious mind is sleeping and your more powerful subconscious mind takes over.

"If you must speak ill of another, do not speak it, write it in the sand near the water's edge."

Napoleon Hill

Success through Happiness

Some people have more talent, some people have more knowledge, and some people have a bit more insight into specific situations or "field training". Despite all of these things, I dare to say that the number one quality that will always draw a fine line between success and mediocrity is one's own willingness to live a life of happiness. The consensus in our socially-driven arena is centered around competition. We compete from the time we are children to the time we are adults. As children, we compete for grades, awards, accolades, and honors in school. By the time we enter into the work force, we must compete for positions that we associate with success. There is nothing wrong with healthy competition; it can drive us to improve ourselves and grow out of our comfort zone, which is a powerfully positive thing. The way most people experience competition is actually through the pursuit of the one thing that will make them not need to compete any further; that one thing is long-lasting happiness. When a rare individual is able to change the equation from success equals happiness to happiness equals success, the results become drastically different.

The drive to acquire tangible things that will result in obtaining the feeling of happiness is irrational on all levels, and produces poor results in almost all cases. When we force ourselves to do something, we are causing friction not only within ourselves but also within the universe. We are building a wall to block off our greater potential we have yet to realize is available. It is astonishing to see all the scientific data that is now confirming what I have always believed to be true, and that is how we feel is vastly more important than simply how we think. I encourage you to sit with this idea for a moment.

We are taught that our thoughts control the gears and switches that turn the wheels that lead to the results we seek. The discoveries coming in are revealing that the brain works in cooperation with the heart, and actually the heart itself is estimated by some to be a million times more connected to the magnetic field of the earth than our own thought frequencies. What that means is exactly what has been said above: if you focus on what brings you happiness and pleasure, then you will be guided to your own personal paradise.

The Institute of HeartMath is a transformative scientific research organization that studies the effects of stress, emotions, heart-brain interactions, and what they call coherence. They believe coherence is the optimal state for which the heart, mind, and emotions are in perfect harmony, similar to when we have reached a deep meditative state. The discoveries that have been made from the two decades of research are astounding in relation to the basic physiological functions of the body and the effects our brain-heart have on our well being. Consider this description from the institute: *"It is a basic fact of physiology that your heart and brain exchange information that governs how you think, act and feel, but studies at the Institute of HeartMath have shown that heart-brain interactions can occur from one individual to another: Your heart can communicate with another person's brain."* The idea that we can communicate with another person outside of linear speech via our emotional state is powerful. The idea of an energetic exchange between two people is not a new concept and have been discussed through out different circles such as martial arts and alternative healing arts. Numerous studies have been done to show that human emotion extends far outside the body and into the electromagnetic field of the earth, showing us that what we think and feel not only effects our experience but the experience of those around us. Heart Math has been able to show that our physical heart exhibits it's own set of intelligence. The most cherished and revered spiritual traditions of our history have eluded to the idea that our personal reality and the world around us is intimately effected by the energetic environment we harbor within ourselves. The science we look to for answers is now confirming these ideas. This implies that the human heart has a language of it's very own, and we can begin to radically shift the results in our lives if only we can learn to communicate with it through our mind.

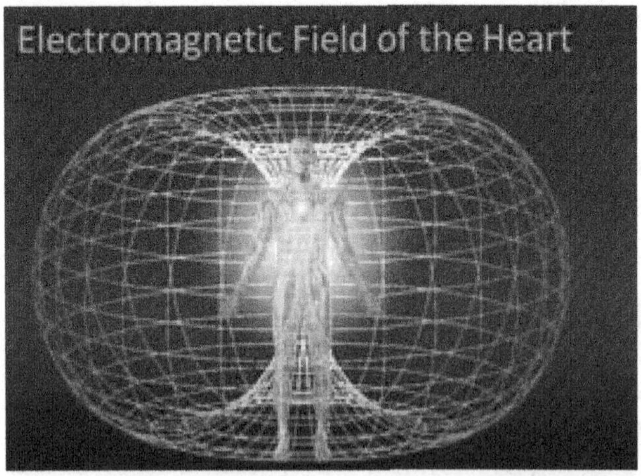

Those that focus their passions on doing what they love, whether they are socially accepted or not, are the same people who go on to create legendary legacies out of their lives. When we are actively engaged in what brings us pleasure, dopamine is secreted in the brain. Dopamine is the brain chemical that helps stimulate a more pleasurable experience in our lives. When we have dopamine flooding our brain, positive feelings in our life are enhanced. When we focus entirely on the mind, we are only participating in one frame of thought, narrowing our human experience and perceptions. When our emotions are actively engaged and we are excited, a whole new possibility for our lives will emerge. Greater imagination, inspiration, and ideas will come about as if they were hand delivered from the "outer realms" as a result of healthy neurotransmitter levels in our brain.

The reason why individuals that seek happiness above results are the forerunners of the future is simply because the majority of the world is doing it backwards. Happiness produces opportunities that are unavailable to those who have their head stuck in a book, even this book (unless it brings you great pleasure of course)! You cannot learn to be happy from literature alone. You must actively pursue what feels good and not focus so much on what feels bad. Engaging too much energy in what feels stressful or frustrating, like a diet program or hectic work load for example, is a clear indication that something is out of alignment. When you use happiness as a way of life and in all situations, you create a huge advantage in terms of staying power in any field you choose. People naturally want to be around positive, drama-free, and pleasant people that go out of their way to uplift others. These people create a better experience for everyone that comes into their presence, and that is how they will be remembered. The more you value yourself, the more you will resonate with giving gratitude. This creates a powerful catalyst to make well thought-out choices that do not contradict this feeling of well being you have become accustomed to. Happiness is truly the edge in life that most are seeking and don't even know it. All the material accolades that so many people strive for are only attempts to fill the void of an empty heart. If you fill the heart first, then all the accomplishments you receive will have true meaning, and you will have the correct formula to create the life you have always desired.

"The more man meditates upon good thoughts,
the better will be his world and the world at large"
Confucius

Communication

"Any problem, big or small, within a family, always seems to start with bad communication. Someone isn't listening."
Emma Thompson

"Effective communication is 20% what you know and 80% how you feel about what you know."
Jim Rohn

"The quality of my life is the quality of my communication"
Anthony Robbins

In our exceedingly fast-paced technological world where unlimited options to any problem are running rampant and confusing more people than ever before, one thing is clear, the more simple, direct, and clear your communication, the better the results in your life will be. The solutions to most people's ailments really are simple enough that anyone can understand and take some form of action on. It is crucial to consider the ways in which proper communication plays into our everyday lives, and also our relationships with others, with ourselves, with our health, with our food, and with our world at large.

Every time we do anything, we are sending out some form of communication to the others around us. Many believe that communication is completely verbal. But in reality, what comes out of our mouth is the least effective way to communicate on its own. The way we use our body, the way we give contact with our eyes, the thoughts we are thinking, the emotions we are feeling, and the ability to silently listen to another speak are all powerful forms of communication with others.

The greatest ways we can affect our ability to heal ourselves is tied in with our communication with the person staring back in the mirror. Since you are the only person living your life, and you are spending all of your time with yourself, it would probably be a good idea to develop an amazing relationship with yourself. It is being shown that the greatest decline in vitality, especially as people age, is in the quality of their relationships, and it all begins with the way you treat yourself.

(Recommended Book: How to Win Friends & Influence People: Dale Carnegie)

Communication with Self

"Death and Life are in the power of the tongue"
Prov. 18:21.

The best place to begin is always with yourself. There is only one person you have complete control over. You have control over all decisions you make, all words you speak, and all of the food you eat. I bet you've never accidentally eaten dinner before, right? It is important to acknowledge your previous communication habits, and if you are not satisfied with the results they have brought, then you should make some changes. This can be difficult because our personal psychology can often get in the way. Generally speaking, most people have a weakened psychology in terms of their own self image. The image you have of yourself will reflect very closely to the way you communicate on the inside.

In the book **Psycho-Cybernetics**, author *Maxwell Maltz* digs deep into the psychological habits of many patients he experienced as a plastic surgeon. Maltz explains how our thoughts of ourselves interact with all areas of our lives, and either sets us up for success or for failure. In this passage, he explains the human "success mechanism":

"In my opinion, psychology during the past 30 years has become far too pessimistic regarding man and his potentiality for both change and greatness. Since psychologists and psychiatrists deal with so-called "abnormal" people, the literature is almost exclusively taken up with mans various abnormalities, his tendencies toward self-destruction. Many people, I am afraid, have read so much of this type of thing that they have come to regard such things as hatred, the "destructive instinct", guilt, self condemnation, and all the other negatives as "normal" human behavior. The average person feels awfully weak and impotent when he thinks of the prospect of putting his puny will against these negative forces in human nature, in order to gain health and happiness. If this were a true picture of human nature and the human condition, "self improvement" would indeed be a rather futile thing.

However, I believe, and the experiences of my many patients have confirmed the fact, that you do not have to do the job alone. There is within each one of us a "life instinct", which is forever working toward health, happiness, and all that makes for more life for the individual, creative mechanism, or when used correctly the "Success Mechanism" built into each human being."

In most cases, we hold the exact answers to all of our dilemmas we face in the palms of our hand. If this is true, then why do we constantly search out others for solutions? Why cant we just tap into our own solution-driven mechanisms inside our brains and simply draw it out? In my opinion, it is because most of the time we are not listening to the answers being given. We avoid the most common sense solutions, believing it should always be more complicated than it needs to be. Since we have an over dependance on outside influences to guide us, we have given our power away. If you listen closely in times of turmoil, the answer could be closer than you ever thought.

I find that most people will actually answer their own questions if you let them. Many health practitioners are very fast to jump to solving the problem, but if you ask someone what they think the problem may be, they will answer it themselves more times than not. The art of silence plays a key role in healing and personal growth because we get confused in the chaos of constant chatter. In the ease of silence, we gain greater perspective. In nature when an animal is injured, it's natural instinct is to find a dark space to isolate itself in silence. The healing power of an environment without distractions is compelling. When we feel out of balance, the first actions should be to release tension and silence the mind. Practice this art in all you do, and find the best solution that fits your situation by following out intuition first.

(Recommended Book: Psycho-Cybernetics: Maxwell Maltz)

The Power of Positive Assumptions

One of most damaging things you can do is make unconsidered assumptions about situations and other people. When you plainly assume something, it can set you up for failure because you are creating a belief that may not be based on any factual basis. We can see this in the mainstream health and diet communities who assume certain advice is good advice because they believe it sounds good. The general assumptions we have been plagued with in science, medicine, politics, and nutrition have created more pain and agony than any theory can reverse.

We have to question all assumptions given by mega industries that may actually be based on nothing more than lazy ideas backed by more well thought-out profit margins. By supporting these ideas without filtering them through our critical thinking process first, it has led us to a place where natural remedies for man-made diseases are looked upon as silly and new-age theories when in reality, these are the healing modalities that have been used by the greatest civilizations to grace this planet. We must exercise cautious skepticism, otherwise we may become like gears in a machine that will ultimately spin itself out of control, destroying all that remains inside.

The way many people communicate with the nature of assumption is generally in the nature of a negative mindset. Human beings have a tendency to assume the worst of things in most situations that call for immediate action. When one slips up, it has a way of snowballing into another slip-up, and as long as someone communicates negative speech patterns or assumes that things will turn out a certain way, that reality is becoming more probable. To assume anything is to predict its arrival in the world. For instance, to assume war is everlasting is to perpetuate its existence, and we can all see the results of such assumptions. The mainstream news is constantly assuming the worst, and urging you to do the same. Fortunately, in the age of unlimited information and untapped potential, you have a choice.

Now that we understand the downfall of unthought-out assumptions, lets explore the flip side of positive assumptions. To acknowledge in our lives that we may not always have all the answers, but must be guided by forces unseen, is true wisdom in my opinion. This is where you can use the power of positive assumptions to your advantage in life. It is my firm resolve that in all situations, there is a profound truth and lesson to be discovered, no matter how bleak or harsh the situation may appear at the time. If you are caught between a rock and a hard place, just assume all is as it should be, and that there is something to be gained from this experience. I know it sounds easier to say than it is to do. But in fact, this is where you begin to communicate this idea to yourself, and over time, it will eventually transmit into the universal intelligence that orchestrates life in ways that we can only assume the best outcomes!

Remember, whenever you assume anything, you are participating in the creation process, so use this for your benefit instead of your detriment. Do not be like 99% of the population that is assuming all is for the worst, driving themselves deeper into the hell on earth they have created through miscommunication with themselves. I assume you are a gifted being of life-force energy that is awaiting your own awakening, and I assume you will assume the same.

Be the Change

"If you want things in your life to change, you must change"
Jim Rohn

"Are you bored with life? Then throw yourself into some work you believe in with all your heart, live for it, die for it, and you will find happiness that you had thought could never be yours"
Dale Carnegie

There is only one true constant in life; that is change. The nature of change is exactly like that of the seasons. When one season reaches its inevitable end, another comes in to take its place. When things in life change, people tend to resist the call to move forward with it. This seems to be the biggest obstacle in the human psyche. If we become complacent for too long, we get comfortable with the way life has been, and avoid the tides of something new, even if we are sick and tired everyday.

I remember hearing from the great success speaker, Les Brown, explaining the mindset most people take when making changes. He said he was walking past a house one day to come upon a dog on the porch. The dog was moaning and groaning in mild pain. He had asked the owner what was wrong with the dog. The owner replied that the dog was moaning because it was sitting on a nail. He simply asked why doesn't the dog just get up and move if it was in pain. The owner replied that the dog was not in enough pain to move. This story perfectly explains the attitude many have in life: even if people are unhappy with their current circumstances, they will not make changes until it is absolutely unbearable, and they can no longer withstand it.

I believe the reluctance to make simple adjustments in one's life is what has led to large-scale issues we face in our world. Instead of taking responsibility for our own lives, we have handed it over to those who are deemed qualified and competent. Instead of taking account of our own health, we appoint others to fix us, as if we were broken. By doing this, we forfeit our power by hanging off of their every word. The truth is, we are in complete control of our lives without a single exception. We are 100% responsible for every event in our lives on some level, one way or another. You should adopt this belief: if it is to be it is up to me!

Another belief that you may want to adopt is that you are fully responsible for everything that happens in your life. Many do not like this mentality because it interferes with the programming of the power structures; it disrupts conformity and passive comfortability. The reason you may want to adopt such an attitude is if you did not create your reality, then who did? Are you merely a puppet on stage, dancing to someone else's direction? Or would you rather be the master and imaginative creator of your own life?

"Be the change you wish to see in the world"
Mahatma Ghandi

It is very easy to see the world in a singular point of view. Since you do create your own reality, it can be very tempting to push your view onto others, even if its not intentional. A very common occurrence in the health and diet world is the constant enforcement of individual ideas and habits upon others, paradigms that may have worked for one but not necessarily for all. I am not writing this book to tell anyone my way of life is the best way; it has worked generously for me up to this point. However, I will do my best to remain open to the possibilities of improving my methods.

If you believe in your message, the best way to deliver it is rarely through words alone; it will be most effective through your own example. This is the key that only a handful of individuals throughout history have grasped and fully embraced. The majority of would-be great leaders are trying to reach others through methods of force and control, using sales tactics to sway their audience towards their own perspective. This is exactly why the most influential minds always face great opposition from mediocre thinkers, as Albert Einstein has so brilliantly said.

If your heart is true, then your message will withstand the test of time when all the maneuvers and tactics we see in politics and false leadership fall to the way side. It is important to not give into the temptation of cutting corners when you are on your mission because, whether you know it or not, there are always people watching you, waiting to see your next move, skeptical but also curious if you are going to finish what you started. Everyone in their truest nature wants to see others succeed. It is the habit of conformity that extinguishes peoples' supportive nature, and that is what creates ill will towards others. Remember, this when others will attempt to sway you in the wrong direction, so you must keep in the direction of your mission by being an example first, and before you know it, those that once held resentment towards you will now hold you in admiration.

We should all exercise personal responsibility for the path we wish to pursue, consider the words of one of worlds greatest humanitarians, His Holisness the 14th Dalai Lama. "*When you think everything is someone else's fault, you will suffer a lot. When you realize that everything springs only from yourself, you will learn both peace and joy.*"

Deconstructing the Die-it

When we lose twenty pounds... we may be losing the twenty best pounds we have! We may be losing the pounds that contain our genius, our humanity, our love and honesty.
Woody Allen

People are so worried about what they eat between Christmas and the New Year, but they really should be worried about what they eat between the New Year and Christmas.
Author Unknown

Dieting is wishful shrinking.
Author Unknown

The biggest movement in the western world has, very likely, been the industry of dieting. Everywhere we look, there is an advertisement for the new cure-all weight loss product, or the perfect diet program from the new health specialist that seems to have the magic bullet. Dieting is a very convenient idea given the nature of society, where everyone is so busy that we must cut a few corners in order to fit everything into our lives. This is where diets come into play because the primary focus is to cut things out, which in most cases, goes completely against human psychology. It is the same idea of telling a child that they cannot have something because they will certainly turn around and find a way to get it.

For years, I have seen people on these restriction "programs", forcing themselves to stay away from the foods they love, and trying to replace it with something they can barely swallow. The biggest reason the die-it industry is still sustaining itself is because it is a perpetually revolving door of "try this try that", "don't do this, do that", and "this is bad for you so do what I say". This kind of approach to health is very misleading in its own nature because in order to successfully change something on the outside you must first change what is happening on the inside. *James Allen* said it best in his book, **As a Man Thinkth**, "*change of diet will not help a man who will not change his thoughts. When a man makes his thoughts pure, he no longer desires impure food*".

From above so below, so if you want anything in life you must be in alignment with it. If you wish for better health and fitness, you must practice the habits and lifestyle disciplines that lead to the results you seek. This is what I call common sense consciousness, where we make conscious decisions that are rooted in common sense, an example being eating food that comes from a garden opposed to an industrial factory.

The deep implications of approaching health from a die-it mentality travels into all areas of our lives, not just what we put into our mouths, although that is the channel from where all energy begins. The word die-it is indicative of nothing other than dying. How can we associate health and vitality with such a word? The words we use as labels should be carefully chosen because they inflict a certain vibe or feeling over time. For example, if you talk to someone who has been "dieting" for an extended period of time, chances are, their feelings about it do not reflect the results they are attempting to gain. When we look to achieve a new standard in life, the action steps towards it should be exciting, fulfilling, and rewarding because it is not entirely the action that gets us there but, in truth, its the frequency in which we resonate during the process of germination, or accomplishment if you will. This idea is perfectly reflected in quantum physics, that which we most identify with energetically and emotionally we will bring about into our reality, with no exceptions and no excuses. So if losing a considerable amount of weight is your goal, it will not be achieved by merely cutting out fats or carbs. That is a superficial idea based on a dumbed down approach to nutrition, which is usually sold as a weight-loss strategy. Many people on diets are adhering to strict guidelines which should give them the results they seek. However, on the core level, they are still thinking the thoughts of an overweight person. They are still feeling the same feelings, and creating the future reality of someone who is unhappy, unsatisfied, and still overweight. This reality bleeds out into the rest of our lives, such as our relationships, our career, and our overall focus in life.

"He wants to gratify his taste for rich and unnatural viands and have his health as well. Such a man is totally unfit to have health, because he has not learned the first principles of a healthy life."
James Allen

I choose to approach a change in lifestyle from a place of abundance, vigor, joy, happiness, and hope because that is truly the only way to reach satisfaction and personal comfort. You can never get to heaven by focusing on hell, so therefore the more one restricts themselves of pleasure by participating in struggle, the more they remain stuck to the ground. This is much more than a food choice alteration because this is a complete life makeover from the root to the fruit. This is an inner journey that eventually leads one to finding their true essence. The biggest thing I see in the health world, wether it be a cheap die-it program or even a whole food or raw food approach, is that many people are treating it simply as a die-it! The focus is concentrated on what one can merely see with their eyes, and rarely taps into their inner guide where true power resides. The goal many times is far too superficial, which will lead to failure when times get tough. Even if you do lose a certain amount of weight, the fundamental changes within have not occurred. The initial goal is accomplished but after that, what's next?

It is my foundational belief that the biggest deficiency in mankind all across the board stems from one thing; one thing we are never taught in school or encouraged in the industrial work force. That one thing is what can take an individual who has lost all zest for life to the pillars of achievement and leadership. This one thing I'm speaking of is your calling in life. Your mission, your purpose, your all encompassing passion for why you're here on this planet is what should guide your food choices. The reason people are disconnected from the food they are eating and drinking is the result of a lack of clarity in direction.

We often put ourselves last on the priorities list in comparison to all the exterior demands of life. No wonder why we are in such a predicament globally, where there are corporate entities monopolizing lands that should be kept organic and sacred. When we put our focus on ourselves in a positive way, and on fueling ourselves with the best food that aids us in our passions and we make that the priority in our experience, then all the outside things begin to change. We can never win with a die-it type of mindset. Instead, we must skip that program all together and teleport to the live-it lifestyle that breeds empowerment and tranquility because that is what we deserve.

(Recommended Book: As A Man Thinketh:James Allen)

The Ability to Choose our Life Style

The most obvious sign of abundance, in my opinion, is the ability to choose and direct our own lifestyle modifications as we see fit. We have every food, super food, nutritional supplement, and informational tool at our finger tips, and to have these things is a luxury few could ever comprehend. We have what our parents never did, we have what our grand parents couldn't believe, and we also have what their parents could never even conceive. The pharaohs and the greatest kings and queens of all time, who witnessed the construction of inexplicable architectural monuments, never even dreamt of the technologies we have access to today.

I believe the idea that we can design a eating protocol specific to our preferences and needs is such a remarkable idea that we actually couldn't imagine life without it. Before the power of the internet and industrial machinery, the options were much fewer, and many died in pursuit of what we have with the click of a mouse. This idea alone is at the center of global importance because without the appreciation for the struggles of the past, we run the risk of falling back into limited thought forms which many are living in right now.

Regardless of the unlimited abundance that surrounds you, if your mind is not in a space to let it in, you will never receive the glory that could be yours for the keeping.

I believe it is now time to lay down the arms of the so called "Diet Wars", and work to find a common ground to cultivate intelligent discussions, and present options for all that choose to take it on. The ways in which many have approached diet education have been very inappropriate and ego driven. If you look behind the scenes of some of the leading health educators, they are not always shining examples of what they teach. This is a mistake that should not be made regularly because others are watching, hoping that we may have something of value that can benefit their lives. It seems we are beginning to move out of the overly fanatical attitudes that has given birth to mass separation, and moving closer to collective consciousness that makes room for everyone.

I personally believe in everything I teach since it comes from my own experience that has so deeply affected my life. I strongly agree with what Bruce Lee once said, which was "we must research our own experience and apply what is useful for our own lives then discard what is not". As a life long martial artist, I have seen the same trends of confinement hinder the progression of so many that could have blossomed into powerful, productive forces in the world but were unfortunately limited to the expectations of another. I recommend that you take everything that is useful for you, consider things you may not understand just yet, and play with new ideas in order to find what works for you the best.

Ultimately a true teacher should be a living testament of his own words, and the best teachers are always the best students. Become a straight-A student in your own life, and as you progress, you will become your own guru! Choose what provides you the most laughter, vitality, strength, and life-force energy. The torch is now in your hands, run with it for you are the forerunner of dreams envisioned by all those that came before...

Variety of Conscious Approaches

There are many different ways in which we can live our lives, and I suggest you look into them as a way to expand your horizons. The more we can open ourselves up to the possibilities that lie far outside of our comfort zone, the more tools we have to use in our lives. I would like to introduce some beautiful ways of approaching a lifestyle that is much closer to nature, which is ultimately adding in more raw organic foods, and there are different ways of doing it. If you allow yourself to experiment in the short term, you will find what works best for you in the long term.

"It is the diet of the times, it is the diet that most specifically addresses the difficulties people are having making their lives work. It's the diet that is best designed to preserve the essence of the world"

Dr. Gabriel Cousens

Vegetarianism

A vegetarian lifestyle is focused on a plant-based diet that may or may not have certain animal considerations, such as eggs or dairy products, but refraining from the consumption of meat. There are different variates of going about this type of approach, such as Ovo Vegetarianism(includes eggs, no dairy), Lacto Vegetarianism(includes dairy, no eggs), and ovo-lacto vegetarianism(includes dairy, eggs, and honey). A vegetarian-centered lifestyle is a beautiful way to live in relation to all living creatures around us. If done appropriately for your own health constitution, it can be an ideal way to thrive throughout life. Many people become vegetarians or vegans(excludes all animal products completely) for all kinds of reasons. Some do it for animal-rights reasons, seeing the destructive horrors of feed lots and slaughter houses can trigger an automatic exclusion from flesh foods in some. For me, this was a big influence. Many find it to be more in line with their spiritual beliefs, and can see the environmental threats current eating habits pose. Whatever the initial reason may be, it should be grounded with the main focus of being on one's health because if we are not strong, vibrant, and in the right frame of mind, then the other reasons do not have much power to express in the world.

Numerous cultures throughout the world have revered vegetarian and predominantly plant-based eating patterns throughout history. In fact, it should be plainly obvious that most major civilizations were mostly not meat eaters, with the exception of those in higher power, which in many cases lived shorter lives with less vitality than many commoners. The practice of vegetarianism is considered by some to be traced back to the Pythagoreans, who were the followers of the ancient greek philosopher, mathematician, and out-of-the-box thinker of the time, Pythagoras. He created a philosophy that was centered around harmonious living through respect for all life which included non-violence and abstaining from flesh foods, believing that the more one eats the meat of a brutalized creature, the more one's own soul becomes brutalized. His ideals are rumored to be derived from different Egyptian(3,000 BCE) traditions that were believed by many to have excluded meat and animal clothing for karmic reasons and the belief of reincarnation.

The traditions of Buddhism, Hinduism, Brahinanism, Zoroastrianism, and Jainism were rooted in the belief of no flesh eating as a way of life for both health and spiritual beliefs. In the sacred Hindu texts of the Upanishads, vegetarianism was highly encouraged and mentioned again in the Rig Veda.

In 1987 *John Robbins*, son and heir to the massive Baskin Robbins Ice Cream dynasty, had put out the book **Diet for A New America: How your food choices affect your health, happiness, and future on earth**. John Robbins had declined his fathers inheritance due to his personal beliefs that were leading him away from the trappings of society, and decided to move onto the land with his wife. This book was such a powerful turning point in the mainstream's food culture, and promoted awareness of the health and environmental repercussions of unethical corporate practices imposed along with the cruelty being endured by factory-farmed animals. This work has sparked many movements and many other books by Robbins. I personally was exposed to **Healthy at 100: The scientifically proven secrets to the worlds healthiest and longest lived people**. This book was a great catalyst that opened me to a new idea, and from that idea has blossomed into a way of life that continues to exceed itself as the days pass.

(Recommended Books: A Diet for A New America: John Robbins, The China Study: T. Colin Cambel)

Fruitarianism

Fruitarianism is a dietary approach which is a branch off of the vegetarian lifestyle. It consists of some nuts and seeds, some vegetables, and dominantly fruits. Some have different definitions as to what defines a fruitarian diet is exactly, but it is mostly 75%

fruit. The ethics and motivation behind this approach varies from person to person. Some people advocate only eating fruit as it has fallen to the ground, believing it is more natural to do so. Others will refrain from eating seeds as they contain the gifts of future fruits. The core belief behind a fruitarian lifestyle is connected to the return of a Garden of Eden type of paradise; the idea that we should live simply and obtain a more harmonious way of eating and living.

In essence this is a beautiful way to live ones life, and the very idea can bring a euphoric remembrance to how life may have once been. The way of least harm is similar to the Jainism belief, which states that pacifism and a centered path of non-violence to all living beings, and the understanding that all life forms have a soul.

We do not know how long into history a fruit dominant diet has been consumed, but there is some evidence that it was popular dating back to our ancient ancestors. Professor Alan Walker, a Paleoanthropologist from Johns Hopkins University, had reported preliminary studies of tooth enamel from early hominoids (existing pre-human ancestors) that showed that they may have had a diet of primarily fruits.

Many authors and health educators have experimented with a frutarian diet having with mixed opinions on it. *Arnold Ehret*, author of **The Mucusless Diet Healing System**, believed that nuts, seeds, and many green vegetables were mucus forming, which would be a disadvantage to good health. He advocated fruits, starchless vegetables, and herbs as the main staple in one's diet. Health author *Johnny Lovewisdom* had originally supported a very strict fruit-based diet until he eventually added in more vegetables, raw kefir, raw yogurt, and avocados. The political and spiritual leader, Mohandas Karamchand Ghandi, had kept up a fruitarian diet for a few years until he had experienced health challenges.

Although the idea of fruitarianism is a enjoyable one and can be very useful in the short term, doing this kind of diet in the longer term is highly discouraged. The nutritional problems that can arise from a diet high in fruits and low in fats and proteins may not sustain a fully functioning body and mind over the course of many years in "most cases". The times we are living in now have created a need to be fully focused on a well balanced lifestyle that fits our personal requirements. The exposure of pollution, radioactive accumulation, pesticides, and stressful byproducts of city living require most of us to have solid fat sources for insulation of our nerve fibers and brain. If one leaves out a lot of leafy vegetables, quality proteins, important fats, and supplemental considerations they may likely run into deficiencies such as low vitamin B-12(Section:**The Raw Naked Truth**), dehydration from too much potassium and not enough sodium(salt), neurological(bain) and hormonal imbalances due to the lack of proteins and long-chain omega fats such as DHA and EPA(Section: **The Sun Food Connection**). The body can be thrown severely off balance because of the acidic nature of most fruits(especially in grocery stores), and from massive mineral deficiencies as all conventional and hybridized fruits today contain little mineral content and high sugar content. Such an imbalance can strip minerals from the bones, causing bone and teeth problems.

To experiment and play out such a diet would require one to be very active to use up all the extra sugar they are intaking otherwise blood-sugar imbalances will come about. If one is dealing with diseases such as candida, diabetes, or any kind of cancerous situation, then I highly advise against a fruit-dominant diet because such sugar in any form will feed these conditions further. I personally believe that the over consumption of simple sugars, which burn up in the blood stream very fast, is a lead cause in many disorders and dis-eases we see in society. Even if it is done completely raw, most people are coming from a situation of highly processed carbohydrates, and artificial sugars that need to be cleansed from the body through highly mineralized and alkaline foods, such as organic vegetables, green juices, super foods, and herbs.

Based on the research I have done, and looking at all kinds of people from a variety of health focused lifestyles, I have to reiterate that no one system will work for all. I have seen people who actually thrive on a fruit/carbohydrate-based diet looking and reporting to feel great. There are slow oxidizers and fast oxidizers(the ratio in which you burn sugar), and depending on where you fall in this spectrum, it can give you a clue as to how much fruit sugar may work for you. If you feel wiped out 1-2 hours after a fruit meal, then you are a fast oxidizer (like me), and would do well to refrain from such a glycemic punch that too much sugar in one sitting can provide. If you feel good, and your body can sustain itself without feeling like your missing something, then more fruit may be appropriate for you.

In our current times, most conventional fruits are genetically inferior strains of their original form. Therefore, I highly recommend people lean closer to the power fruits such as edible organic/wild berries of all kinds. Fruits such as goji berries and noni fruit contain polysaccharides, which have positive effects on blood sugar levels, promote the immune system, and are highly mineralized. Also, high-fat fruits such as avocado, durian, and olives to support our raw plant fat needs.

Breatharianism

Inedia is the latin term used to describe fasting or those who live without the consumption of food. A word that describes a dedicated lifestyle to sustaining oneself without food or water is breatharianism. Those that abide under this way of life believe that they are able to fully harness the energies of the sun, earth, wind, and nature in order to fulfill their needs for nourishment in every way. Some may view this idea as a new-age concept, but truth be told, this has been done far longer than we have been eating foods made from human hands. Breatharians come from all walks of life and cultures spanning across the globe, and each with a different story that led to such a dramatic shift in lifestyle.

I have been made aware of many living examples of breatharianism, both short term and long term, which has given me a wider outlook as to view new and incredible possibilities. For example, Wiley Brooks, who was introduced to the world in 1981 on the television show, That's Incredible, by showing his strength by lifting 1100 pounds ten times for the audience, is a breatharian. He started the Breatharian Institute of America, and accepts a handful of "qualified" students to teach his ways of conducting this lifestyle. Jasmuheem, who is possibly the most well known breatharian, wrote the book, **Living on Light**, and is an international lecturer who spreads her message of living on the prana(cosmic energy) of the earth. Jasmuheem speaks on many topics. But one, in particular, that I think is very relevant is the idea that our brain waves run on certain beats, and our bodies will require various forms of nourishment based on the frequency of that beat. She says most people in society are running on a "busy beat" or beta beat wave which leaves the person depleted of energy and constantly reaching for food. We begin to experience the alpha and theta brain wave frequencies once we slow down the chattering of the mind by living moment to moment and practicing meditation daily. I have noticed over the years that her idea makes a lot of sense, and plays out in my own life as I live in a more meditative, intention-focused state. I also require much less food, and the food I do eat is 100% conducive to my health and happiness. The idea that what we eat or don't eat, in this case, has deep implications on the way we process our own reality through brain activity, and can be seen in another section in this book. (See Chapter **The Scientific Method**)

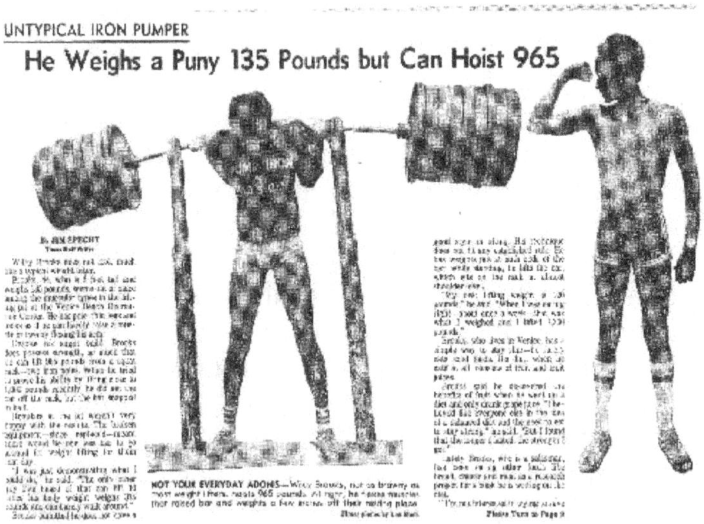

UNTYPICAL IRON PUMPER

He Weighs a Puny 135 Pounds but Can Hoist 965

NOT YOUR EVERYDAY ADONIS—

A powerful example of the breatharian way of life is a man named Genesis Sunfire. Genesis is a fitness trainer who has shared his story with many people throughout the world, and more information about him is available online. Genesis Sunfire is a former professional rugby player who has gone through a long process to reach a state of not eating food or drinking liquids. He was a fruitarian after his athletic career, eventually moving onto consuming only liquids(liquidtarian) as his source of fuel. After liquidtarianism, he moved to becoming a watertarian (drinking only water), and eventually became a fully committed breatharian who is being powered by the energies around us. Genesis's example breaks many of the health and nutritional paradigms we hold, simply because he consumes no food at all. How does he get his protein or carbs? Perhaps the human body can fully sustain itself on by it's own resources, and food acts as a detriment to the fully expressed potential of the human experience. In most cases, I would say the food we are eating definitely holds us from becoming all we can be.

It is important to note that all experienced breatharians such as Jasmuheen and Genesis Sunfire have stressed that this lifestyle is not for everyone, and must be approached with caution. The idea that living on little food, or none at all, is popular in the raw food lifestyle as we shed away the density of foods we may have grown up with that hindered us from reaching our higher potential. The phrase, "the less we eat the longer we live", definitely plays a major role in our health journey, and I leave it to you find where that fits in your current lifestyle.

(Recommended Book: Living on Light: Jasmuheem)

Honoring Tradition

The unique and grand innovations this generation has been blessed with are the direct results of the previous generations who had less to work with while having a greater vision to aspire for. It is the role of the youth to take what has been passed on, decode it, and ultimately uncover the message so that they may communicate it in a language the new world can understand. Although I have "deconstructed" many of the paradigms and traditional thinking of the past for you in this book, in no way do I wish to ridicule or embarrass them. The common attitude in western thought is to assume that each current generation holds the "missing-link", and therefore disregarding the lessons our ancestors worked so hard to preserve is justified. We must move forward in our thinking and action steps as well as cherish the ideals of past efforts for a more prominent future.

When I was originally given the responsibility of leading a martial arts academy, I felt a strong sense of leadership and the need to do right by the traditions that gave birth to my art. Many things have changed as these valuable art forms have been passed among leaders throughout the ages, including the techniques, the curriculum, the educational settings, and the traditional philosophy. As I became more exposed to the masters and grand-masters as a result of my position, I was given a deeper understanding of the heart behind the physical expressions of my art. I remember at times feeling resentment towards the older generation; I felt they were too rigid and unwilling to embrace the change in times. It was only as I became more mature and was leading hundreds of students that I began to realize why the values of tradition were so critical to upkeep. The reason why many of the older generation were rigid and sometimes unwilling to accept change is because they inherited these teachings from their instructors from the old country. They could see the effects of innovation without respect to the core fundamentals that drove their art, which is why they respected their tradition as much as they did their lives and wanted to pass on the same values. I suspect this same analogy could be applied to the vision that the pioneers of the raw food movement uphold- it is unsettling to have to adjust their core beliefs in an ever-changing world.

I ask that we do not forget the past and the originators of the healing field as we embrace the future. Every generation is building a brighter future on the back of its pioneers. Weston Price opened our eyes to the drawbacks of a processed and unnatural food system. Herbert Shelton showed us the science and fine art of fasting. Ann

Wigmore inspired countless individuals worldwide by saving her own life through vegetable juicing. Viktoras Kulvinskas detailed how to survive into the 21st century while co-founding the Hippocrates Health Institute which has passed onto Dr. Brian Clement. Patricia and Paul Bragg toured the country teaching audiences on the power of natural eating. Dr. Gabriel Cousens integrated spiritual awareness with the raw food philosophy, dubbing him the grandfather of raw foods. John Robbins made a single choice of morality that resulted in our changing the way we look at our food choices forever. These forerunners, along with many others, must not go unannounced as the movement grows with greater momentum. If we easily forget where this information first came from, then we may easily forget where we are intending on going.

Allowing Intuition to Guide You

"All spirituality is about relieving suffering"
Buddha

The key idea behind the live-it lifestyle is allowing our intuition to guide our lives in the direction that feels good for us. All suffering in the world is a result of people giving their power away, entrusting their lives and their families welfare to doctors, lawyers, gurus, banks, corporations, and governments, all of which are guided by their profit margins, and not our health. In order to truly live, we must speak, act, and move in the direction of where our internal guidance system is leading us. The conventional food choices are of a 3D nature, keeping us stuck in a conventional reality. As we shed these layers, getting back to what is natural and effective, we create a new relationship with ourselves, and guiding ourselves to a new destiny all together. We do not need a host of people telling us what to do about every little thing we encounter. We have the answers within ourselves, and to trust that inner knowing is to live in alignment with our authentic purpose.

The reason why some kids drop out of high school and become massively successful in the field of their choice is because they followed their intuition. The systematic routines of society are breaking apart under the pressure of bad results and hollow theories that seem to lead nowhere. You have complete control of where you go in your life. You control what goes into your mouth, and you have complete control of your health. The live-it lifestyle is a way to give you choices to choose from. You are the captain of your own ship, and this book acts as a reference point for ideas to help assist you along the way.

Whether you decide to become a 100% raw foodist, mostly raw and some cooked, or whatever the case may be, let it be a personal decision and not because someone said you should. I have seen all kinds of diet approaches work for a great number of people. I do not, in any way, advocate that there is only one way for everyone; that will never be the case. However, there are common themes and approaches that seem to work for a great multitude of people. If you feel a calling towards something specific, answer the calling without guilt or fear because there will be a message inside that only you can encode. Others, like myself, can assist you if needed, but ultimately, only you can answer the call!

Change Your Approach

"For everything you have missed, you have gained something, and everything you gain, you lose something else"
Ralph Waldo Emerson

"There is nothing wrong with change, if its in the right direction"
Winston Churchill

"Change is the essence of life. Be willing to surrender what you are for what you can become"
Unknown

The ability to adapt to change and re-access yourself are skills shared by all great achievers in life. If you decide to do anything in your life, you will be met with various obstacles that require a different set of solutions. Albert Einstein left us with this great quote, "insanity: doing the same thing over and over again and expecting different results". The solutions to the problems we have not yet faced, but most likely will, cannot be found in the same thinking that created them. We must change our approach when what we are doing is not working.

In *Maxwell Maltz's* book, **Psycho-Cybernetics**, he explains the procedure of a heat seeking missile relentlessly pursuing its target. It will go through twists and turns, readjust and recalculate its approach, all while moving forward in order to get to its pinpointed destination. That is exactly what our brain does when we define what we want. It sets up every possible situation for us to get there, but the desired outcome is completely dependent on our own willingness to adjust to unforeseen circumstances that might pop up. The brain is the most advanced machine on earth, capable of sending signals to our nervous system that allows for all human function. But remember that you are not a machine, and you are in complete control of this machine, and you may program it in any way you choose.

In the grand scheme of things, life is really just a constant flow of energy moving from one point to another. This energy is rarely ever sitting in one space, always being transferred and interacting with its environment, and influencing all who it touches. To clearly understand this idea, just spend some time next to a river. The flow of water is always moving without resistance, adjusting to all challenges that may attempt to disrupt its motion. Even a dam cannot hold the flow of water in motion because eventually, the forward motion will find a crack, and the water will find its way through. This is a key metaphor to use for approaching life: always moving forward, adjusting simultaneously in order to get to the decided result. Once you stop in your tracks, you halt the momentum and lose your power.

When you are pursuing your health journey, it is so important to stay in constant communication with yourself at all times. One day you may feel absolutely amazing, like nothing can detour your enthusiasm for life, and the next day you could feel zapped, fatigued, and emotionally subdued. This can be a detoxification response, but it could also be a host of other things as well. It could be a nutritional deficiency, such as not having enough B vitamins, demineralization, or lack of proper omega fatty acids. Many times, the ailments of the body are responding to ailments of the soul. Sometimes the deep-seated issues we suppressed can arise unannounced. This is very common on a primarily raw food lifestyle, mainly because you are naturally clearing out junky matter from cooked, processed, and contaminated animal products which can keep a lot of these issues locked away until they surface later, usually in extreme ways if not dealt with appropriately.

Learn to maneuver through your life experiences gracefully, like a dancer executing movements of agility and coordination with the fluidity of the wind. Take a non-resistance approach to life, and be amazed at the miracles that come about. It is our resistance to change and our hesitation to make adjustments on the spot that keeps us separated from the life we are meant to enjoy. As a martial artist, the greatest skill is not one of power or technical prowess, but that of adaptation. If you can adapt to your opponent's strikes and redirect their energy, you will always remain the victor. Survival of the strongest is a much outdated and false idea. It is not always the smartest, fittest, or that who has the most money that survives. Instead, it has always been, and will always be the one who can adapt to arising situations as they happen and move with the current of life.

Find your sweet spot, the place where you lose sight of all obstacles, and the only thing that appears in front of you is the result which has captured your attention. In sports, we call this getting in the zone. It may take time to adjust from mistakes, but thats ok. We are all striving to be professional mistake makers! If you are on a treadmill, there may be someone to your right and left, there may be music playing in the background, but as soon as you move into the zone, all of those things begin to fade away from your reality, and all that you can see is your intended goal. When life gets the toughest, that is when you need to dig down deep and give it everything you have. Do not give up on yourself until you have given it every ounce of energy you have.

As *Eric Thomas*, author of **The Secrets of Success**, said, *"if what you want is not in your comfort zone you need to get out of your comfort zone to get what you want"*. No one said it was going to be easy to be all you can be while you're on this planet, but that doesn't mean it cannot be fun either. In fact, to be all the creator has in store for you should be the most exciting and transformative experience possible. Imagine losing all the excess weight that has been holding you back from your potential, and doing it with laughter and joy in your heart. Imagine reconnecting with your children who may be separated from you for whatever reason. Imagine having a powerful influence on the lives of children everywhere! Imagine educating one parent on how to provide better nourishment to their own child, and now imagine that child fulfilling their life's purpose because of that seed planted from your tree of prosperity.

I want you to imagine all of life's possibilities as you change and rearrange your approach to obstacles, and do it with a smile knowing that the best is always yet to come. Each and every day before us is an open invitation to unleash magnificence into a world that needs a little more of that stuff.

Leaving Excess Behind

"And I figured out that the reason I couldn't get through the day as well as I can now is because I had too many things on my mind, on my plate, you know, for one person to have. So I started to eliminate some of the things that were too heavy to carry and unnecessary."

Erykah Badu

The effectiveness of moving into a new place in life is greatly dependent on how much of the old life you are willing to let go of in order to gracefully move forward. Your health journey is one of great discovery into the depths of who you are and who you can be. There are no limits or restrictions in how far you can take this if you truly apply yourself. In order to successfully reach the next level in your progress, there are a number of things to consider. It is never as easy as what appears on the forefront. You must dig a little bit because the more you do, the more shadows of the past will present themselves for you to look at.

I think the biggest obstacle people experience is their own unwillingness to face the darker sides of their lives. With the positive always comes the negative, and vice versa. We live in a universe governed by duality. Life is much like a sea saw in this way, and we must acknowledge both sides in order to get to where we are trying to go. The old adage that says "you must face it in order to erase it" is a perfect mantra to ingrain into your personality when you come across personal resistance. Often enough, when you do openly and honestly face it, you will find the problem removes itself from your life completely. The biggest effort comes in finally taking a look at what is going on.

The list of chronic conditions and physical dis-eases so many people deal with are usually two sided. The body is responding to a much deeper crisis that is of a spiritual nature, usually. There is an unsettling emotional that must be released before true healing can begin. To focus on the symptom and ignoring the root cause is what has delivered the results we currently have. It is time to get back to basics, which is considering the person as a whole being and not just a mechanical entity.

Lets take a journey into your own transformation!

Fasting

The idea of fasting is one that has been misunderstood, in my personal opinion. There are many different approaches and ways to look at this topic. Within the health food community, long-term fasting is extremely popular, and can be a very uplifting and powerful experience for many people. I want to present what I believe fasting is designed for, that being to rest and recharge.

Our body, mind, and spirit require rest from the stresses of life and the different influences around us. In order to effectively rest the body, abstaining from certain foods for the short term is very helpful for your digestive powers to reclaim themselves if they have become weakened from years of improper food abuse. Obviously, some foods should be removed for the long term as they serve no productive purpose and do not have anything to do with a healthy lifestyle. The mind needs to break from certain activities that could be causing other problems, such as negative thinking patterns and over analysis. Sometimes the best way to uncover a problem is to write it down, put it out of our mind, and go to sleep because a clear mind is much better at resolving issues than a cluttered mind. The way in which we rest spiritually is different for different people, but simple things such as surrounding yourself with nature, positive friends or family, and definitely being around children is a way to deeply connect yourself into the healing powers of laughter and joy!

Fasting, in general terms, is about taking a break from food in order to replenish the entire human being, which is what the act of sleeping does for us. In the section **Sleep Less, Live More**, I speak about many of the stresses that interrupt the bodies ability to effectively recover even if we are sleeping longer. One of those obstacles is the body not properly resting during times of sleep due to the process of digesting foods that have not yet been broken down and dispersed throughout the body. This can take a lot of energy from the body, depending on the density of the food, and the closer the meal is eaten to the time you sleep, the harder it will be to efficiently recharge your energy. This helps explain why there is great wisdom in the way our ancestors lived. They did not have 24 hour access to food as we do, and because of this, their meals were much more spaced out, which allowed for greater recovery of the body along with improving mental and emotional health.

In the biblical tradition, a day of rest was advised for each week of work. This tradition was referred to as the sabbath, which translates in hebrew as "to cease". This term was originally derived from the story of creation where the creator spent 6 days putting together the heavens and earth, and taking the 7th day off for rest and replenishment. Fasting can be approached from the very idea that we all live fast-paced lives, and yet we require adequate time to rest, recharge, and re-evaluate the week thats now past, all while creating the week that is to follow. Once a week, anyone can take a break from heavy foods. It would be of great service to your digestive system to take a day to only consume liquids instead of solid meals. If you feel up to it, take a day to abstain from food all together, drink only water, and see how generously your body thanks you.

After looking at many different approaches to fasting, I personally agree strongly with the idea of *Intermittent Fasting,* which is the idea of fasting in intervals. This means to create space between your last meal and the time you sleep, and fasting throughout the morning until you "Break Fast". The term breakfast really means to break a fast. We have grown up to believe that eating your biggest meal early in the morning is ideal. This idea seemed very intelligent as a competitive athlete, but now I can see the problems it can pose over the long term. As you awaken in the morning, your body is still in detoxification mode as it is attempting to eliminate all the waste from days prior. The best way to help your body do this is to drink high quality water, preferable with magnesium and/or sea salt to help with bowel movements. Hydration is the number one key to optimal health, so to prepare your body this way early in the morning will create a biological environment that is much more self sustainable over time. As you go through the morning, you will eventually "break fast". A great way to do this is with some form of exercise, seeing as how your body has truly recovered and stored energy, so its time to use it. Combining these two disciplines in such a strategic way has been shown to increase growth hormone production by eating less and exercising relatively close to each other.

After your work out, you should reintroduce high quality and easy to absorbe foods back into the body. I personally create a super food drink that is combined with high quality protein, carbohydrates, and some fats to help me rebuild and sustain me throughout a portion of the day.

Theres healing clinics around the world that specialize in helping guide and monitor individuals through fasting safely. Long term juice, fruit, and water fasting can be extraordinarily healing, especially in the case of a healing crisis where measures must be taken in order to save a life. I highly encourage those interested in long term fasting to seek out the professional care of a highly skilled fasting specialist who has an expertise in raw food nutrition and detoxification.

Cleansing

Herings Law of Cure

"We heal from the top down; We heal from the inside out; We heal in the reverse order in which we took on our health challenges."

Constantine Hering

The word cleansing means to clean, and in the terms of this subject, it is to clean out the body. Cleansing is absolutely critical in our modern world where we are so open to toxins coming into our bodies. We need to open up the back door to let these toxins out. There are many different methods of cleansing out there. From 21-day cleanses, gallbladder cleanses, liver cleanses, and many others to look into. They are all important because our bodies take a tremendous beating over the years of socially suggested living patterns. Depending on your own situation, I would recommend you look into a cleansing specialist, and do your own research before purchasing any type of cleansing product because most promise more than they provide.

What people must understand about attaining true health is that it is not a quick fix project that can be worked on for one month and left behind the next. It is an ongoing process of learning and adjusting. When you dedicate yourself to clearing out the "confusion" in the body, there will be detox symptoms that occur, and you must be prepared for it. The effects differ from person to person. If you approach it with a fast track immediate result mentality then I can assume your symptoms will become severe, especially if you are coming from a standard diet void of nutrition. If you learn to approach cleansing in a way that is gentle, with a long-term vision in mind, your symptoms will be lessened. However, that does not mean there will be no speed bumps, but the drama of it all will be much easier to accept.

I personally believe for someone coming from a less-than-ideal lifestyle looking to clean up their health, going towards a more raw food protocol is the easiest and best bridge to transition into a healthier life pattern. Most people's health problems are directly related to being nutritionally deficient, and living foods fills that hole. A one-time cleanse will not plug the hole of the ship that is sinking. The journey is what we should place our focus on. The word cleansing broken down is clean-sing, so enjoy the process of becoming clean. If you are green on the inside, you will become clean on the inside, so make sure to incorporate as much raw organic plant foods as possible to start with. Green leafy vegetables, specifically, have high amounts of fiber that will help break down old food residue that is clogging the intestine. This will be a major relief on the rest of the body, now it can do what it was designed to. If you are in a situation where you may have some bad digestive issues, bloating, or stomach cramps, you might be better off with doing green juices because it removes a lot of the fiber that you may not be ready for. You will need to test the waters a bit to find your perfect medium, but ultimately the more plant foods you add, the better of you will be, guaranteed!

Foods rich in sulfur are great for detoxification of toxic residues that are stored in our body, our lungs in particular, because that is where our immune system is activated from. When we are in a toxic state, the harmful substances will attach themselves to the thyroid gland in our throat. Foods such as garlic, peppers, ginger, red onions, sunflower seeds, cabbage, kale, hemp seeds, spirulina, and asparagus are all great sources of sulfur. Look into MSM(Methyl-Sulfonyl-Methane) in the section **The Sun Food Connection** as a primary source of adding sulfur into any cleansing strategy.

Cleansing is an art, and must be practiced diligently to tune up your body to its highest potential. The cleaner your body is on the inside, the more it will show on the outside. A very good indication of someone's health is by the quality of there skin and energy radiating from their personality.

As important as cleansing is, do not get carried away with making it a complete approach to life where you must cleanse all the time. This can create a series of problems physically and mentally. The theme is similar to someone who is addicted to cleaning their house. Even after it is almost immaculate, they are still cleaning for fear of it getting dirty again. The same idea exists in the health world where many people are obsessed with doing cleanses, believing that anytime there is a physical or energetic disturbance, it is due to being toxic, and they must then clean house. Whether this is completely true or not, I will not get into details. What I will say is that at some point, it is time to move on from a catabolic state(break down) and get into a more anobolic state (growth) by adding in more building foods that help provide full spectrums of nutrition. This is why I recommend a living foods approach that is harmoniously balanced with your personal needs.

The way you choose your surroundings throughout your day can be just as powerful as the foods you take into your body. As you go through the journey of cleaning out the obstruction from the inside, emotions that are tightly knotted will come out as well, and these can show up in different ways. Make sure you have a core support system, preferably friends or family that can help ease the pressure that this transition may cause temporarily. Ask them to hold your hand and aid you emotionally and physically when needed. It is important to use this time to create new habits to go along with your new direction, such as removing old material items that are taking up space, deleting phone numbers that no longer serve you, spending more time in nature, and creating a journal to unfold your thoughts either to yourself or loved ones you may have unspoken words with. I remember when I first went through my major transition, I found myself spending much more time barefoot in nature, running the hills, hiking, calling up people that I felt needed to hear my voice, and selling old possessions that were taking up space.

The experiences we go through in life are completely unique to us and our own personal needs at that time, but we can relate with one another by opening the doors of communication. I highly recommend connecting with other raw food enthusiasts and those who have been where you are so that you can receive the benefit of their experiences.

The Pancreas

The pancreas is one of the various hormone-producing glands in the human body. This indispensable organ serves two major functions, one of which is for hormonal production involving insulin, somatostatin and glucagon, which regulate metabolism. The other purpose is to act as a digestive organ, secreting liquids known as pancreatic juices that contain digestive enzymes. The health of our pancreas is a priority for vibrant and vital living. If this organ becomes stagnant, our entire life will follow suit.

The proper balance in blood sugar is dependent largely on the intelligence of the pancreas. If you or anyone you know is dealing with a diabetic or pre-diabetic condition, invest time into studying the chapter **Symptoms of Society, Diabetes**. The pancreas is located behind the stomach, and attached to the gallbladder and small intestine. Blood sugar levels are regulated when insulin is secreted, helping to escort glucose(sugar) into our cells so we can produce energy. The pancreas's ability to secrete digestive enzymes is crucial for the metabolism of nutrients. If there is too much undigested fat or protein, for example, it can interfere with glucose entry, creating hyper blood-sugar disorders.

The variety of minerals in our diet is another factor that is critical, and one I mention all throughout this book. Out of all the organs in our body, the pancreas draws in the most abundance of minerals required for enzymatic activation upon reaching the small intestine. There is a strong correlation between pancreatic distress and heavy consumptions of cooked foods. Foods that contain the most minerals also contain the most enzymes, which reduces the work load of the pancreas. This is why raw plant food is the number one choice for internal cleansing and maintenance. When food is introduced to high heat, mineral integrity is lost. Something else I find very interesting is that rocks contain heavy concentration of minerals but we are not biologically designed to break down rock sediment. However, plants are capable of doing this, and the minerals become a part of the plants that we make a part of us. This is one more indication our ideal choice of food is, and has always been, raw plant foods.

Foods specific for the Pancreas:

- Cucumbers (Water rich, alkaline, helps relieve indigestion and heart burn)
- Celery (Potassium/Sodium balance, lowers blood pressure, calcium, dietary fiber)
- Heirloom Tomatoes(Lycopene antioxidant, fiber, vitamin c, potassium, chromium)
- Ripe Peppers(Sulfur content)
- Olives (important oils, oleic acids, anti-inflammatory, polyphenols for cellular health)
- Okra(fiber, vitamin a, vitamin c, magnesium, folate, folic acid, potassium, calcium, helps intestinal lubrication improving digestion)
- Beets(blood building, blood detoxification aid, contains betaine, flavonoids, contains methylation compounds that have been linked to decreasing cancer cells)
- Sea Weeds(The high concentration of oceanic minerals)
- Turmeric(anti-inflammatory, neuro-protective increasing cognitive function, defends against oxidative stress)

The Liver

The liver is the largest glandular organ of the entire human body, and it is responsible for many different functions. The liver deals with protein synthesis, converting amino acids into usable proteins. It deals heavily with our metabolism, producing an alkaline compound called bile which helps with our nutrient absorption. This vital organ aids our body in its ability to metabolize fats, important vitamins, and carbohydrates which are turned into sugar(glucose) as immediate fuel for red blood cells and the brain.

The liver is the great filtration unit in the body, separating out toxins from the blood stream. All the food we eat is given to the liver to convert into usable nutrition or store for later use. All toxins that are ingested pass through the liver, and are turned into a less toxic form. Throughout one's life of consuming dense cooked foods, animal products, alcohol, and pharmaceuticals, the liver becomes less effective, resulting in the potential for problems.

Living foods will greatly aid in revitalizing the large amount of liver cells that may have been damaged in the past. Even if the liver is functioning at a very low level, it can still carry out the task of healing if given the right tools to work with. The way in which someone deals with cleansing the liver should be soft and gentle at first. If the liver is very toxic, the organ will be more sensitive to heat or spices, so we want to work with foods that have a cooling effect such as cucumbers, dandelion root, celery, apples for their malic acid, lemons, and beets. All these foods can be juiced as much as you want in replacement of solid foods, but should be taken slowly to not put too much strain on the liver during the healing process. Make sure to drink at least 1 liter of clear water each morning with a spoon full of MSM inside.

Foods specific for the Liver:

- Garlic(in moderation) (Helps activate liver enzymes for cleansing, antibacterial, antimicrobial, anti-parasitic, also contains omega 3 fatty acids)
- Camu Camu Berry (Highest Vitamin C content food world wide)
- Grape Fruit (Vitamin C & antioxidants)
- Goji Berries (Extremely high in Caratonoids, Beta-Carotene, extremely high in antioxidants)
- Chlorella(10% Chlorophyll, aids in detoxification)
- Avocados (Nutrient dense food that is easy to digest, meat & cheese replacement)
- Apples (Contains high amounts of pectin, malic acid, helps aid in digestion and cleansing)
- Cold Pressed Olive, Hemp, Flax, & Avocado Oil (Can suck up heavy toxins from the liver, aids in regenerating liver damage, easily assimilated into the body)

The Kidneys

The Kidneys are the two bean shaped organs that rest in the back-middle of our back, directly underneath the rib cage, one on each side of the spine. The kidneys primary task is as a filtration system, processing around 200 quarts of blood in order to filter out excess waste products and extra water build up. The waste along with excess water is turned into urine and exited out of the body by our gall bladder. Waste products can build up in our blood stream through food particles and scar tissue from the break down of our muscles. The body uses the nutrients from our food for energy production and maintenance/repair. A healthy kidney will successfully extract the excess waste given off from unneeded calories. A unhealthy kidney will not be able to perform this function efficiently and that is when problems can arise.

Diabetes is a nutrition and mineral deficiency syndrome that can impair kidney performance. High blood sugar levels due to the body not producing enough insulin or not being able to use available insulin adequately has been suggested as the number one leading cause of kidney disease.

The long-term usage of over the counter drugs or street drugs are directly involved in kidney problems. The popular calcium supplement industry may be one of the most dangerous supplements for this reason among others. A kidney stone is the production of bad calcium(false-calcium) formations or excess calcium from artificial foods that contain synthetic forms of calcium used as preservatives. City water and well water are notorious for containing calcium-forming-organisms which creep into our tissues and organs. Study the section in the back of this book, **The Calcium Theory**, chapter, **The Scientific Method**.

When detoxification occurs the body will utilize the four main channels of elimination which are the bowels, the lungs, the skin, and the kidneys. The state of our urine may be a reflection of the state of our blood. If there is disturbances in our blood it will show up in our urine as detoxification is occurring. When our urine is clear this is indicating that our blood is clean at that moment. When we are in a high-detoxification state we may find ourselves urinating 4-5 or even more times a day. It is important to keep hydrated so we do not fall into a dehydration situation.

Foods Specific for Kidneys:

- Raw Cabbage(Vitamin K & C, fiber, folic acid, phytochemicals)
- Red Onions(chromium(balances blood sugar metabolism), high sulfur content, flavonoids including quercetin.)
- Cranberries(antioxidants, has been known to aid in bladder health and baldder infections)
- Fresh Berries(Antioxidants, high vitamin concentration, wild berries contain high mineral counts, phytochemicals, extremely effective in inflammation reduction)

The Lymphatic System

The most commonly associated medium for circulation in the body is through our blood via the arteries and veins. Less commonly known is another mode of circulation called the lymphatic system. It is sometimes explained that if our bodies were like a city, then the lymphatic system would be the garbage company, sewage system, and police force all comprised into one system. The lymphatic system is composed of organs, ducts, and nodes that assist in the transportation of lymph fluid released from our blood plasma and recycles it back into the blood. This fluid helps with the circulation of blood in order to drain fluids from the cells and bodily tissues along with sending out immune cells through out the body. The blood delivers oxygen and nutrients to the cells while the lymph fluid removes waste products from the cells. If you can imagine a natural river washing away trash, then apply this same concept to our bodies. The lymph is bathing our cells and washing the accumulated waste so long as the body is kept in high regard. The Lymph system acts as a drainage system, using lymph vessels to extract excess fluids from the body tissues. Swelling will occur when there is chronically too much Lymph fluid built up in one area of the body. This condition indicates a blockage of blood and lymph transportation, usually resulting from a poor diet and/or scar tissue from old injuries. It is crucial to keep our lymphatic system in top condition. When lymph fluid builds up excessively like this, proteins, lipids, and other molecules leak out of tiny capillaries into nearby body tissues.

There is an estimated 5.5 gallons of lymph fluid in the human body- that equates to almost 3 times the amount of blood in the body. The lymph fluid circulates through the body unidirectionally(one-direction) up to the neck area. Women must pay special attention to this information as they are more susceptible to this issue due to menstrual cycles. An excessive loss of blood can lead to anemic conditions which is a lower than normal red blood cell count, usually leading to iron deficiencies among other complications. The quality of our lymphatic function will determine the quality of our blood and intracellular communication among cells.

One of the main functions of our lymphatic system is the regulation and optimization of our immune system. We have lymph nodes, an oval-shaped organ, that reside along a network of lymphatic vessels distributed through out the body. These nodes are designed to filter out foreign particles or molecules to maintain the performance of the immune system. The lymph nodes contain white blood cells called lymphocytes that produce certain antibodies known as natural kill cells(NK cells) that attack infectious microorganisms. These NK cells serve as a component of our "innate-immune-system", influencing the fortification of our health and defending us from dangerous infections. The other types of lymphocytes are called T cells and B cells. These lymphocytes are specifically related to our "adaptive-immune-system". The T and B cells serve to identify an "invader" and immediately create cellular responses that are specifically designed for the elimination of the offending pathogen (virus, bacteria, fungus, etc.).

There is a form of exercise known as rebounding that stimulates the circulation of our lymph fluid through out the entire body. Although fresh organic fruits and vegetables are a great way to detoxify and cleanse our lymphatic system, our lymph fluid does not move unless we do. Rebounding has been shown to effectively stimulate every single cell in our body, creating a cascade of better functioning cells that communicate with one another. This form of exercise is basically a small trampoline that we bounce on and perform a wide variety of exercises in order to activate every muscle group. We are literally doubling the effects of gravity with zero strain on the body as we jump up and down on a rebounder. Nasa has done numerous studies and testing on rebounding, confidently stating that "Rebounding exercise is the most efficient, effective form of exercise yet devised by man".

We must allow our lymphatic system to keep circulating fluids through out the body in order to maintain good health. The most effective way to re-balance a stagnant lymph system is to alkalize, and allow the detoxification process to take place. The standard high-fat high-protein diet is responsible for blocking oxygen exchange in our blood and stagnating the lymph fluid's ability to escort toxic waste from our cells. For this reason, moderate cardiovascular exercise is the prerequisite for lymphatic circulation.

Foods specific to the Lymphatic System:

- Black Seeded Grapes (Antioxidants, Anti-aging Resveratrol, Tannins within the seed, Polyphenols, and Short-chain Fatty Acids)
- Grape Fruit (Anti-inflammatory, Vitamin C, Fiber, Potassium)
- Citrus Fruit (Oranges, Lemons, Clementine, Tangerine-The most detoxifying fruits)
- Black Seeded Watermelon (Magnesium within the seeds, high-fiber and high-water content)
- Vegetable Juice (Alkalizing, absent rough vegetable fiber means all nutrition, increases hydration, helps the blood and lymph circulate)

- High-grade Algae Oil & Marine Phytoplankton (Essential Omega-3 Fatty Acids)

The Lungs

All of our organs and glands are tremendously affected by the foods we eat, and none being more susceptible to toxins than our lungs. We must concentrate the majority of our attention on our breath because the breath is where all of life is. If we are unable to breath naturally, then we will lack in all other areas of bodily health. The number one most common cancer in the world is lung cancer. The lungs are extremely sensitive to environmental damage, which causes oxidation. The lungs were designed to open up to the atmosphere to take in fresh air, but because of the pollutants, heavy metals and toxins in the air, this causes problems if we do not detoxify these dangerous compounds.

The lungs' ability to transport oxygen from the air we breath into the bloodstream, and then release carbon dioxide from the blood out into the atmosphere, is critical for respiratory health. The function of breathing is done primarily from the diaphragm muscle, which indicates that we need a strong cardiovascular system through exercise and proper eating. The health of our cells creates oxygen for our blood, which travels to all areas of the body, and much of it must passes through the lungs. The best way to purify the blood is through green juices such as sprouts and leafy vegetables. The chlorophyll(See chapter: **The Sun Food Connection**) content in organic dark green vegetables is exactly what our blood requires for easy transportation of oxygen. Vegetable and sprout juices are the easiest way to make an immediate impact on the cellular level because there is no digestion needed; it is pure energy!

Those involved in endurance sports and activities that require heavy lung function are being turned onto super foods and herbs to increase respiratory strength. One example is the root vegetable, maca, which grows at the highest altitudes in the world. According to the research, maca can double ones oxygen intake based on the environment they are in. The very fact that cultivators have to climb up the greatest mountain tops to obtain it should tell you something: the area in which a food is grown speaks highly of its power. Since the lungs are easily affected by oxidation, we want to make sure we consume a vast amount of antioxidants. A diet rich in colors, such as all kinds of berries, lots of different organic vegetables and fruits(with seeds), cacao beans, and coconut products are incredible tools for lung health.

Foods specific to the Lungs:

- Oranges (Vitamin C, Iron, Antioxidants. Increases oxygen support)
- Green Vegetables- Kale, Dandelion, Mustard, Arugula, Spinach, Collard, Lettuce, Chard, Cabbage, Cauliflower, Brussel Sprouts, Broccoli, Bok Choi, Chinese Savoy, Lamb's Quarters, Miners Lettuce, Cilantro, Coriander, Fennel, Mint, Water Cress(Extremely Alkaline, minerals, nutrient dense, easy to digest, fiber, water content, enzymes)
- Pineapple (Bromolean enzyme)
- Coconut & Coconut Oil (Stimulates thyroid & metabolism, saturated fats buffer heavy toxicity built up in the throat, lauric acid)

- Raw Honey (Soothes the throat, highly enzymatic)
- Lemon (traditional throat remedy)
- Cayenne Pepper (Ramps up metabolism, anti-viral properties,)

The Adrenals

The adrenals are endocrine glands that sit directly on top of the kidneys, acting as our bodies natural battery packs. These glands are activated in response to stress, releasing certain hormones such as cortisol and epinephrine(adrenaline). Cortisol helps with our metabolism of glucose(sugar), immune function, and helps with the fight or flight responses that can become overwhelming in our culture. Cortisol release is really about relaxing the body, especially after heavy stress or panic situations. Throughout history and small pockets of the world in modern times, the fight or flight response would be triggered by something such as a wild animal or bandit, creating an immediate life threat. In such a situation, adrenaline kicks on, boosting heart rate, constricting blood vessels, and creating oxygen pathways to the lungs in order to aid in higher alertness and rapid performance. Adrenaline is also a neurotransmitter, having a substantial effect on the health and sharpness of the brain. A big reason why so many people are breaking down so rapidly is because their adrenal glands are in high demand far too frequently, a physical response reserved for a life or death potentiality is being activated for every day occurrences, like losing your keys or locking yourself outside the house. This amount of stress is pounding our entire glandular system, starting with the battery packs. Once those become sapped out, the rest of our body begins to fall apart, leading to adrenal fatigue or adrenal insufficiency.

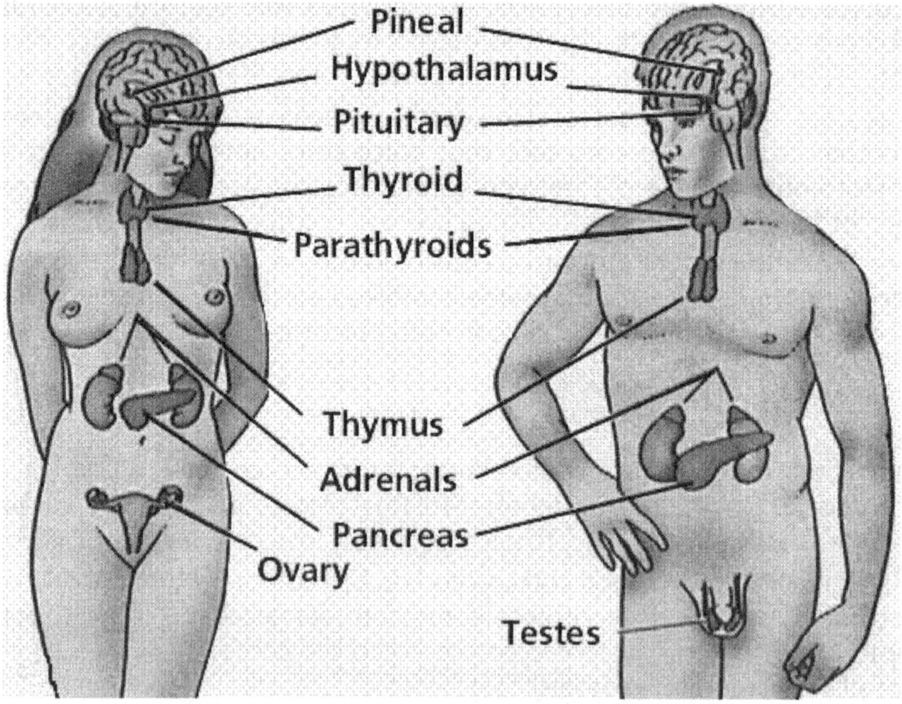

The male & female Endocrine system

Effects of weakened adrenal glands can be grouped together, such as consistent fatigue, light headedness, physical aches and weakness, having trouble getting up in the morning, etc. These are all signs that there is a problem that should be addressed, and taking proper care of these glands will make big improvements. *Dr. James Wilson* discovered the condition he named his book by, **Adrenal Fatigue**. On his website, adrenalfatigue.org, he lists what he believes to be the biggest culprits in perpetuating this condition.

Examples of lifestyle factors that may contribute to adrenal fatigue: (Most of these are within your control.)

- Lack of sleep
- Poor food choices (white flour, low fiber, sugar, few vegetables or fruit, lack of raw food, etc.)
- Using sweet or salty food and sweetened or caffeinated drinks as stimulants when tired
- Staying up late even though tired
- Feeling/acting powerless
- Constantly driving yourself
- Trying to be perfect
- Staying in double binds (no win situations)
- Too few of enjoyable and rejuvenating activities

This seems to be one of the most common problems of the industrial age in terms of health challenges. If one is constantly in a state of anxiety, stress, fear, and ingesting artificial substances, they will experience this road block. Fortunately, like a high-quality car battery, it can be recharged, and the way to do that can vary. Adrenal difficulties can result in low blood pressure, which means you will need to make a big lifestyle adjustment. If you are under the influence of any stimulants, junk food, or conventional animal products, you should begin removing them from the diet immediately. Whenever you eat anything at all, it creates a blood sugar increase. All food is a stimulant in this way, and because of that, mineral deficient fruits should be consumed moderately as the simple sugar content burns too fast. It is suggested by Dr. James Wilson to avoid putting off your first meal of the day past 10:00 AM in order to maintain regular blood sugar levels. The best foods to consume are a wide variety of organic vegetables, grasses, adaptogenic herbs, and moderate nuts and seeds. If you consume cooked foods at all, the most ideal food choices are whole grains, such as brown rice, oats, quinao, buckwheat, millet, and barley. Someone in such a condition may do much better to include these small portions of cooked foods as a balanced caloric source as doing the living foods lifestyle is not about perfection but always about health first.

Including super foods and herbs can jump start the body in a way that can produce enough energy to supply the glands to do their job. Certain herbs can be of great assistance because the role these plants have is to tone our organ system, which literally means to take our organs through a workout. An herb of particular interest is the Ayurvedic plant *macuna*. This herb is a tropical legume that grows in different areas of the world. The properties that make this plant stand out among others is specifically in its L-Dopa content. L-Dopa is the direct pre-cursor for the neurotransmitter dopamine. Dopamine is essential for the well being and alleviation of stress in our body, and it works in conjunction with serotonin to make us feel good. The increase of artificial stimulants results in the decrease of dopamine in the brain as it becomes overwhelmed and sapped out of the brain. The magic of macuna is that the L-Dopa(dopamine precursor) penetrates the blood brain barrier effectively, stimulating our dopamine reserves, and allowing us to increase our feelings of ease. Macuna is a restorative herb that has powerful effects on our sympathetic nervous system, and has been shown to be effective in treating the defects of Parkinson's disease.

Foods specific for the kidneys/adrenals:

- Red Bell Peppers (Vitamin C, A, B6, contains the antioxidant lycopene)
- Colorful Berries (Blue Berries, Cranberries, Rasberries, Strawberries, Black Berries, Goji Berries, Mulberries, Golden Berries, Cherries, ect.)
- Sun Dried Raisins (antioxidants, boron, tartaric acid, polyphenols, fiber, pectin)
- Coconuts/Coconut oil/Butter (Healthy Saturated Fats, MCT's, increases metabolic efficiency)
- Cinnamon (Antibacterial, anti-fungal, improves digestion, known to have blood thinning efficacy for clotting)

Colon Hydrotherapy

The colon is the long intestine that is responsible for completing the phases of digestion. Over time, the colon can become extremely burdened by the food products of society, picking up toxins, voc's(volitile organic compounds), plastics, parasites, and fecal matter. The practice of internal cleansing or colonics(colon hydrotherapy) has been administered in different forms dating back to the ancient Egyptians, and adopted by the Greeks afterwards. The idea behind modern day colon hydrotherapy as an alternative healing practice is based on a term called "autointoxication". This condition is believed to be caused when too much food matter has filled up inside the colon, causing decomposition, which then leads to many circulatory problems.

In *Victoria Boutenko's* book, **Green for Life** she cites the great health and nutrition pinoneer *Dr. Bernard Jensen* who had this to say in regards to the health of our colon

"Any cleansing program should begin in the colon...In the 50 years I've spent helping people to overcome illness, disability, and disease, it has become crystal clear that poor bowel management lies at the root of most people's health problems. In treating over 300,000 patients, it is the bowel that invariable has to be cared for first before any effective healing can take place."

The purpose of doing colonics regularly is to clean out the bowels so that our colon is able to operate efficiently. The build up of toxicity over the duration of ones life, in most cases, causes a breaking down of the internal organs. Colon Hydrotherapy helps speed up the detoxification process, escorting harmful backed-up matter out of the body within a session instead of over weeks or months. In 1991, an article in USA TODAY stated, *"most people have 5-10 pounds of matter stored in their Colon...According to autopsies, John Wayne had 40 lbs and Elvis had 60 lbs."*

Engaging in colonics from an experienced practitioner for 3-6 times a year could keep you out of the doctor's office indefinitely. The immediate release of fecal baggage built up over the years of one's life can lead to extraordinarily powerful emotional releases, ranging from any number of extremes. The connection between our physical health and emotional health is joined together in perfect harmony. When our body becomes clear of corrosive matter, our emotions are allowed to flow free. Read the section below in this chapter called **Forgiveness** for a clear understanding of what to expect from this experience.

Outside of engaging in regular colonics perhaps the most important health practice we can participate in is more effective eliminations when we go to the bathroom. The modernized toilet seat poses an anatomical problem due to it being positioned higher then our body is meant to sit when eliminating. When we sit in an upright position whats called our anal-rectal-angle is bent partially, closing our rectal canal and not allowing us to fully eliminate fecal matter. Since the beginning of time humans have squatted in a hole and because of the invention of the uprising toilet seat most westerners have rarely had a complete bowel-movement. A large amount of people have been known to die on the toilet from what is called a "Valsalva manoeuvre", this is when additional pressure is placed upon the intestines and our colon from pushing too hard during attempted eliminations. When pressure is increased in this way our vena cava vein becomes pinched off and blood circulation to the heart automatically stops. Constipation is a serious problem that effects most Americans and leads to long term health stresses such as hemorrhoids and diverticulosis. When going to the bathroom we want to be in a squatting position, you can place a small box under your feet allowing your knees to raise and back facing forward.

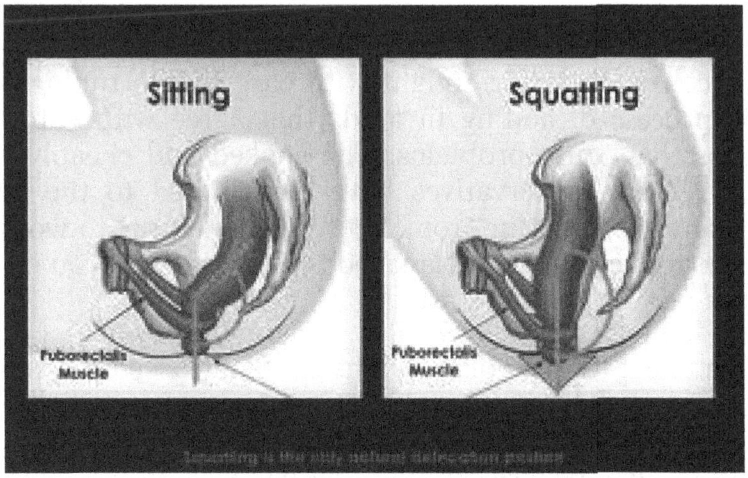

It is a good idea to begin changing your eating habits right away if you are anticipating a colonic. The goal would be to make your experience as easy and effective as possible. Raw plant foods are the best foods for improving digestion by far. Consume as much leafy green vegetables, fresh organic fruits(with seeds), and as much clean water as possible. Below is a short list of foods that are especially powerful for digestion, and can act as laxatives to help get things "moving".

Foods Specific for the Colon/Digestion:

- Ginger (Anti-inflammatory, contains compounds that bind to serotonin receptors decreasing anxiety and stress)
- Cacao beans(Magnesium, soluble fiber, vitamin c, laxative)
- Aloe Vera Gel (Polysaccharides, anti-inflammatory, digestive aid, skin cell healing aid, 200 active phytonutrients)
- Noni Fruit/Extract (Polysaccharides, anti-inflammatory, digestive aid)
- Prunes (vitamin a, potassium, iron, dietary fiber, known remedy for constipation)
- Raw Apple Cider Vinegar (pectin, malic acid, helps improve bowel movement irregularities)
- Pumpkin Seeds (Amino Acids, Vitamin E, Zinc, Fiber)

Metabolism & Weight Loss

Being mindful of the efficiency of our own metabolism is where the future is headed in health and nutrition. Since each person has their own unique metabolic code, and requires a different ratio of foods, no one person is identical. Therefore, the general idea of dieting for long-term health and weight loss is a lost cause. It turns out through the years of doing all the wrong things, we have stumbled onto the most effective and ideal way to approach weight loss, which is eating foods closest to nature, unattached by a stove or ingredients you cannot pronounce. The great thing with living foods is the only ingredient is the food itself, so your body knows exactly what its getting. Nutrition as a field is still an immature science in it's entirety. We are still discovering the key's to optimal nutrition so by adding in whole raw plant foods your body is obtaining the nutrients science has yet to uncover.

Overall, all the keys to losing weight with ease is fine tuning your metabolism, which is a simple process of adding in foods that agree with you, which eventually pushes out the ones that cause problems. The cooked and cheaply processed animal foods filled with artificial preservatives have contributed to the production of the excessive weight many are suffering from. Truly, the only way to work your way out of this situation is to introduce as much plant foods as possible. If you do not normally eat salads, then that is a perfect place to start.

The best foods to eat for dropping weight are plant-based foods, specifically green leafy vegetables, because they contain a large amount of nutrition with virtually no calories. The problem with diets that preach cutting calories is that most people cut all their nutrition, and in turn, receive nothing that will sustain them over the period of a day. This is why living foods is the obvious choice for fast-track weight loss. The methods of weight loss are in line with those of cleansing because, in reality, you are cleansing yourself of the extra fat that is full of toxic substances that prolong weight gain. If you can develop a regular habit of adding in one green juice or smoothie a day, then you will see major changes. As your body gets cleaner, you will notice increases in energy, which will encourage you to use it! Many programs work to force one to exercise, failing to understand that if there is a lack of energy, then there is a bigger problem than what the eye can see. We are truly a creature of unlimited energy in our most natural physiological state. Too much exercise can be counterproductive if the body is not running on clean-burning fuel, so the first step is to begin from the inside out, as I always say.

Cooked foods, hybridized grains, artificial drinks, and conventional animal products create stress to our digestive system over time, which causes disturbances in our metabolic intelligence. The more efficiently you can metabolize food, the easier it will be to reduce useless weight, and in turn, maintain your natural body type. Study the section **The Sun Food Connection** & **The Raw Naked Truth** in order to get a clear idea of certain food groups you should be focusing on, and what you should cut out immediately.

If your goal is to reduce weight with the least amount of resistance, then there are certain raw foods that should be either minimized or left alone for a period of time. Nuts such as macadamia, cashews, almonds, pistachios, and walnuts are very fat-containing foods, and can be easily over eaten in place of the old foods that we were used to. Seeds are a much better substitute because they generally have a better fat-to-protein ratio, and can be digested a little easier. It is a good idea to give the body a break from heavy fats since the body has been overloaded with dense foods for so long. The healing process will be accelerated by eating less and drinking more. If you do feel a need for more sustainable calories, then I suggest leaning towards avocados because they are a soft and gentle source of fat. Olives are fantastic as well, and can be very satisfying along with promoting weight loss.

Lemons are a vastly underrated food that require minimal effort to procure, yet yield tremendous results. There is a popular weight loss strategy referred to as "The Master Cleanse", which focuses mostly on using lemons as the base for your nutrition. This sour yellow fruit is well complimented for its value of vitamin C and citric acid. Lemons are most beneficial in our morning water, this will not only help hydrate us but also allow our body to flush out the lymphatic system which vastly influences our ability lose excess weight.

A highly unconventional strategy that may actually influence more metabolic shifts than just our food practices is that of "grounding". This is the act of connecting our bare body (feet, hands, head, etc.) to the bio-electric field of the earth in order to "recharge" our biological battery (adrenals). By disconnecting ourselves from this field not only have we cut off our most superior supply of energy, the exceedingly high amount of electromagnetic pollution coming from cell phones, phone lines, computers, internet broadcasting, televisions, microwaves, kitchen, and bathroom appliances disrupt the cells in our body from functioning optimally. The practice of getting barefoot on the grass and/or dirt regularly promotes weight loss simply because it aids in the decrease of inflammation. When our cellular structure within the body is inflamed, our body must work twice as hard to yield half the results which eventually will result in a breaking down of the entire system. (See Chapter: **The Triangle of Life, Earthing & Peak Performance**).

If someone is working diligently to lose weight on a raw food diet by focusing mostly on greens or juices, and has refrained from fat sources for too long, they can develop nervous conditions such as jitteriness, irritability, extreme sensitivities, and anxiety, which is why many people will go overboard on nuts in order to ease these issues that can arise. Quality fats and oils can act as a delivery system for other nutrients to come into the body and ease our central nervous system because they give the nerve fibers a buffer from stress. Adding in an avocado to a green smoothie can be a great way to keep your body in balance and keep your mind from shifting towards heavier caloric sources.

I continue to see more and more people relieve themselves of every layer of body fat that was once holding them down. The story of *Angela Stokes-Monarch,* author of **Raw Emotions**, is one that many raw food advocates have drawn on for inspiration. Angela shares her story of going from a typical girl growing up to becoming over 300 pounds, suffering from an under active thyroid and food addictions. She was moving towards a fate that many never wake up from. Fortunately for her, she found a book called **The Raw Family**, and she decided to take on the raw food lifestyle the very next day. Angela completely changed her life, returning to her perfect body weight and has enjoyed a completely raw plant based diet for many years. Her story is not an isolated incident. People from all over the world, literally on a daily basis, are being positively effected by the knowledge of living-food nutrition and natural healing methods.

Forgiveness

Perhaps the single greatest factor in cleansing ourselves of toxic residue built up over the years comes from accepting factors in our lives that we cannot control, and forgive those that we can. As we go through life, the most powerful experiences we have are stored in our body, which either promote well being or create stress, leading to physical inefficiencies. If you research the root cause of almost any major illness, it can usually be traced back to a relationship crisis. A disconnection from a loved one can lead to a personal disconnection, and that will always lead to suffering. I encourage all those who are feeling the weight of the world, whether it be from stress, chronic pain, digestive atrophy, or any other symptoms, to begin analyzing their relationship health immediately.

In our Chakra system(bodies energy system), each layer has a specific purpose that always translates from the inner body to the outer body. In her book, **The Synthesis of Healing**, *Judy Jacka* details the many connections between our body's ability to perform optimally in relation to our state of being associated with the chakra system. I was personally fascinated with the *solar chakra*, which is considered by many to be where our power lies. In martial arts, the core of our body(solar plexus) is where our greatest energy(QI) exists. Consider this statement from her book.

"It is no wonder that when we get emotionally upset the solar plexus shuts down and we cannot digest anything or it becomes so over-stimulated that we might get stomach ulcers. All the digestive organs are conditioned by the state of the solar plexus-the stomach, the liver, gall bladder, small intestine, and most of the large intestine"

It is time we fully recognize the body and light body(spirit) are beautifully intertwined, and must be respected as such. The superficial way of diagnosing an ailment with standard medicine is comparable to kindergarden arithmetic; its very immature. Whatever emotional state one is in, it will always impose upon the body in one way or another. My own experience has confirmed this to me, as I have gone through my own stages of releasing resistance.

I find that in most cases, its not always someone else that we must forgive that stops us, although that can be a good starting point. It is actually ourselves that we have beat up and abused over time. We have discredited our own worth, and the child of God inside of us knows the difference and is calling out. It is up to us to hear that voice as it speaks. This is where the key to all good communication comes into play; listening not just to others but also to ourselves. Often times, we acknowledge what others have to say but we rarely give ourselves the same attention, and that is where I suggest one should start in this healing path. Remember, if you are not your own best friend, you will continually be disappointed with others, and that will lead to the problems that contribute to toxic build up.

The environmental and dietary pollutants are remarkable easy to deal with once you deal with the emotional pollution going on within your own soul. It is my firm and unwavering belief that we were placed here with a purpose, and the further we move away from our purpose, the closer we move into pain, disease, and agony. These are not punishments for our sinful behavior but are actually signs that we have moved away from our divinity and must now realign back with our power.

Begin to trust yourself in all things, and adopt the habitual patterns of the healthy radiant being you know you are, and watch the healing you desire take place!

"In forgiveness lies the stoppage of the wheel of karma"
The Law of One

The Sun Food Reality

"With all the conflicting information on diet, what makes sense? Pesticides, herbicides, fungicides, larvicides, genetically modified organisms, chemical fertilizers, microwaves, pasteurization, homogenization, hormonally injected animals, color dyes, artificial additives, and high fructose corn syrup? Or raw, organic, sun-ripened plant food"

David Wolfe

"Nothing will benefit human health and increase the chances for survival of life on Earth as much as the evolution to a vegetarian diet."

Albert Einstein

"In general, mankind, since the improvement in cookery, eats twice as much as nature requires."

Benjamin Franklin

"Everyone has a doctor in him or her; we just have to help it in its work. The natural healing force within each one of us is the greatest force in getting well. Our food should be our medicine. Our medicine should be our food. But to eat when you are sick, is to feed your sickness."

Hippocrates

"As custodians of the planet it is our responsibility to deal with all species with kindness, love and compassion. That these animals suffer through human cruelty is beyond understanding."

Richard Gere

Each day that is presented to us provides awesome opportunities to showcase our value in the world. Each breath we breath is a blessing of the highest order. The emotions we feel should be acknowledged and understood to the depths of our soul. The thoughts we think should be positively focused in the favor of our deepest convictions. The actions we take should be made consciously and ethically at all times, rarely wavering in the face of counterproductive temptations. The path we take should be calculated, heartfelt, and in alignment with the betterment of the planet we have been entrusted to occupy.

There are many avenues in which to carve out a life for ourselves, none of which are actually right or wrong. The concept of right and wrong is something that has created more suffering and confusion than anything else in world history. All of the wars since biblical times until now, which were seeds of the ego promoting false ideas, were most likely issues of self-esteem and arrogance. We are all unique in our differences, and deserve respect despite our scope in which we view life. The path we choose is ours to decide, and the results of our choices will come to bear.

The path of a sun foodist, in my opinion, is unique among all other dietary, spiritual, and lifestyle disciplines for a great number of reasons. I have seen many case studies of people, along with personal experiences, overcoming detrimental illnesses one by one on live foods alone. This lifestyle plugs you back into the great mysteries of the world, making you become a researcher instead of just a spectator. It enhances relationships by centering your spirit and grounding your mind. Everyday gets better as progression takes place and frustration fades away.

As with any path in life, there are a host of things to look at with an intelligent curiosity and mild skepticism. Just as you should not buy a packaged food without considering the ingredients, you should not adhere to any lifestyle without considering all factors involved. As with anything, there are always misconceptions coming from different opinions, and there is always contrast, which is why we are going to explore all sides.

There is tremendous beauty here for you if you so choose to accept it, so let's take a detailed look into the world of the living sun food lifestyle.

Better living through common sense

All throughout history, we have transitioned from era to era changing ideas, philosophies, social appearances, and ways of life. We are social creatures who enjoy the interaction and stimulation of new ways of doing things. The creativity and imagination we have is what makes humans unique among all other living creatures. However, when a new concept of how things should be done rapidly emerges in popularity, one very probable thing usually happens: chaotic insanity.

In the last few hundred years, we have steamrolled through more changes in lifestyle than any other time in history. Our environment has changed, our family structure has changed, our physiology has changed, our dietary intake has changed, our relationships have changed, and our primary needs for self and group sustainability have dramatically changed. Human beings really are simple beings like all creatures but we were given the gift of free will, which is the blessing of our creator and the downfall of our ignorance.

The way we fuel ourselves is an absolutely key aspect on how we experience our reality. The livings foods cut through the facades, the role-playing, and masquerading of mainstream culture. The society as of now has worked hard to promote many ideas that have been suspect from the beginning. We have seen better living through fear and dogma. We have seen better living through control and conformity. We have seen better living through chemistry, better living through antibiotics and pasteurization, better living through fluoride, chlorine, chemtrails, genetic modification, and nuclear technology. Or have we? All of this has brought us better living through degradation of self-esteem and artificial entertainment. These methods of living have all delivered their results, and the evidence is conclusive. This just will not suffice, so I have a much needed alternative: how about we try better living through common sense.

The ability to live in our bodies present in each moment is the greatest gift we have. It's time to do away with all of the outside interferences that sabotage our true talents, gifts, and vitality. The sun foodist of a new era is endowed with the thoughts, disciplines, and clarity of a true super hero. When you dedicate yourself to the addition of a dominantly plant-based lifestyle, the kind of energy you feel is indescribable. The chlorophyl from the plants fills your blood, the heat from the sun fuels your heart, the electricity from the earth activates your nervous system, the breath of the wind strengthens your lungs and the consciousness of living spring water sustains your life force. The energy you feel at all times is actually transmuted to you through you being consciously connected in each way; it activates your full potentialities, which will allow you to become a force of massive healing and prosperity for the planet.

Clarity

For me the greatest beauty always lies in the greatest clarity.
Gotthold Ephraim Lessing

The kind of euphoria-like enthusiasm for life that can rush the flood gates of consciousness is inspiring. I have seen people in massive pain on a completely acidic diet bite into a fresh fruit or drink a blended coconut cashew cacao smoothie, and become totally transformed. I heard the great quote, "the subtle energy of your food becomes your mind", and I was actually transformed from that moment on. I immediately got the message, and ever since then, my life has been getting better and better. The clarity of everyday life that comes over you may seem small at first, or it could be dramatic, but if you are in chronic pain, what will end up happening is that you will forget you were ever in pain over time. This realization alone can cause someone to become a powerful force in the world.

Clarity is the ability to see yourself as you truly are; centered and aligned with your purpose in front of you, relieving all notion of doubt or fear for the future. Our food choices have such a pivotal role in our ability to focus from one thing to the next, our stream of energy from fuel, and our actions so we can actually accomplish what we are setting out to do in the most effective way possible. If our focus is on life-force energy, then we will become that. But if our focus is on artificial, refined, flesh-based, and severely processed foods our energy turns stale and one day our bodies will become stale as well.

A lack of clarity on one's life is what will drive someone to hand over all of their power to someone else in exchange for a sedentary lifestyle. That is more comfortable for those waging war, in what could be called "inner civil conflict". Everyone wants health but few are willing to open themselves up to the possibilities. Their focus is off target, and they view health as giving up pleasure. I believe the true definition of sacrifice is giving up something of a lower nature for something of a higher nature.

You can think all the happy thoughts, do all the affirmations, and pray as much as you'd like, but if you are fueling your body with junk, then you are going to produce junky results in your health quest. I have met many beautiful people who were not anywhere near raw foodists, and I am not implying that their worth is somehow devalued, but what I wish to say is because of certain habits, the positive energy they have is not being fulfilled because they are making decisions with their lives from a place of lack instead of abundance. The living foods will undoubtably open someone up to energy reserves they never knew existed, and that is what fuels the complete capacity of human ingenuity. The easiest way to build a bridge from the mind to the heart is through the foods of mother nature, and I have seen this happen instantly in my own life and in others almost everyday. Remember the body follows the mind, but by the same token the mind follows the body. When we are in pain physically our mental attitude is much more likely to go into pain as well. Raw plant foods helps to tune us into the removal of painful attachments from our lives. When we feel better, we think better, and this allows us to do better, in all that we choose to pursue.

Animal & Human Bond

Genesis 1:26. Then God said, "Let us make man in our image, and let them rule over the fish of the sea and the birds of the air, over the livestock, over all the earth and over all the creatures that move along the ground."

When we were placed on this earth, I do believe we were designed to be the caretakers of it. As humans, we have developed points of view that are most often formed from self-interest of how to best proceed with our plans for the future. We must stop and deeply consider the implications of our choices and where it has led humanity. If we are the stewards of nature's beauty and vibrance, then we have seriously gone backwards. The destructive nature that we all have inside of us has been widely exploited, and because of it, we turn our backs on our most sacred companions: the animals.

What is it that allows us to hold dominion over all life, and decide whats going to live and whats going to die? This is a question many are very uncomfortable with, and for good reason. The effects of inhumane factory farming practices have become full blown, and the majority of meat people are consuming comes from sick, feeble animals that had to live out their lives knowing very well that they were going to be slaughtered. The vibrational deposits of this energy play major roles in the decisions people are making everyday. I find it interesting how we have grown up with animals, calling them our pets, but on the other hand, we have no similar attachment to the animals we eat. We would never consider eating our own dog, yet many may eat another's pet unknowingly. Human beings separate pets, those who we show love to, from live stock who are shown the most grotesque examples of disrespect and cruelty anyone will ever witness.

Ezekiel 34:17-18. As for you, my flock... Is it not enough for you to feed on good pasture? Must you also trample the rest of your pasture with your feet? Is it not enough for you to drink clear water? Must you also muddy the rest with your feet?

The animals have so much to teach us about ourselves that I am actually inclined to believe their main purpose is to show us the deeper layers of ourselves. We all share a deep knowing of the invisible field of consciousness that surrounds us. This is how we are able to communicate with the animal kingdom, not only through our minds or mouths but also through our hearts. The animal to human bond is crucial for the progress of mankind since we all work together in different ways. What ends up happening as a result of going towards the raw living foods is your relationship with wild life improves dramatically. Animals become less hesitant to be around you, probably because they can sense you don't want to eat them, and you no longer become a strange creature to them.

Gabriel Cousens, in his famous book, **Spiritual Nutrition and the Rainbow Diet**, speaks about the SOEF (Subtle Organizing Energy Field) we and all creatures of the planet have been endowed with. We all interact with one another from this subtle energy, expressing itself through every thought, word, and action. The earth, the plants, the elements, the animals, and all of us are spun together in this web of creation that should be considered in all decisions we make.

If you remember the story, **The Jungle Book**, originally inspired in 1894 by *Rudyard Kipling,* you know that Mowgli, a boy who was separated from his family as a child and wound up in the jungles of India, was found and raised by a pack of wolves. He grew up completely oblivious to the fact that he was somehow different than all the other animals in the jungle up until the point of adulthood where he ventured outside of the jungle, finding the British settlement. The British people had occupied India, caring little for the cultural traditions or "laws of the jungle". When Mowgli had arrived, he was seen as a savage, treated with embarrassment, and even mild neglect, like a stray animal because in their eyes, that is exactly what he was. Eventually, Mowgli was embarrassed of the human behavior, and went back to the jungle to reunite with his family, who happened to be animals. This story, in my opinion, greatly shows that the nature of the thinking behind human superiority, and how animals, in many cases, can become much better companions for people than people are for each other when compassion is lacking.

To further the deepening of this pertinent subject take a moment to ingrain the words of one of the worlds most successful entrepreneurs, philanthropist, author, and peace activist, **Russel Simmons**, *"The number 2 use of oil, besides the army, all the water, all the grain, the destruction of the ozone layer, all the cancer, sickness, and the worst karma in the history of human kind is the animals and the abuse of them".*

Recommended Book: (Spiritual Nutrition: Gabriel Cousens)

The Life Force Principles

The concept of life force energy has been discussed and theorized all throughout history by some of the most sophisticated and systematically advanced civilizations. As a student of the chinese herbal medicine approach, I have grown to understand the different views on healing based on the philosophy of the great masters. In the chinese understanding of the life force principles, they drew heavily on a concept known as the Three Treasures. According to the Taoist teachings these treasures consisted of compassion, frugality, and humility. The traditional chinese medical teachings consist of Jing, Qi, and Shen, all of which philosophically parallel each other. These treasures govern our overall vital life force, determining how we experience life in direct proportion to the thoughts we think, the food we eat, and the activities we participate in.

The western methods of identifying illness is packaged as scientifically advanced, yet in reality, it is very much in the embryonic stage of maturity. The most popular ways in which a doctor might approximate a diagnoses is through standard blood testing. According to many masters of chinese herbology, this method is extremely limited since blood testing has no way of determining the energetic disposition someone may be in, which in fact is the root of illness. The physical ailment just happens to be a symptom of a much deeper problem. For example, the western approach to healing and nutrition may focus entirely on one organ such as the liver, and the immediate approach may be to only detoxify the liver. In chinese medicine, it is more focused on directing the energy through not only that specific area of the body, but also through all of its connective components that are related to the functionality of it. This is not to imply one is better than the other, it is to show the difference in approaches so that we can create a broader view in our understanding of what we consider to be the fundamental life force principles.

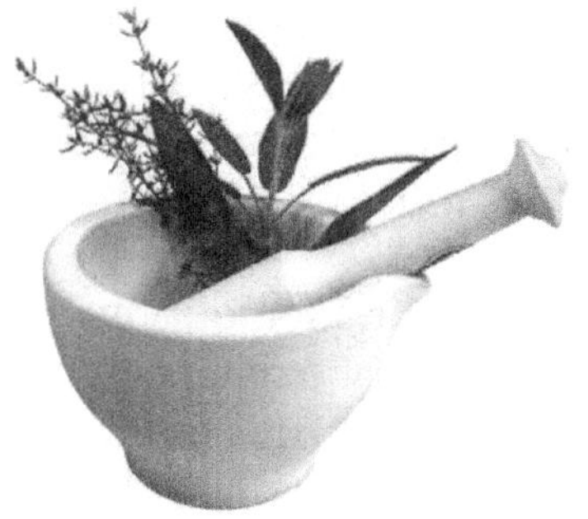

Qi: The energetics most closely related to the concept of Qi are the warming energies of the body. Qi is the animated force in our body that allows us to move in any which way we choose. Our ability to produce instant energy is based heavily on our ability to produce daily Qi, and this is why this life force principle in particular is most identified with the element of fire.

In the western world, initially in many people, there appears to be a surplus of Qi. Western civilization is very well equipped with a core "fire power". This can become depleted if we do not contribute in the lifestyle factors that supply our body with Qi energy, which also show the western world is sorely lacking by the consumption of caffienated beverages. By entertaining artificial substances excessively, we end up tapping into our longevity store house which is known as Jing.

The physiological attributes that are associates with Qi are directly related to our lungs, our blood flow, and our spleen(digestive system). In exploring these three factors, diet becomes absolutely the critical influence in how we produce Qi. By consumeing nutrient-dense foods that are easily recognizable to our digestive system, we are able to absorb these nutrients more readily, which converts into energy packets for the production of our blood. If we consume pasteurized juices or processed candy containing refined sugar, for example, we become unable to create the appropriate streams of energy in which Qi exists. This activity alone will begin to draw out energy reserves from our long-term life force. The reason people become addicted to energy drinks and substances of this nature is because they provide an instant stimulation which mimics our natural Qi. This momentary stimulation is desired only in the depletion of our core energy. We will lose all desire for artificial stimulation when we fulfill our nutritional needs and participate in positive activities that promote our three treasures.

The act of deep breathing throughout the day increases our potential for cultivating Qi. The stomach should expand a bit when we breath naturally through the diaphragm, allowing oxygen to build. At the top of the breath, we let the air from our lungs slowly out. This also allows oxygen to flood our cells and helps create healthy blood flow. I was educated on the importance, for women in particular, to develop healthy blood due to their menstrual cycle where blood is lost every month. Nutrition for women must be identified individually in terms of building back blood after the cycle has completed. If a women is constantly passing over her nutritional demands month after month and year after year, she will very shortly tap into her central energy reserves. This idea alone is very important for vegans/vegetarians to investigate as restrictive dietary protocols are in many cases not adequate or are improperly done for the production of healthy hormones and blood. (See Section: **The Sunfood Connection, Supplementing for Pregnancy**)

Jing: The idea of our Jing is based on the primordial life force that exists at the center of our very existence. When we are born, in the Chinese herbal understanding, we not only inherit the life-force energies of our mother and father, but we also transmit the energies of the heavens and the earth. Our Jing essence is our stored energy that we are born with and either cultivate through our lives or deplete, depending on the lifestyle choices we make. In the raw food understanding, a similar concept would be that of metabolic enzymes which each one of us is gifted at birth, and must use intelligently throughout our lives. Unintelligible use of our enzyme reserves we will cripple our longevity.

In western culture, the concept of life force energy is only vaguely understood at best. When phrases such as "I'm fried", "I'm burnt out", or "I'm wiped out" repeat themselves, this is the result of chronic adrenal fatigue brought on by excessive behavior. Jing energy is stored largely in our kidney/adrenal glands, and when these vital organs begin to fail, every aspect of our lives will fail as well. It is said in the Chinese understanding that anything that has to do with stress has to do with loss of Jing.

The emotional and mental states we experience daily are a reflection of the care in which our Jing or life force is being utilized. If we constantly experience or entertain negative thought patterns, as well as emotional disturbances, we will break down the protective layers of our core essence, at which point our precious Jing energy slowly seeps out of our body- much like the air in our bicycle tire once it's punctured. George

Lamoureux, Master Tonic Herbalist, states that women must be very attentive in their mental and emotional states, especially during the months of pregnancy. The mother's own core Jing literally translates into her babies "genetic potential" for everything it will be upon the moment of conception and there on after. According to George Lamoureux, Jing is pure potential in a human being; it is everything they will ever do, ever think, and ever become. Jing blossoms into who that person becomes in the world. If you follow out this logic, then it becomes obvious that all of our collective Jing force will shape what the world becomes.

Shen: The Shen is essentially a subtle energy that circulates throughout the body, relieving us of our unnecessary doubts, worries, and emotional baggages. Through the combination of the Qi and Jing forces, Shen becomes awakened in our overall being. Shen is what allows us to envision a bigger and broader picture of our lives, and it is what alleviates the stress in order for us to become inspired by our innermost desires. This may appear on the surface to be more esoteric in nature but this life force principle is related to the idea of positive thoughts breading positive results. When someone has a positive outlook on life they radiate from the pores of their skin, they may even give off a glow. When you see someone who has clear white eyes, attentive focus, and clear communication that means they have an abundance of Shen energy.

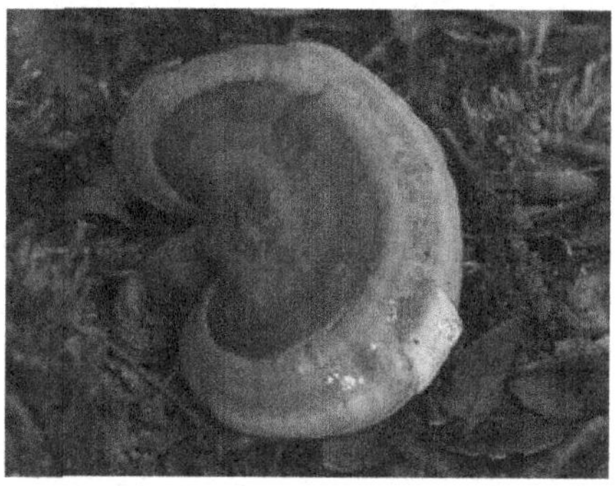

The depletion of Shen in our lives can be correlated with the amount of negativity we allow in our space. Shen is extremely powerful in the sense that if we use up excessive Qi and even Jing energy, but have a positive attitude, it can help make up for these other factors for a certain duration. The other two treasures are there to be utilized as investments into the cultivation of our Shen energy. When we have strong Qi force, we can go out into the world with will power and make things happen. When our Jing is strong, we have great reserves in which to draw on when needed. These two factors combined create the building blocks for our Shen essence, which in my opinion merely translates into our purpose for our time on this planet.

The Doctrine of Signatures

The Doctrine of Signatures is an approach to healing the body through drawing an association with the foods found in nature resembling individual parts of the body. This concept has been adopted by herbalists and nature-based healers for centuries using simple discernment to apply food-based remedies. The modern day allopathic approach considers this to be pure superstition with little to no scientific data to support it. The fact of the matter is that those who study raw food nutrition will soon find that this approach is scientifically validated through identifying basic foods and studying their nutritional properties. Theologians found this idea useful and assumed the position that the creator must have set up signs in nature upon the various means of curing disease. In the early 1500's, the alchemist Paracelsus developed the idea of this doctrine and published writings on it.

This Doctrine of Signatures is a profound wisdom that calls for innocent perception and a reconnection to simplicity that the ancients understood very well. Every natural food such as vegetables, fruits, herbs, nuts, and seeds express patterns that seem to resemble a particular human organ. This concept extends beyond the physical attributes of food, associating the smell and environment the plant is grown to identity its health-giving qualities.

Let's take a look at some interesting examples of the Doctrine of Signatures:

Kidney Beans: The name is given to this bean because it looks anatomically identical to our kidneys. Kidney beans are known to lower cholesterol levels and aid in preventing heart disease as well as chronic kidney disease. If you consume a high raw diet but not entirely raw, kidney beans are a great addition.

Walnuts: Walnuts are perhaps the most obvious example. Their outer shell resembles a skull, and within the shell is the edible walnut which looks identical to our physical brain. The walnut further resembles our brain by resembling the right and left hemispheres and even the wrinkled folds! It is no shocking discovery that we find walnuts as a great brain food, containing omega 3 fatty acids (important brain nutrient).

Carrots: Raw carrots have been heralded for being a great food for eye health beacuse of their concentration in beta-carotene. You will notice the cross sections of a carrot look just like the pupils, iris, and outer lines of our eyes.

Figs: This delicious fruit hangs in two's and is full of viable seeds which look similiar to male testicles. Figs are known to increase male sperm counts and are an excellent aid in male fertility.

Sweet Potatoes: Sweet potatoes seem to resemble the shape of our pancreas and are excellent for balancing blood sugar levels. Sweet potatoes are much preferred over the conventional potatoes because they are low on the glycemic index whereas conventional potatoes are very high in sugar and can imbalance individuals with sugar sensitivities.

Maca: Maca is a cruciferious vegetable that is known as a potent adaptogen. Maca is the highest altitude crop grown in the world which seems to grown in areas where the temperature can fluctuate rapidly from forty degree's up or down, making it adaptable to extreme climates. Maca is known to improve the adaptability of people who consume it, including regulating bodily temperature. It improves one's ability to adapt to an extreme environment, especially in cold climates.

Olives: Olives are one of the great longevity substances in the food realm that look like a womens ovaries. An Italian study found that women who's diets included generous amounts of olive oil had a 30% lower risk of ovarian cancer. It is suggested that the oil of olives may suppress cancer promoting cells. The longest recorded living women in the western world (122 years), Jeanne Calment, attributed her longevity to three foods: chocolate, port wine(grapes), and copious ammounts of olive oil, which she consumed and rubbed all over her skin. Black olives are related to the Chinese understanding of longevity known as our Jing essence. Dark black foods seem to have an affinity to our kidney/adrenal glands and supporting core energy which promotes long life.

Tomatoes: A tomato has four chambers which resembles the heart, which has four chambers as well. The shape and color of a red tomato has a resemblance to the heart. It is known in nutrition that tomatoes are indeed a heart and blood supporting food.

Synchronicity

"Though we can't always see it at the time, if we look upon events with some perspective, we see things always happen for our best interests. We are always being guided in a way better than we know ourselves."
Swami Satchidananda

The links of life are so intricately connected in such an infinite way that it is absolutely invisible to the human eye. The more we try to see it, the more it escapes our vision. But those that have developed their inner vision, and their true knowing unlike any indicator given on the outside, are the people who remain connected to the magic of life's expected surprises.

Synchronicity is what happens when you are in complete alignment with your preferred path in life. The joy, happiness, and profound abundance that is naturally circulating in your veins is the same exact force that will guide you all the way to your dreams. The sometimes subtle and sometimes major clues that the universe will drop in your lap are your indications whether you are on the abundant path or not. Life is funny. Sometimes an event can present itself in such a way that it may lead one to assume the worst, only to find soon after that it was the greatest catalyst for growth needed to advance into the next stage.

It has been my experience, and that of countless other raw food advocates I have met, that the clues of life become much stronger on a primarily raw living foods lifestyle. I do not want to say it is a requirement because cultivation happens in many ways, but the sensitivity one will gain over their entire energy field physically, spiritually, and everything in-between heightens to amazing degree's, even if only practiced periodically as a cleanse. I do believe that the raw living foods approach to diet is the surest way to maintain what is known as the "flow": a string of events that continue to show up in our life, pointing us in the direction of our desire or destiny.

When someone is introduced to a raw food diet, they essentially begin to cleanse their body of residue from past behavior. Even if only introducing a salad, it begins to break down unwanted particles and fermentation that can have a clogging effect not only on the organ and digestive system, but also on a person's ability to feel the world around them from a place of connective certainty. This is exactly the reason why so many people feel uncomfortable in their own skin. It is because they are backed up on the inside, and need to release this congestion. Digestive issues are some of the worst experiences because it interferes with the pleasurable experience of living. It puts a block on the flow of positive energy that wants to express itself through you and yet it is unable. Consider this: what is happening on the outside is a reflection of what is happening on the inside. If the world around you looks like madness, chaos, disorganized, and scary, then just imagine the environment living in you.

"When we're interested in something, everything around us appears to refer to it."
Paulo Coelho

The fact you are reading this information could be a massive clue to your next move. The experiences that lead you to finding this book could have been the starting point that may lead you into the greatest adventure you never saw coming. I know for myself that when I pick up a book I was drawn to, it propels me into a new world of imagination and insight. I have had this experience many times. I have acted on innocent hunches to go to a health food store, seminar, or farmers market, and have been introduced to someone who had set up a string of events I could never have predicted. We are given ideas, inspirations, and clues as to what action to take step by step. It is our job to be in tune with these ideas, to open ourselves up to inspiration at all times, and to refrain from the dulled down systematic patterns of everyday routines. Engaging in mundane routines is no way to experience life; we were meant to experience abundance on the greatest platforms of possibility. Next time you get a hunch to act on an idea, do it! Next time you get an inspired notion to take a walk or make a call, do it! Next time you second guess yourself, hang up that doubt, and do what most never do: take action!

Sleep Less, Live More

The idea that we needed to sleep almost half our lives had never crossed my mind until I realized I was needing less and less sleep as I become more involved in live foods. This is a common experience for many people who spread out their food intake with a multitude of fresh vegetables and fruits as their caloric foundation. I have reviewed many theories and studies on the requirements of sleep, and the effects it places on the body. Although it goes without question that proper sleep is essential for repair of the body, nervous system, proper hormone production, and emotional health, I have been a bit skeptical of some of the claims stating that we need 8-10 hours of sleep every single night. If you do the math, that adds up to almost half of ones life span. Lets investigate this idea!

There is a lot of information stating specific demands of the body for sleep. For example, some researchers believe the body always repairs from 10 pm-2 am, and the mind repairs from 2 am-6 am. Although this seems a bit rigid(and unrealistic to goal achieving individuals), in my opinion, it could be because of our natural sleep cycles or **circadian rhythms**. When we go to sleep at night, the **Pineal Gland**(See Chapter: **The Scientific Method**) in our brain secretes a chemical called **Melatonin**, which signals sleepiness, and as we rise in the morning, this function is turned off. Our natural sleep patterns are to awake as the sun comes up, and to begin the process of calming down and going to sleep as the moon comes out. The majority of peoples sleep cycles are completely upside down, and I will explain why that is, along with providing some interesting information that could lead you to need less and less sleep while gaining more and more life.

The average person in society is getting far less adequate sleep than they should, even if they sleep more. Take a look at these statistics from the National Sleep Foundation:

1 in 6 US Adults have chronic sleep and wakefulness disorders
1 in 3 woman uses some type of sleep medication a few times a week
Over 2 million children suffer from sleep disorders
The use of sleeping pills among children and very young adults rose 85% from 2000 to 2004

The general lifestyle is one full of disruptive frequencies and stimulants that lead to the depletion of your body's ability to heal itself over time, leading to accelerated aging, frail bones, cloudy thoughts, and poor assimilation of food. One area of concern is the environment you sleep in. If this area is full of electromagnetic devices, your body is going to be affected. This disturbs the body's ability to repair and fully relax in the state of sleep because it is never fully at ease. This is one reason why someone may end up waking up multiple times a night, especially if there is any kind of light in the room. The room you sleep in should be pitch black to put you into a proper sleep state. Using the phone or alarm clock is detrimental over time because your body is the best alarm clock, knowing exactly the amount of sleep it requires. Your body will not allow you to sleep past its ability to repair. Any time spent forcing yourself to sleep after this process can actually work against you, so sleeping in is not always a good idea. As you become more in tune with your body as a result of adopting a raw food lifestyle, your sleep needs will become easier to discern.

Getting barefoot as much as possible on the earth is the best way to reset your natural circadian cycles because the energy(negative ions) pulsing from the earth is what your electric body craves and actually runs on for optimal function. Since we are disconnected from the earth's concentrated field of energy most of the time, we are suffering from malnutrition of an electrical nature. The sun plays a big part in our ability to absorb nutrition and keep our fuel intake cleaner burning. It does this while putting us in a more relaxed state throughout the day so that as night approaches, we are more balanced with our energy levels instead of the extreme fluctuations. Study the chapter **Triangle of Life!**

The role food plays in our sleep cycles is crucial to understand if you are to maximize your rest time. Getting the best quality sleep in the shortest possible time is key to extending the amount of living you are able to do while awake. This is achieved by your body's ability to metabolize the food it is processing. The cleaner the environment, largely meaning the more clean oxygen the cells have, the more efficient your body can digest food. Each person's metabolism is constantly trying to determine which substances are going to be used as a nutrition source, and which are considered "poisonous" and need to be excluded. Your enzymatic(enzymes) bank account, so to speak, plays such a big part in your bodies ability to process food, repair itself, and function, that it brings new light to many ideas in regards to sleep. It would seem many of the rules about what and when to eat at night are completely centered around a cooked-food lifestyle. (See Chapter: **The Sun Food Connection: Enzymes**).

Cooked food is completely void of all enzymes it may have had at one point, and makes your own enzyme reserves work harder in order to digest this food. The amino acid **Tryptophan**, which helps induce sleep through Serotonin, Melatonin, and dimethyltryptamine(DMT) production, is extremely heat volatile, and loses much of its efficacy in secreting these neurotransmitter hormones when cooked. So much of the suggestions from many health advocates about eating turkey, and any kind of meat late at night, which is supposed to be high in tryptophan, is not accurate. If falling asleep is the only goal, it may be helpful mainly because of the stress it will place on digestion, but it will not be the restful sleep you truly need. In many cases, eating conventional meat will stimulate you more because of the artificial hormones injected into it.

The big culprit in our ability to get the most out of our sleep, or lack there of, is digestion. When we go to sleep, our digestive system is using this time to clear out residue from past meals. The more our body has to process, the less our body can engage in quality rest. This can easily explain why you may habitually toss and turn at night, and wake up through the night and feel unable to go back to sleep, even when you know you need more rest. There is an adage all raw foodists I believe are familiar with: “the less you eat, the longer you live so the more you have to eat”. This is directly related to the amount of energy you have. The less time you spend eating and compounding layers of food into your digestive track, the easier your body can process, assimilate, convert nutrients into fuel, and discard unneeded excess. High water-soluble foods, like green leafy vegetables, and juicy fruits and berries, are ideal for late-night cravings because they have the water, which is another aspect a mostly cooked diets contends with: dehydration. (See Chapter: **The Raw Naked Truth: Cooked Food**).

The length of sleep does not determine the quality of sleep. This idea, I believe, was the catalyst that led me to question why some people sleep for over 10 hours but wake up feeling unfulfilled while some people sleep for 4 hours, or even less, but wake up feeling fully replenished! Going beyond the importance of nutritional practices for sleep quality, other areas can be explored as well. The benefits of taking “power naps” has been brought up in many research studies and athletic recovery methods. It is a means to recalibrate the brain’s ability to store and let go of information. The habit of napping was taken on by many historical innovators such as Thomas Edison, John F. Kennedy, Albert Einstein, Winston Churchill, Bruce Lee, and Leonardo DaVinci. The habit of napping can become a replacement for the get-up-and-go coffee at the work place. Make space to take a 20-30 minute mind nap, and you may be surprised at how alert and focused you become as a result. It seems that most of the fatigue and sleeping people do is a byproduct of the extreme use of artificial stimulants to stay productive at work, which comes at the expense of health(See Chapter: **Leaving Behind Excess: The Adrenals**).

Two more valuable tips would be to begin sleeping without a pillow. The spine can become misaligned due to unnatural pillow usage, which disturbs sleeping patterns and negatively affect long-term nerve/skeletal health. Also, keep the window open a bit for fresh air to come through. Most houses are filled up with dust, and needs to be flushed out. Air can help us breath better and sleep sounder.

One main interest of mine on this subject is to maximize the life in my years, not only the years in my life. I figured out early on that If I could sleep one hour less each day, that would be 7 hours less each week, 30 hours less each month, and 365 hours less spent sleeping each year. That is 12 extra days of living each year! Imagine how much that could be over a life time. Over a span of 50 years, that is an extra 600 days of fully fledged life from 1 less hour of sleep each day. The desire to explore this area of research, of course, is completely dependent on ones own temperament. I tend to be extremely driven and single minded in my pursuits, which attracts this type of information to my door step. I wish to write all the books I can, read all the books of the past, and explore the possibilities at every waking opportunity.

"I was dead 4 million years before I was here and I will be dead 4 million years after i'm gone"
Michael Franti

Abundance

"Everything you need you already have. You are complete right now, you are a whole, total person, not an apprentice person on the way to someplace else. Your completeness must be understood by you and experienced in your thoughts as your own personal reality."

Wayne Dyer

"Be generous! Give to those you love; give to those who love you; give to the fortunate; give to the unfortunate - yes, give especially to those you don't want to give. You will receive abundance for your giving. The more you give, the more you will have."

W. Clement Stone

Everything that exists in our heart and travels through our mind, forming an image we can clearly identify with, is already available and waiting for us to receive it with open arms. The idea of lack and poverty is an extremely false projection of what the world really is, and is delivered by a fear-based consciousness that has chosen to not flip to the other side of the coin of life. If you look only with your eyes, then this is a reality many face, but this reality is based on the choice to live life on a lower frequency than what is available for all of us.

An attitude of gratitude can be obtained and concentrated by anyone of any age at any point in time, regardless of current or prior circumstances. If you are facing dramatic relationship issues with a spouse or lover, tap into appreciation right now, and learn how to stop the flow of negativity. If you are having financial issues, then now is the time to release the pressure that is holding your abundance from flowing to you. If your health is failing, then step back from the madness of self-doubting and disempowering energies. Take a barefoot walk or stroll in nature while taking in deep breaths of gratitude for the new connection you have with the healing power of life force rushing through your cells.

All too often we focus on the lack, the limitation, and the pain in our lives, all while walking right past the solutions to the problems. They are all around us, trying to knock on the door, yet half of the time, no one is home to answer. People go through their lives in tunnel vision with the blinders up, blocking out everyday remedies for lifelong distresses. If you are one of those people who are in a rush to work every day while having to drop off the kids to school, and has to hang up the phone before you answer, then this is your wake up call. The majority of heart attacks happen on Monday morning while being on the way to a job that most people can't stand! Abundance is all around you, but you must first open yourself up to this abundance before you can receive the magic.

When you tap into the power of living foods, you are seemingly overcome with a rush of invigorating energy and vitality that no cooked or processed-food product can provide. The forces of nature are fully enriched in the deep unseen energies that our bodies were really made for. It provides clean oxygen to our cells, it helps restore damaged enzymes to our digestion, it cleans out sludge in our intestines, it smoothens out the filtering process of the liver, and it relaxes the cardiovascular system to aid our blood in reaching the heart. We actually receive the minerals that our entire system requires, the ones that have been absent in conventional diets. Our thoughts then become crystal clear, allowing us to become the electrically-charged beings we were designed to be, and providing us with the ability to attract love, sunshine, fulfillment, all around stability and extreme abundance.

We all have choices all around us at every turn of the corner. If you feel deprived of nourishment, look around for the solution, grow your own sustenance, or at very least get a small pot and start the act of creation from there. One small act of kindness can spark a multitude of options where you thought there were none before. Life is very interesting in this way. The forces of the universe thrive on life, and I believe it is our imprinted responsibility as active creators to actively create more channels for life to thrive.

The more you give, the more you open yourself to receive. Make it a habit to take a a pass on the grocery store and go to organic farmers markets instead. There is a law of exchange that we should all take part in. This is the idea that by including others in the game of exchange, we are also putting ourselves in a much higher vibration to receive all that we need. If you practice the law of exchange with those who deserve it, then most of the mega corporations that need your energetic stamp will lose their footing and will no longer be able to sustain themselves. They will the be forced to invest their money into the people who need it most. This can happen if that is what we choose to focus our attention on.

The flow of all that is good and fruitful in life is drastically weakened when we dismiss abundance in all it's forms. A powerful idea to consider and contemplate is that of consuming less translating into receiving much more. In terms of what we eat and how we live, one of the biggest indicators of lack and deep seeded fear is the participation in gluttony. The habits we carry with us tell the story of our inner most thoughts and beliefs about our lives. Those who carry obese forming food habits, meaning the excessive consumption of substances that they are fully aware will lead to a negative outcome are operating out of selfishness. Many would soon enough claim that it is their body and they can do anything they choose with it. In one sense this is true, on the other hand this excuse in no way excuses their actions from leading to destructive consequences, not only for them but all those that surround them. A mother or father who carries the responsibility of leading a family may work till exhaustion to "pay the bills", taking in sugar and caffeinated beverages to keep a fatigued engine running. Once that individual burns out, the entire family suffers the burden of that parents personal actions. A teenager who sneaks out, indulges in parties, junk food, drugs, alcohol, etc. rarely can see the effects of their actions which are heavily weighing on the same parents who become burdened by stress. A critically important concept to perpetual abundance is taking full responsibility for our own actions and understanding how the simple decisions we make day to day impact everyone around us.

In order to actively experience abundance, it is necessary to give up all attitudes and feelings of greed. Greed is like the angry troll that lives under the bridge. It is hidden in the shadows, and only comes out when you're least paying attention. Subtle energies of greed can seem unnoticeable. What seems minor up front may have a way of building up out back. If we respond to another's good fortune with signs of jealousy or dissatisfaction, be mindful because it only takes one thought to start the process. All great would-be leaders have been halted from their goals by the wall of greed. The ability to treat all circumstances with a light concern is indicative of someone who owns their mind and is open to anything. If you look at the problems of any individual, team, business, relationship, or environmental, it can be traced back to actions of negative self-centered agendas. Every single pesticide, herbicide, farm fence, and poisonous spray were designed to keep animals and insects from participating in the cycle of life, and it is a sure sign of scarcity. The BGH(Bovine Growth Hormones), the antibiotics, and forced milking of factory farmed animals are the results of strong attachments to a state of fear, pain, disconnection, and control issues. The detriment of greed must be strongly opposed by the uplifting perspective of abundance. To know you have all that is needed, and more, is always on the way would remove the need to always concern yourself with trivial matters that lead into worry and lack.

(Recommended Book: The Science of Becoming Rich: Wallace Wattles)

Invest in Yourself

The best investment you could ever make is always towards your own growth. There is no such thing as a resource spent on your personal development that will go wasted. We all have choices in life, and to deny this fact is to live a life of quiet desperation. We are constantly surrounded by an overwhelming array of options, and it is entirely up to us to choose from the menu of the universe as to what reality we want to experience. This may sound like a nice theory but if you carefully study the patterns of your own life story, you may come across a similar conclusion. The details of life are always changing, shaping themselves according to our deepest desires, thoughts, and personal interactions. The reason most people are experiencing the same results is because they are depositing the same investment in their life account.

The deposits we make in our lives are numerous, ranging from the financial resources we spend, the food we eat, the liquids we drink, the relationships we engage in, the time we have, and the seeds we plant. I have come to the conclusion that good honest integrity-based attitude towards life is the general nature of people. We are all doing our best with the tools we were given to carve out a life for ourselves. I have come across many people with good hearts that could be powerful forces in the world, but yet they seem to fall short. I wondered why this was for many years, and came to the understanding that it is all about how we invest in ourselves. Many people are so consumed with spending their time and energy on other people's needs that they lose sight of their own. They are fastening someone else's life support system and ignoring their own, pretending that it is selfish to turn inward when others are in need. This is a noble idea that I respect, but a misguided idea nonetheless because it relieves another of their own responsibility to their life, and it distracts you from yours. To help others in need is important, but to carry them across burning coals when their feet are untarnished is sabotage, for both you and those you intend to support.

I encourage you to look deep inside yourself and find out what you need to create to allow the abundance you deserve, for yourself and for those you love. Every minute of our time is an investment. It may not seem like it in the regular flow of things, but you have to consider that you will never get that time back, so you use it wisely. Whenever you have an extra five or ten minutes in between projects or appointments, direct your attention to the most conducive activity at that time. This is why I always carry a book with me wherever I go. Even if I only have a minute of idle time, I like to open a book just to skim through the pages and attempt to saturate my mind with positive ideas. Reading is so critical for the positive outcome of your life. The ideas of those that came before are sealed in the pages of time. There really is no problem or dilemma you could ever go through that someone before you has not experienced themselves, and I can almost guarantee it has been written down in a book somewhere! Make it a point to donate time to flipping the pages to uncovering the solutions.

When we spend money, we are investing our time, effort, and resources into that which we purchase. It is not merely a matter of spending money for the sake of receiving something, it actually becomes an indication of where our true values are at that moment. We must be selective of how we use our resources in these times. If we regularly spend our money on frivolous things, then we will breed that of a similar or identical nature into other areas of our lives. If we focus on material gains, then we will cut corners where it is most important. I have seen those who make large sums of money skimp on their health practices, and not because they couldn't afford it, but because the right values were not instilled. The continual practice of focused and attentive investing in one's life will produce results that will steer one in the direction of their choosing. Those that spend money while looking in another direction will end up somewhere they never intended to be.

If you make a habit of investing in those things that will serve you most, then you will reap the rewards that life has set up for you. If you let things that do not serve you fall away, and increase your standards for your own life, then you can be surprised at how new options rise up for you. Choose to invest in the food you eat. Choose to go 100% organic, unwilling to settle for inferior food that contributes to the life you have left behind. Choose to invest in the people that support and encourage you, the ones that compliment your life. Choose to invest each minute of each day to the constant and ever expanding progression of the life you have only yet embarked on, you are worth it!!

"Your economy has always been about the exchange of human energy: As contrast produces a new idea within any human consciousness, the Nonphysical Energy to supply it flows forth. The economy expands proportionate to the idea. There is no shortage of anything. Those who believe there is shortage, hold themselves over in this place where they

disallow the Energy from flowing to them. And so, in their resistance, they have it not. And then they say, "I am proof that there is shortage. And that man over there that is awash in money is the reason I don't have any." He has nothing to do with your shortage. He is evidence that there is abundance."

Abraham

The Raw Naked Truth

"We must adjust to changing times and still hold to unchanging principles."
Jimmy Carter

"Your descendants shall gather your fruits."
Virgil

We have entered into a new frontier in the human experience, one that has opened the flood gates to all educational technologies available. As a result of our predecessors and as our children's caretakers, we have been hand delivered an awesome responsibility to ensure the prosperity of our future. The generations that came before us had their chance to uplift this planet decade after decade. We can all see the results of their actions towards freedom and fruitfulness. We hold the torch now, blazing a trail for our children to one day inherit. It is time to begin planting the seeds of a desirable future. It will be up to each one of us to ensure those seeds will be capable of bearing fruit.

As we approach more innovative ideas, we are being presented with an astonishing truth that can no longer be ignored. The wisdom of the ancients still holds true today and, in most cases, overrides the conventional wisdom of the world we are inhabiting. Although it has been persistently ignored, the understanding that the food we put into our mouths has deep implications on every aspect of our lives, including the entire world, is becoming more accepted.

The brightest minds have all confirmed that in order to get ourselves out of a hole we have dug ourselves into, the solution is not to keep digging until we have no way back to land- the solution is to start building a ladder. I personally believe the mass emergence of raw foods over the last few decades is the result of society carelessly swinging the pendulum too far over to one side, focusing on profit and supplying short-term gratification.

We have been lost in the midst of chaos and smoke, most of it coming from the completely irresponsible use of viable resources. It is time to reveal the truths that have always been with us.

Food Psychology

The importance of our food choices is found most evident in our own mental attitudes. It is becoming common knowledge that the majority of all mental conditions, if not all, are the result of nutritional deficiencies and toxic substances. The paradox of this situation is that our daily choices are being "fueled" by our fuel intake. Therefore, if our "fuel" is contaminated or dirty, it will cloud our judgement, further perpetuating the vicious cycle of making more poor decisions that lead to poor results. There are some great questions we can ask ourselves to shed a much brighter light on this subject, and will we usually get back good answers when we ask good questions.

- Why do people give up their freedom for a sedentary lifestyle?
- Why are people increasingly irritable and angry?
- Why is there a continued decline in literacy?
- Why does the media promote primarily doom & gloom reports?
- Why is there an increase in divorce rates?
- Why are less and less parents actively involved in their children's lives?
- Why is there so much chemicals, petroleum, chemtrails, pesticides, and plastics in our environment?
- Why is obesity, heart disease, inflammation, and cancer on the rise with so much funded research in these areas?
- Why do our "leaders" continue to make more destructive decisions?
- Why does 1% of the population dictate what the other 99% of the population does and is allowed to do?

These are only a few of the questions I began asking as I felt that the stressful situations we face must have answers that are more reasonable than the typical shove-it-under-the-rug responses we have been getting all this time. The absolute truth of the matter is the standard American diet that most of us grew up with actually retards human capabilities in ways that lead to laziness and passiveness, as well as decrease in focus, reduced enthusiasm for life, and continually exhausted energy levels. If there is a leakage of energy, then all of our abilities will be compromised. This jeopardizes our mental cognition with regards to making intelligent and precise decisions, focusing on tasks, and working effectively with other people with varying perspectives.

As I have covered in more detail in the chapter, "The Scientific Method", author Tony Wright describes in his book, **Left in the Dark**, the more we have traveled away from a natural raw plant-based diet, the more we have become increasingly left-brain dominant. Left-brain dominance is the very strict, rigid, and calculating mindset associated with making decisions based entirely on analysis as opposed to intuition or creative expression. This perfectly explains why we continue to find ourselves in wars, why people continue to think in terms of profit instead of sustainability, why many find themselves working a job that they cannot stand, and why people are taking medications that undermine their right-brain activity even further.

When anyone decides to implement more organic fruits, vegetables, super foods, sprouts, seaweeds, and herbs into their lifestyle, the immediate changes are sometimes subtle and sometimes massive. I have seen time and time again that even though many people who initially adopt this lifestyle don't always have a vested interest in the environment or animal rights, their attitudes greatly changes after just a short time. The heightened awareness that natural raw foods can bestow on our world and our personal lives is profound; it has the ability to compel someone on Wall Street into the middle of a rain forest. It took me from becoming another single-minded professional athlete to a fully fledged raw food advocate, speaker, and promoter of all sustainable operations worldwide.

In the book, **Blatant Raw Foodist Propaganda**, Joe Alexander describes an interesting experience many people have when going raw:

"My experience has convinced me that cooking converts the life-force or orgone energy in foods to what Dr. Reich called DOR or deadly orgone energy, a stagnant and inimical form of energy which Reich said created a desert when it was present in abnormally high concentrations in the atmosphere of an area. You see, as an artist, when I ate cooked foods I painted bleak and dull, muddy colors; I was a creator of deserts in my art, but when I became a raw food eater, all of a sudden I began to paint instead, vibrantly alive pictures with lush abundance of healthy shapes and brilliantly beautiful colors, like the sort of lush jungle growth that Reich said was created by a strong concentration of healthy orgone energy in the atmosphere of an area."

Cooked Food

There are numerous debates and theories on when and why humans started using fire to heat their food. These theories can persist until the end of time, and no definitive answer will ever surface. Obviously, ancient man came across the discovery of fire in order to alter his environment as a way to keep warm and see in darkness. Tribes from all over the world adopted this practice throughout the ages in ceremonial gatherings. I would imagine that people began to use fire as a means of cooking animal meat as it probably tasted better than eating it raw, and also as a way to preserve food. Nobody knows for sure, but one thing I am certain of is this: the moment we started cooking our food is the moment everything in civilization changed. In his deeply fascinating work, **The Origins of Human Diet & Medicine**, *Timothy Johns* points out that "*the primary contribution of cooking may have been in controlling the microbiological toxins associated with the increased use of meat*".

Fire, like all the elements, must be respected in its use. Fire has allowed us to progress and evolve in ways where we would have been hindered without it. However, it is also destructive in nature. Fire does not produce life. In fact, it only takes life away from everything it touches, much like how the candle wax that is used to light ones path will eventually burn out. If you put your finger in a flame, the flame will damage your finger. If you put your finger in cold ocean water, the water will heal your finger. When you add fire to a seed, the fire will instantly kill the seed. If you add water to a seed, the water will make it grow.

The assumptions surrounding cooked foods is that there is something wrong with nature, and therefore we need to alter it. It instills the mindset that we need to de-nature the plants in order to digest them because we are imperfect beings on our own. Whenever you consume cooked food, you are essentially consuming a molecularly altered substance that creates some form of stress on the body in mostly all cases.

A diet high in cooked and processed foods is extremely dehydrating. Cooking food strips off all of the hydrogen molecules immediately. Your body is mostly water, and it requires your food to be convertible into liquids for digestion and absorption. I am convinced the two biggest ailments in the western world are directly linked to a dominantly cooked food diet: fatigue and dehydration.

The cooking process completely wipes out the life force of our food. Raw organic plants have an abundance of light radiating through and around them. This example is shown beautifully in *David Wolfe*'s book, **Eating for Beauty**. The display of energetic differences between cooked foods and raw foods is shown through **Kirlian Photography**. Kirlian technology, discovered in Russia in the early 1900's, has the ability to reveal the ultraviolet light that is emitted from all things where the human eye cannot detect. The indication of electricity or life force is profoundly different in raw organic food than it is in a cooked food. In my opinion, this is enough evidence to discern whether I should be eating living foods or dead foods.

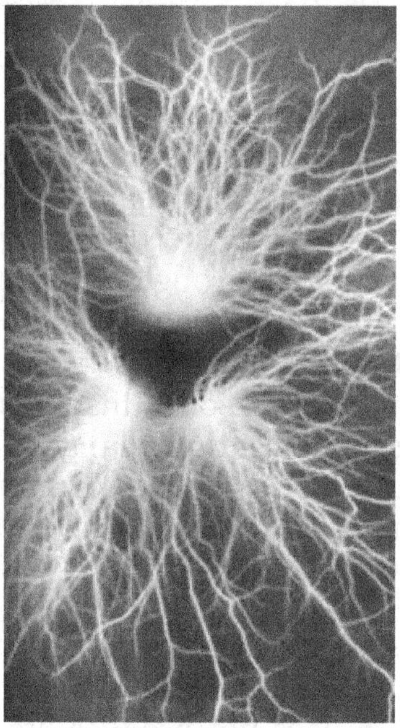

A electrical current of one raw Goji berry is revealed through this Kirlian photo!

This idea of life force energy or "mana" can also be described as biophotons, which is a term brought to popularity in the scientific community in 1974 by *Fritz-Albert Popp*, a German biophysicist. A biophoton can be described as an electromagnetic wave of light in the optical range of a living organism. All living organisms, ranging from plants, animals, and humans, emit biophotons that are not visible by the naked eye but do exist in living cells according to the original research data dating back to 1923 by Russian medical scientist, Professor Alexander G. Gurvich. A great deal of this research and experiments were done to show the importance of our food selections from a purely energetic perspective, which opposes the entire mainstream nutritional paradigm as we have known it. In the early 1900's, the pioneer of what is known as bio-frequency medicine, Dr. Valerie Hunt was born. Dr. Hunt is responsible for introducing the idea that the physical problems people face are not due to the body itself, but are linked to a disturbance in their electromagnetic field or biophotonic resonance. She has spent most

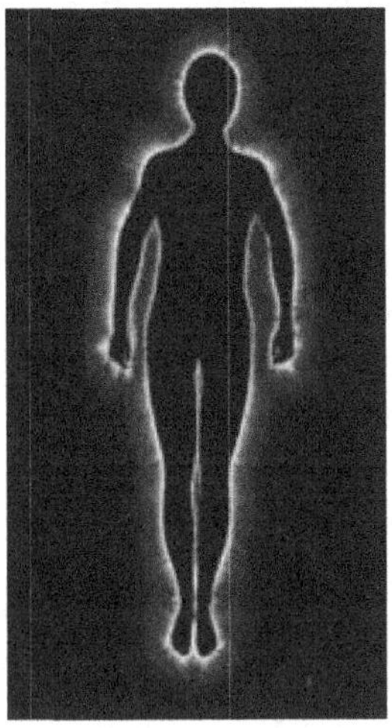

likely more time than any human on the planet promoting this idea, and has done numerous studies clearly showing how outside influences dampen our energy field, especially outside influences such as food. Dr. Hunt performed an experiment doing ultraviolet motion filming with an athlete. The subject athlete first consumed a traditional fast food meal consisting of soda, fries, and a hamburger, resulting in the significant dampening of his field. Ten minutes later, he consumed fresh raw plant foods. While measuring his field, the light of his body increased immediately! You are what you eat is not just a catch phrase; it is a biological reality that each one of us is experiencing, whether we are conscious of it or not. Valerie Hunt is now 95 years old and remains extremely active in the world. She believes that humans do not die by default but rather it is a decision we all make.

People on the standard diet are falling deeper and deeper into nutritionally deficient illnesses by the day. Cooked food is very dense, and will leave a charred-ash residue in the intestinal lining as well as the colon over time. The extreme use of cooking methods has led to more and more people needing colon hydrotherapy. The toxic build-up starts to inhibit your digestion, continuously making it more difficult to break down food and convert it into clean-burning fuel. This will cause corrosion in the pipes as the aging process becomes accelerated. Aging, in terms of breaking down as we mature in life, is a very inaccurate theory which has everything to do with the fuel that runs this magnificent and self-sustainable vehicle we call the human body.

Furthermore, the nutritional properties of food is greatly reduced by the use of heat. The temperature that heat begins to greatly damage the nutritional value of most foods is between 118- 125 degrees Fahrenheit, and many foods are effected at even much lower temperatures. It is true that some vitamins retain their value after heating, but an important idea to remember is that regardless of a nutrient's individual role(lycopene in tomatoes for example), the synergy of the combined nutritional value is weakened. The true power in food is not the isolation of nutrients but the balanced combination that promotes the healing process. Many vitamins are fat soluble and must be delivered into the body through a fat source. Most fats convert into trans-fats when cooked under high temperatures, which can wreak havoc within the body. Saturated plant fats, such as coconut oil/cream and cacao butter, are significantly more heat durable than their monounsaturated and polyunsaturated counterparts.

All cookware leaches into the food, regardless of what material is used. Even the best equipment will degrade under the conditions of heat eventually. Do not forget, the application of fire is to break down solid materials; there is no exception to this rule. Heavy metals from cooking pans are introduced into the body through the leeching process, creating free radical damage, especially with the addition of oxidized cooking oils that are rancid in many cases. This leaves the immune system more vulnerable to opportunistic organisms. When food is cooked at high temperatures, a carcinogenic toxin known as acrylamide is created from the combustion of oils and carbon/hydrogen bonds. According to the WHO (World Health Organization), acrylamide is used primarily in the formation of polyacrylamide materials which are used to make glues, paper, and many cosmetics. Acrylamide has been linked to cancer in both animals and humans, and nervous system disorders have been found as a result of the accumulation of this known toxin.

Cooked foods are very addictive for a few reasons. A highly cooked diet degrades your intuitive perception of taste over time, making it harder to fully engage in the experience of eating. There is a process in nature known as the allostatic taste change that occurs when our taste perception changes due to our bodies no longer desiring food or the same category of food that is being eaten in excess. Raw food provides this taste alteration whereas cooked food does not. A sweet fruit, such as a pineapple, can become sour or even burn your lips once the taste receptors signals for you to stop eating. Impulsive eating, usually on cooked/processed foods, is the most obvious cause of obesity. I have never seen an obese human being that binges on raw plant foods before. Cooked foods can be very addictive because it causes extreme malnourishment at the cellular level. The cells, which are the building blocks of our physical template, require adequate building materials that a cooked diet will not sufficiently supply. This is what causes a desire to keep eating way past the physical needs- the cells are 'hungry' but the body is overwhelmed. A high amount of toxins in the body are then stored in your fat cells and thyroid gland(throat area), resulting in an increase in excess weight and the bodies desire to keep feeding it.

In the 1930's, research was conducted at the Institute of Clinical Chemistry in Lausanne, Switzerland under the direction of Dr. Paul Kouchakoff. He did a test on the effects of cooked food on the immune system, and how the body responds immediately after eating it. What Dr. Kouchakoff found was that as soon as someone ate some kind of cooked food they would immediately experience what is called "digestive leukocytosis", otherwise known as a white blood cell reaction. A white blood cell response is due to signals in the body alerting that there is a foreign compound in the body requiring the immune system to react. The same experiment conducted on raw foods did not trigger the same reaction. He discovered that if the diet consisted of a higher percentage of raw foods than cooked foods, the it would help neutralize the acidity of cooking. So one does not have to eat 100% raw foods to reap extraordinary benefits. It is important to note that Dr. Kouchakoff was not arguing for or against cooked food or raw food- he was simply researching the effects of the experiment.

"Let the reader consider that a human baby, like an infant animal, is given raw foods having a full complement of enzymes, from the breasts of its mother. If it needed cooked food for survival, it would have been provided with it. A cooking stove, which is a human invention, does not come permanently attached as a part of the anatomy of a newly born infant!"

Dr. Edward Howell- Enzyme Nutrition

Going Organic

The awareness of making better choices with our health and nutrition is gaining greater momentum as people realize the benefits of upgrading their lifestyle. When we step into the world of raw living foods many more doors of learning begin to open up, exposing us to information we may have never known before. One of the doors we all need to step through is the growing organic movement. The importance of going completely organic, either step by step or right away, cannot be overlooked by any conscious health advocate. Organic foods are grown without the use of synthetically sprayed materials such as pesticides or chemical fertilizers(NPK), are non-genetically modified, are not irradiated, and should contain no industrial residues or food preservatives.

It is common to get caught into the excuse making trap, which usually is a financial concern, regarding purchasing organic foods. It is true in "most" cases that organic foods may cost a little more than conventional food. However, do consider that a sports car sits on a higher price tag than a commuter vehicle, and it depends on ones value system where they will put their money. A change in perspective is helpful for this because, in almost all cases, we do not consider the vast amounts of money we literally throw away on a daily basis. Health assurance opposed to "health insurance" is substantially less expensive if the average American held back a fraction of what is spent on bills and invested into their food. The trips to the doctor could stop for good! The cost of going to the hospital for one day is a far greater financial burden than the cost of eating organic for over six months or more! I found in my life that the money I saved on night clubs, alcohol, junk food, frivolous dating, and entertainment to plug in the holes of boredom was outrageous. When you upgrade your nutrition everything begins to turn on, and you will find yourself involved in activities that no longer seem to burn a hole in your pocket.

Wherever someone is in their lifestyle pattern I always suggest they work to make gradual upgrades, and the best place to begin is moving into organically grown foods. There has been misinformation stating that there has been little evidence shown to differentiate the health effects of foods sprayed with pesticides, herbicides, fungicides, insecticides, and rhodenticides, and the health effects of organically grown produce. Not only is this absolutely false, but the consequences of consuming chemical-sprayed foods has long term effects that are easily neglected in the short term. The idea that we can just remove the skin from a fruit to avoid the chemicals is naive, and is in part a way of devaluing your own worth as it shows you are not willing to invest a little extra in your own well being. The chemicals seep into the flesh of the fruits and vegetables, rendering them completely unfit for human consumption.

Dr. Alan Green, a pediatrician from Standford's Packard Children's Hospital, did a study measuring the blood of babies immediately after they were born found an average of 200 industrial chemicals. A babies immune system is undeveloped and unable to defend against toxins. This is the reality we face when we choose to cut corners on the quality of our food, and no amount of money we save in the short term will create the value we may enjoy for a lifetime. As Dr. Green so brilliantly states, "every bite of food is an investment into your body or its a debt your bodies taking out".

"On Average a child eats or drinks something contaminated by pesticides five times a day"
Discovery Channel - The Truth about Organic Foods

We are bombarded with the exposure of toxins every day, which leads many to believe it makes little difference whether they consume chemicals or not. The good news is that the more organic fruits and vegetables you can include the more it will buffer much of the toxicity in the body and help to escort it out. It is a commitment to live a cleaner, and more attentive lifestyle. If you strive for quality, the rewards will far outweigh the cumulative efforts. When you taste a freshly picked strawberry or peach from the farmers market it tastes completely different than whats in the stores. It invigorates your taste buds, influencing new thought forms that eventually leads one to a new way of being.

I highly suggest that we do as little shopping in the supermarkets and take our money to the people who deserve it the most: the local organic farmers. The produce in the stores is, in my opinion, always a last resort due to the exposure of many human hands, and foods picked out of season. I prefer to go straight to the person growing my food whenever possible. The ethical farmers in charge of our organic industry strive so hard to provide us with the best possible quality food and, because of this, they deserve every bit of support we can give. I always like turning on others to the farmers market. If you live out of town from one, then take the family and make a day out of it.

If it is hard to afford to go completely organic 100% of the time, then consider these foods in particular that have the highest rate of chemical sprays when grown conventionally. These foods are considered the dirty dozen and should always be purchased organic: apples, celery, strawberries, peaches, spinach, nectarines, grapes, bell peppers, potatoes, blueberries, lettuce, and kale.

Hybridized Foods

Hybridization is the process of cross breeding two sub-species of foods, usually from, but limit to, the vegetable or fruit kingdom. There has been a vast difference in speculation on whether hybrid foods are appropriate for human consumption, usually from an emotional basis in defense of certain dietary preferences. Many philosophers, lecturers, archeologists, and raw foodists believe at one point in our history humans were primarily fruigivores(fruit eaters) but have migrated away from this set point due to dramatic landscape alterations that have been created over the centuries by human intervention. The truth as I see it is not that our biological needs have drastically changed but that our feeding habits have. In following unnatural patterns of eating, we began to develop imbalanced living conditions.

Plants occurring in their natural ecosystem have been known to hybridize on their own through cross pollination. These plants commonly develop extreme traits that neither parenting variety contain. This can allow for increased durability during environmental shifts which ultimately leads to the extinction of the original phenotypical expression of the plant(the parenting plants). All plants, animals, and humans, to some degree, are hybrids of their ancestry. As time has moved forward so has the gap between all species, increasing the tendency to mate with one another. There is a strong commonality of infertility in hybrids in the plant world, making them unable to reproduce. This seems to be dependent on whether a hybrid species inherits an even or odd number of chromosomes to create their genetic material. We will revisit this concept below as it relates to the popular notion of consuming a large amount of "sterile" foods.

The cultivation of hybridized food crops and most fruit trees seems to be a method in yielding the most quantity of food production in exchange for monetary value, not necessarily for qualitative purposes. Certain crops are hand selected by cultivars for cross breeding in order to increase taste and variety, and therefore expand their market value. Although it would make little sense to initially grow crops that are incapable of producing seeds, this is an attractive quality for many people, and therefore the surge of seedless fruits has emerged in the world. Hybridized plants have short term appeal while lacking long term sustainability and virility. In order for a plant that contain "no seeds" or "non-viable seeds" to survive, it requires a protective environment set up by human hands. The capacity to endure in wild nature has been lost due to its genetic weaknesses, resulting in these strands(seedless) being ill advised for long term consumption. If the cosmic mantra, "You Are What You Eat" is accurate, then the Doctrine of Signatures must be seriously considered. A food found in nature will show its traits by its very nature. If we ingest substances that harbor certain attributes such as infertility, lack of minerals, and vital energetics, then we run the risk of taking on these same attributes.

There are those who have decided to make a lifestyle out of hybrid fruits(modern day/store bought frutarianism) in the raw food community, claiming the warnings about such approaches are just fear mongering and propaganda. I have no intention to dissuade someone from their chosen lifestyle. My words come from long term research from those who came before me and my own simple observations. It is well observed in the evolutionary records that sweet foods such as honey and fruits were a crucial source of nutrition; there is no dispute to that here. The modern day idea that a dietary philosophy based on 75% and above "man-made" fruits serves as an experiment at best, and in no way is it a proven method of long term health that a large sum of individuals can implement into their daily lives. Extremely hybridized foods lack the proper endocrine system, nervous system, and reproductive system of their original counter part. We also know without a doubt that an overconsumption of simple sugar molecules feed yeast, mold, and fungus overgrowth. I find that those who choose to defend their dietary philosophies to the point where it becomes irrational and abusive share similarities with alcoholics. Excessive drinking has been directly related to sugar addictions, and this combined with a drastic lack in minerals can create personality disturbances.

One factor for the continual usage of chemical pesticides for intensive farming is because the unnaturally high sugar content of hybrids becomes an easy target for bugs, fungus, microbes, and insects to feed on. These foods do not contain the bitter

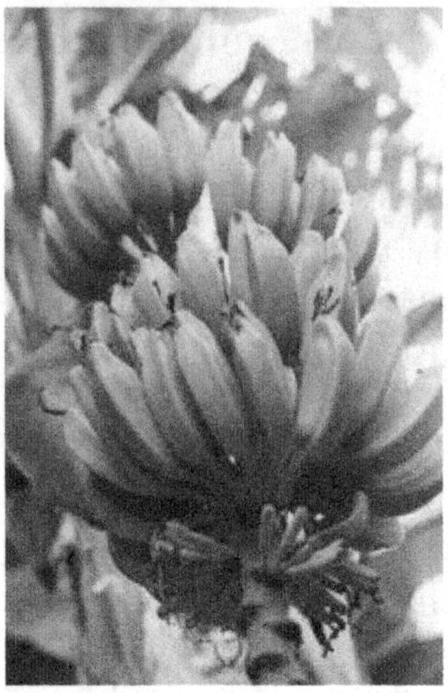

alkaloids(protective medicines) that wild foods contain, and therefore there is no intelligence/immune system left over to ward off outside invaders, making pesticides, herbicides, and chemical fertilizers a necessity in this type of agriculture. Fruits in general are designed to be a seasonal foods. Through agricultural impositions on nature, we have force bred many favorite selections to show up in shopping markets year round. We live in such expansive abundance in modern times that discernment for naturalistic lifestyle becomes nearly impossible for most.

Some of the most iconic fruits such as the watermelon, banana, pineapples, cucumbers, grapes, oranges, dates, kiwis and strawberries are commercial hybrid varieties. These are some of the most popular fruits in the modern world which are fantastic selections when their seeds are intact. When fruits are consumed "seedless", they become less of a substantial food source and become closer related to nature's "candy bars", and should be treated as such. The traditional yellow cavendish banana that has been themed as the worlds most natural food has in fact been excessively hybridized into a concentrated sugar magnet. These particular strands are facing the fate of extinction due to the extreme demand and inability to reproduce itself. I was exposed to bananas that came from Asia that still contained edible seeds. It was so filling after eating one that I couldn't possibly think of eating another.

It is not meant to be implied that "all" hybrid fruits are a bad choice in the big picture of this conversation. The accessibility of varying food options is different everywhere. Therefore, I implore everyone to do the best they can. Almost all store-bought fruits are hybridized to some extent, and as long as it contains viable seeds and is closer to its natural size(I.E. wild blue berries are pellet sized compared to enlarged commercial berries), then you should be able to enjoy these foods with little worry. Such fruits are avocados, heirloom tomatoes, figs, cherimoyas, grapes(seeds), watermelon(seeds), apples, nectarines, and durian to name a few. I completely understand the strong attachment towards easily accessible fruit- it is the most attractive food in nature, stimulating our taste buds towards pleasure. Fruit is beautiful and in is many ways nature's most irresistible food so long as it comes from natural derivatives. The insatiable taste of biting into an apple, a pear, or a ripe juicy peach straight from the tree is an experience that is hard to match, especially if that tree is growing in your very own back yard!

Hybrid foods are not limited to standardized fruits. According to *Dr. David Jubb & Annie Padden Jubb, m*ost of the foods that people are eating in general comes from a plant that is "missing vital electrics", meaning its assimilation into our body is not fully recognized. In their book **Secrets of an Alkaline Body**, it is stated that "*a hidden cause of disease has to do with how the body handles hybridized and cooked food, especially acid-forming flesh, starch, and simple sugars that raise insulin*".

Food addictions from a nutritional standpoint can be traced to the dominant consumption of highly bred plants that have been relieved of their core fundamentals(nutrients/alkaloids). Foods such as rice(grass seed), bread(wheat-gluten), chips(corn), potatoes/french fries(starch), carrots(juice), and bananas are all very sugary and come from severely domesticated sources. Food sensitivities are a serious problem for most Americans following this eating pattern. In my opinion, excellent health and robustness simply cannot be sustained on this program.

I want to state, for the record, that my health substantially increased when I switched from a cooked-food paradigm to mostly hybrid fruits and vegetables. In the initial stages it is not always about what you put into your body but what you leave out. I had reached a new stage in my health journey which felt fantastic, but after a while I hit a wall and needed to explore a little more in order to find new options. As I begun to upgrade my nutrition protocols the effects of excessively hybridized foods, mainly fruits such as bananas, began to upset my stomach as well as impair my mental clarity shortly after. I used to eat the sterilized banana most of my athletic life in bunches, and it took me a short period to move away from it. Since then I have never looked back.

(See Chapter: **Raw Philosophy, Becoming Raw**)

It is possible to make hybrid foods work for you in the most appropriate fashion possible. We all must work with what is available while being aware of our surroundings in order to make better choices. Focus on organic vegetables for increased chlorophyl, fiber, and alkalinity when purchasing produce in stores. Certain varieties like the Cruciferous(Brassica) family contain many wild plants and hybrid plants that have been domesticated in order to produce wider range of food such as turnips, kohlrabi, cabbage, kale, cauliflower, broccoli, brussels sprouts. A wide variety of foods are suggested when dealing with commercial hybrids in order to expand nutritional value and avoid negative reactions that can occur when consuming too many foods of the same variety. When looking for greens that are minimally bred, focus on bitter plants such as dandelion greens. Bitter foods still contain those original compounds found in their progenitors. It is always a good choice to shop at the local organic farmers market as the food is fresher, and the chances of chemical sprays are minimal. Also, you can communicate directly with the farmer to get a feel for their integrity of food production. In order to make hybrid foods work review **The Sun Food Connection** chapter to gain a complete perspective on additional food choices that can provide the needed balance to stay in optimal health.

Meat

"It's actually quite obvious why heart disease and cancer 'run in the family.' Everyone in the family has their legs under the same dinner table!"

Unknown

It is becoming much more wide spread the dangers of consuming meat on a regular basis. The ever growing problems associated with a diet high in cooked animal foods are becoming more apparent. As a result, many people are choosing to lower their meat intake or completely leave it alone. The benefits of reducing meat consumption are numerous, including greater clarity over your thoughts, increased functional brain chemistry, less anxiety and aggression, more flexibility and elasticity of joint, muscles, and ligaments, and a massive reduction in modern day agricultural influences such as pesticides, depleted uranium(radioactive particles), calcium-forming organisms, chemical fertilizers, and chemtrail residues (just to mention a few).

There are many myths in the health world concerning our nutritional requirements regarding animal flesh. We have grown up with the mass assumption that we need meat for sustenance. Meat was preached to be the prime source of protein, iron, and even source of energy in the sports world. After studying some exceptional athletes who turned vegan and vegetarian after years of eating their standard diet, I was inspired by their stories to make the transition as well. The results have been nothing short of personal confirmation that the transition was valid.

The massive demand for animal products has not only resulted in the accelerated decline in health but has also created the factory farming industry to raise animals in their unnatural environments in order to keep up with the increased demand for meat consumption. Most meat being sold come from factory farms. Support of this industry results in not only detrimental karmic repercussions(See Chapter: **The Karmic Bank Account**), but also environmental catastrophes and horrific health defects. The animals in these farms are being exposed to all kinds of hazards that is the result of extreme unconsciousness from those that maintain these operations. The animals are not only bunched up in confined spaces, they are also fed food that is unnatural to their own individual needs resulting in sickness. They are administered antibiotics as a result of this, which kills all forms of bacteria, good and bad. In turn, consuming these animals also means you consume these same antibiotics.

The environment these animals are raised in is easily comparable to that of the holocaust victims. If you read the book **Mans Search for Meaning** by *Victor Frankl*, a holocaust survivor who vividly portrays the conditions of his experience in concentration camps, then you may find many strong correlations between the concentration camps and factory farms. I have no doubts that a factory farmed animal would feel it is receiving identical treatment as the Jews did in World War II. Also, many of the animals are injected with Bovine Growth Hormones in order to increase the animals size in a shorter amount of time. This finds its way into our bodies as we eat the flesh of these creatures. In his book, **Diet for a Poisoned Planet**, *David Steinman* reports that 95 to 99 percent of the poisonous chemicals in food come from meat, fish, dairy, and eggs.

A factor that is less talked about is the fear factor that plays a major role in this equation. Adrenaline is a natural chemical response in the body when it senses danger or stress. Factory farmed animals specifically are subject to massive secretions of adrenaline rushing through their body as they knowingly anticipate their fate. It isthen stored in the tissues of the animal and remains there when it is eaten. According to *Dr. Robert Morse*, author of **The Detox Miracle Sourcebook,** the adrenaline that is pumped out of the adrenal glands of the frightened animals is the exact same substance that makes meat eaters feel energized. The accumulation of adrenaline from meat consumption over timecauses the adrenal glands to become weak, resulting in issues such as low blood pressure, high blood pressure, and high cholesterol levels. Many people will say this particular issue is only subject to factory farmed animals but I personally believe any animal that is killed has this biological response, and it is only more prolonged in animals that can anticipate it through the duration of their lives.

The bio-accumulation of environmental toxins are by far the most prevalent in the fatty tissue of farm-raised animals. According to David Wolfe, every single animal that has ever been tested for chemicals contains the pesticide DDT. DDT is an insecticide used for its effective killing power of insects. The greatest exposure of DDT is through food because it is fat-soluble and is stored in the fat of humans and animals. DDT breaks down slowly, releasing into the urinary track and the breast milk of mothers. According to the IARC (International Agency for Research on Cancer), DDT has been found in virtually every breast milk sample tested. The effects on human health have indicated that there is a strong correlation over the last 20-40 years between this pesticide and reproductive abnormalities. This applies to farm animals, aquatic life forms, and other wild life as well. The evidence that a diet higher in animal fat increases the chances of cancer are strongly influenced by the concentration of dangerous chemical substances which are imbedding themselves into conventional flesh foods.

An observation I have gained over the years is that the more meat one consumes, generally speaking, allows for the increase in a wider assortment of socially accepted draw backs. The heavier the density of meat products such as beef, pork, and steak one eats the easier it becomes to participate in stagnant behaviors that detract from the self liberation process.

Fish:

There is a lot of debate on where to draw the line when it comes to including fish in one's diet. This question may arise frequently for those that choose not to consume heavy flesh foods but still consume fish. The current story on fishing for food has two sides to it that deserves special attention for benefiting the greatest number of people. Fishing has been a core staple in most dietary practices throughout the last few thousand years. The Okinawans of Japan, one of the current cultures noted for their impressive longevity, ate a very balanced diet with minimal meats where fish was the main staple in that category.

In comparison to the standard meat line up, fish is generally a much better source of protein. I know many long term vegetarians/vegans who have expressed feeling out of balance until they added fish back into their diet. Whether they were eating appropriately on a raw food or cooked vegan diet is an entirely different question but this is a reality many people experience nonetheless. The biggest factor fish is touted for right now is the bio-availability of Omega-3 fatty acids (See Chapter: **The Sun Food Connection, Omega Fatty Acids**) that are crucial for alleviating cardiovascular diseases, macular-degenerative diseases, excessive blood pressure, and many arthritic conditions. The literature regarding health conditions improving due to the inclusion of fish or fish oil products would suggest these be the best sources of this nutrient. Some people are able to metabolize fish and meat better than others; this is a clear fact.

The problems from my perspective are vastly beginning to outweigh the benefits of consuming any kind of flesh food. The benefits of concentrated omega-3's begin to compete with the hazardous effects of industrial chemicals and heavy metal toxicity that all oceanic foods are subject to, none more than those resting at the top of the food chain. Mercury(heavy metal) and PCBs(Polycarbonated biphenys) are two major toxins finding their way into the fish people are purchasing at the supermarket. When cooking fish the omega-3 fatty acids(unsaturated fat) content is liable to oxidization and flipping into a rancid fat. For this reason, low-temperature cooking or smoking is recommended for fish consumption(raw fish is never recommended!).

The aggressive fishing companies have placed a huge strain on the environment with little concern for the future or ocean-life sustainability. The quantity of viable fishing regions continue to decrease each year, leading us to source out alternative options. Many fish products on the market are now coming from factory farming operations where fish are raised from seed in a incubation tank. These fish are fed factory farmed cow by-products which makes them a potential carrier for numerous health dangers. Since these fish are bred in a completely unnatural environment and fed synthetic food substances, they do not possess an immune system, and therefore if one were to eat the flesh of these fish they would stand at a higher risk of contracting sickness.

Although I am personally a vegetarian, I feel pescetarianism (no meat except fish) is a much better choice than consuming heavy meats as it is a closer step towards a vegetarian/vegan lifestyle. If you are going to place yourself in this area, then it is up to you to resource the best quality you can.

Eggs:

Eggs over the years have taken a lot of punishment from competitive marketing and scientific biases. The truth is that eggs that come from healthy and properly treated chickens may be one of the more important foods for many people going into the future. This, in my opinion, is not a question of ethics as much as it is lifestyle of sustainability. I certainly do not think consuming eggs or any other animal derived products is a requirement for everyone but if someone wants to put themselves in that caloric safety zone then this is a great way to do it.

There has been many scares about high cholesterol content contained in eggs with the assumption that our cholesterol levels determine our level of health. This idea we have about cholesterol levels indicating overall health is not accurate and originates from a pharmaceutical standpoint. It presents the perfect opportunity to prescribe "medication" as opposed to healthy food. High cholesterol long with the witch hunt on saturated fat was derived from whats called the *lipid hypothesis* theory that was theorized in the early 1900's as a way to explain the spike in cardiovascular disease. This idea had gained popular notion throughout the twentieth century with little to no scientific evidence connecting saturated fat and cholesterol to cardiovascular disease. This began the great "cholesterol controversy", opening the door for many legal drugs to supplement a lifestyle that, most likely, is out of balance with natural eating habits. We require an adequate amount of cholesterol in our diet to stay in hormonal balance and keep our cells protected from oxidation. This is an area where many vegans and die-hard raw foodists can get into trouble if ignored for too long. In his book **How to Eat, Move, and be Healthy,** Holistic Health Educator *Paul Chek* lists these important details regarding cholesterol:

- Gives Cells stiffness and stability
- Precursor to steroid hormones and vitamin D
- Needed for proper function of serotonin receptors in brain
- Low cholesterol levels have been linked to aggressive and violent behavior, depression and suicidal tendencies
- Role in maintaining health of intestinal wall

"Cholesterol production in the cell membrane is a part of the cell's survival system. It is a necessary substance. It's excess denotes dehydration"

F. Batmanghelidi, M.D. - Your Body's Many Cries For Water

The source of eggs will determine if it is fit for consumption or should be left alone. With all foods in our world(especially animal foods) we want to pay close attention to where we are getting it. If at all possible, I suggest you exclusively purchase your eggs from a farmer either at a local market or find someone who procures eggs from their farm/home in order to bypass the commercial standards of grocery stores. All eggs should be free range, fed a natural diet, and kept unrefrigerated. Refrigeration causes a temperature change which may not make a big difference short term but according to farmers I have spoken with it is not ideal.

Eggs should be consumed raw and whole for maximum nutritional value. The popular strategy of eating excessive quantities of egg whites is a good way to increase inflammation in the body. Egg whites contain enzyme inhibiting factors the same way many nuts and seeds do, which is designed to keep one from consuming more than is needed. Eggs are seeds that have the capability to bear life or provide nourishment for supporting life. The benefit of approaching egg consumption with a vegetarian perspective is to use only what is necessary, make wiser uses of our resources, and consider the animals which the eggs come from.

When consumed in the whole natural state, eggs contain important raw fats for lubricating the nerves, brain, and organs. They also contain high quality proteins and important omega-3 fatty acids. Be careful not to purchase eggs with Omega-3 on the label though, as this is usually a sign the manufacturer has introduced unnatural compounds in the chicken for marketing purposes.

Animal Protein:

"Where do you get your protein?" This is the question I get most often when I decided to leave meat completely out of my diet. The myth of protein needs is one that has been widely blown out of proportion, especially concerning cooked foods and animal products. It turns out most peoples cravings for "animal protein" is actually a fat and/or salt craving. Meat is a concentrated fat source, not an adequate protein source.

The Max Planck Institute for Nutritional Research in Germany found out that 50% of the bio-availability of protein is immediately lost when we cook meat due to the cooking process damaging the integrity of valuable amino acids. The important amino acids that help form hormones and neurotransmitters are very heat sensitive. (See Chapter: The Sun Food Connection, Section: Protein)

Meat requires an extended duration of time to digest which, I would theoretically imply, reduces the proportion of protein assimilation in the body after it has been cooked. The effects of cooking appears to coagulate proteins and interrupts the absorption process. Research published in the September 1982 issue of **The New England Journal of Medicine** states, "undigested protein must be eliminated by the kidneys. This unnecessary work stresses out the kidneys so much that gradually lesions are developed and tissues begin to harden".

I personally feel that the excessive requirements for protein in the mainstream world of nutrition is completely based on a cooked-food paradigm and, based on the evidence, is completely inaccurate. Generally speaking, Americans are suffering from either one of two conditions in relation to protein: a protein deficiency resulting from poor sources or way too much protein from excessive build up in the colon based on the inability to process properly in the human body.

In my many attempts to review information from a strictly objective viewpoint, I continually discover challenges in doing this when hearing the mass claims that we require meat for superior protein when in reality these statements are based on assumptions at best. In *Dr. Joel Fuhrman's* book, **Cholesterol Protection for Life** he provides a detailed chart of the nutrient density of broccoli, romaine lettuce, kale, and a sirloin steak all at 100-calorie portions. The sirloin steak was shown to provide the least amount of nutrition in every category but, most specifically, as a protein source. We can see that the protein content of the steak in comparison to kale was abysmal, only being able to account for half the density of this super green food.

One of my missions is to educate young and professional athletes on the truth about the fabricated protein facts and how to excel on a plant-based lifestyle. When an athlete is able to remove high-density animal products from their diet and move into a high-raw plant-based diet, they will most likely notice their body snap into their ideal weight over a few months, allowing for increased levels of performance and clarity. The long time heralded image of huge muscles and professional body builders in, my opinion, is very unnatural to the physiological design of the human body. The excessive intake of coagulated animal proteins promotes inflammation along with cellular oxidation to follow shortly after. As athletes, we want to make every attempt to decrease inflammation in order to recover and repair from the demands of heavy exercise.

Animal & Supplemental Iron:

A major debate surrounding meat consumption is the argument for meat being the best source of iron because its iron content appears to be more bio-available than plant sources. Many people associate vegans or vegetarians with having iron deficiencies(anemia) because they are regarded as having much lower iron absorption than meat eaters. There are two types of iron: heme iron which comes from the blood of meat and non-heme iron which comes from plants. If you look at the numbers, it is true that heme iron is much more absorbable than non-heme iron, and with good reason why this is so.

It has been shown that iron in excessive dosages can be very toxic to the body. The reason why non-heme iron in plant sources is of a lower absorption rate is because the human body is not required to absorb large amounts of it. Inorganic forms of iron from supplements, for example, cause tremendous stress because they are not easily recognizable to the body and actually act as free radicals. I have actually heard people in the mainstream nutrition field suggest cooking with cast iron pans to get iron! Many people look purely at numbers and assume because the absorption rate of iron is better in meat or a supplement, so therefore it must be better. This completely disregards the actual needs of the body, which does not adhere strictly to mathematics; common sense must be applied to nutrition.

According to *Dr. Jameth Sheridon*, author of **Uncooking with Jameth & Kim** and the co-founder of **Health Force Nutritional**, non-heme iron(plant based) is only less absorbable in the blood than animal or isolated products when your body has enough iron already. Dr. Sheridon points out that many supplements in the past that were isolated with iron had to be labeled "accidental overdose in iron containing products is the chief cause of fatal poisoning of children under 6".

All plants have blockers that restrict the release of certain nutrients in the body so that they are not consumed into extinction, and we do not over absorb any one nutrient in order to avoid imbalance. This is the intelligence of plants that many fail to understand. Iron in isolation can have adverse effects such as liver damage and heart disease, and excessive iron absorption is linked to Haemochromatosis. It has been shown that only about 10% of iron is required from food for bodily needs, which is exactly what you get from plant-based sources, while animal iron absorption is somewhere around 30-40%. According to Dr. Robert Marshal in the 1940's, an inorganic form of iron was added to white flour in order to "enrich" it, thus creating enriched white flour. He states that at that point in time 1 out of 300,000 people were diagnosed with having excessive iron accumulation in the body. Now in 2012, Dr. Marshal claims 1 out of 300 people have excessive iron accumulation. It is obvious that the increased emphasis on ingesting more iron has played an adverse role in public health over the last century.

When moving into a vegetarian lifestyle your body must adjust its ability to absorb iron from nutritional sources. The body may be accustomed to receiving iron entirely from meat sources, which can make it difficult to adapt immediately to consuming strictly plants in some people. AFA Blue Green Algae is an amazing super food that can increase the bioavailability of iron in those who may experience difficulty transitioning away from a meat-based diet.

For example, Vitamin C works in direct conjunction with iron and is needed for optimum absorption. Vitamin C is completely absent in all cooked foods. Cacao is a power house source of iron and has significant amount of Vitamin C. Spirulina, Chlorella, Kale, and most green vegetables contain adequate servings of iron as well without negative side effects.

Raw Meat:

The raw meat approach to diet and lifestyle in my opinion is attempting to merge the abstinence from cooked foods with the idea of how our ancestors may or may not have survived in the past. I do believe that our ancestors originally consumed meat as a survival method when all other options had been exhausted in short-term situations and this trend carried on. The idea of consuming raw muscle tissue seems blatantly ridiculous to most people today but we do know that civilizations contributed in this behavior at certain points in time. The common arguments that we should revert back to common dietary practices of our long passed away ancestors always seem a bit naive to me, mostly because we live in a far different world than they ever considered their children would. The obvious negative environmental factors, including toxic exposure of all kinds, are fully present in uncooked meat. Despite what some believe, I feel that all meat products are contaminated to some extent, whether they are free-ranging grass-fed or raised in the most extreme factory farms. The karmic perspective is very interesting because it is believed by many to soften the spiritual repercussions of heavy animal consumption when the meat is cooked. The belief is that by indulging in what is essentially a rotting carcass that is not shielded(cooked) from the environment, there is a much stronger energetic connection between the human and what is perceived as food.

Raw meat is notoriously contaminated with parasites or tapeworms that can create massive disruptions in the body. The unsanitary conditions that most factory farm animals are raised in guarantees the infection of tapeworm eggs inside the meat that is sent off to the market. The popularity of raw sushi (fish) worldwide is a cause for concern as parasites are known to be present in many sea food, especially if hygiene is not top priority. The most common tapeworms are the pork tapeworm, beef tapeworm, and the fish tapeworm. These parasites usually burrow themselves in the stomach or intestines of the person who ingests them. Most worms can grow an entire foot per year and can live to 20 years! While many worms will pass through the stomach, being deposited out with the stool, some attach themselves to the intestinal lining where they create a new home. The thought of having a large snake-like creature inside our bodies seems outlandish and unthinkable but, the reality is, more and more people are being reported of having just that. Parasites have been stated to suck out the B-12 vitamin in its host, which leads to extreme energy depletion and anemia-related conditions. The only way to deal with a tapeworm infection is by terrain modification. This means cleaning the body from the inside out through all the strategies discussed in this book.

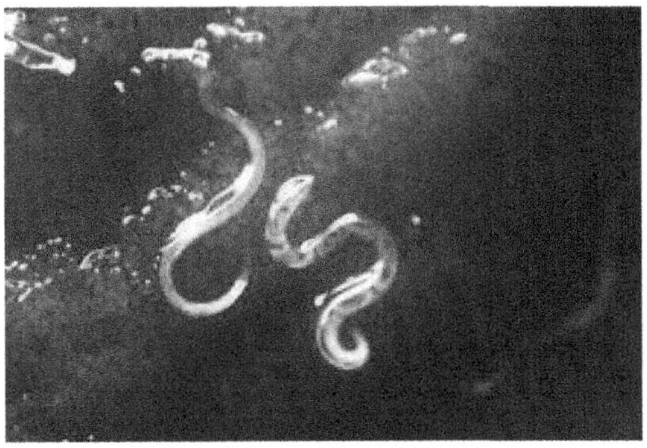

Tapeworms can also find their way into the brain which they are known to lay eggs while showing no short-term effects but causing long term neurological problems and even death in some cases. It is also important to consider the fact that a parasite of any kind strives to use a host as a remote control and we now know that many of the food choices being made are not entirely coming from the person making them, chew on that idea!

(Book Recommendation: **ParasiteRex**, *Carl Zimmer*)

The inclusion of raw meat for many is, in my opinion, very misunderstood and a misinterpretation of the valuable live-food information for healing. Dr. Brian Clement, head of operations at the renowned Hippocrates Institute for Healing, has made the point that raw meat is in no way the same as a bio-active raw plant food. As described above, raw plants have a much higher electromagnetic field than cooked food. This fact is also true about plants when compared to meat; raw or cooked. Raw meat is definitely much more concentrated with the viable energetic imprints of the dead animal and, because of this, it is my belief that we absorb this into our own field of energy. If someone feels they need to consume any kind of animal products, for no reason should raw meat be an option.

Vitamin B-12:

Something I have noticed in the "carnivore-focused community" is the overarching statements opposing a completely plant-based diet. I personally feel that many well-intentioned people gather snippets of information that confirm their own ideas and make a run with it. After looking at much of the research and meeting so many long-term raw foodists, I have to believe that the issue of Vitamin B-12 deficiencies among non-meat eaters is extremely misrepresented. Dairy products and meat do contain traces of Vitamin B-12 but are not natural sources due to the fact B-12 comes from bacteria that usually comes from the soil found in wild foods. The best sources of food to eat for Vitamin B-12 are going to be organic unwashed vegetables, root vegetables, wild foods, and some algaes such as Blue Green Algae (E3Live). The reason animal foods can contain B12 is because they are eating microbes from the grass they eat. Animals are not being fed a natural diet in conventional farming practices. They are fed corn, wheat, and soy, in addition to consuming unused parts of other animals. Whether or not meat was once a prime source of B-12, our current situation has drastically changed.

Vitamin B-12 (Cobalamin) is a water soluble vitamin containing the trace mineral cobalt which is at the center of its molecular structure and has a very low recommended daily intake requirement. Vitamin B-12 is naturally occurring in the human body and is stored in the liver, kidneys, and muscle tissue. It has been shown that up to 75% of the vitamin is re-absorbed into the body instead of depleted. Vitamin B-12 helps protect nerve fibers with fatty insulation that maintain your nervous system, aiding in neurological health. Deficiency in vitamin B-12 can cause fatigue, nerve damage, decreased mental cognition, trembling, and pernicious anemia.

It is now coming to light that the majority of people who end up with B-12 deficiencies are meat eaters at large, most likely because most of the world eats meat.

The main culprit of such deficiencies stems from poor absorption. Those with poor digestion will have difficulties absorbing adequate levels of B-12, especially the elderly. Also, the cooking process will damage all vitamins and hinder proper absorption and availability. *David Wolfe* states in **The Sunfood Diet Success System** that Raw Vegans with powerful digestion actually absorb more vitamin B-12 from reabsorption from the bile from liver secretions than they do from external food. Our bodies are truly designed to activate nutrient responses to maximize nourishment. The idea that we must get all of our building blocks from "food-alone" is somewhat out of touch with the natural rhythms of the body. The human body does indeed have back up reserves like a USB card that can be used, assuming the body is clear of corrosion and is running on optimum fuel to keep the machine performing efficiently.

The ability to process B-12 can be affected by smoking, excessive alcohol consumption, high animal protein intake, and chlorinated water which destroys good bacteria in the digestive track. Malabsorption is commonly a gastrointestinal disorder since B-12 is absorbed directly from the lower regions of the intestines. There have been those who have said B-12 production is far too low in our intestines to properly absorb the vitamin. However, *Elaine Nicpon Marieb* clearly states in **Human Anatomy and Physiology** that we do absorb vitamin B-12 in this way. Vitamin B-12, which contains the largest molecular structure of any known vitamin, is produced in our gut. If we have damaged our intestinal lining and digestive capacities then we will be unable to properly create vitamin B-12 reserves.

Lets get down to earth in regards to the popular theory that only vegans or vegetarians are at risk of B-12 deficiencies. Many of these groups (vegans/vegetarians) are still taking antibiotics, participating in toxic behavior such as smoking, constant exposure to chlorine, and cooking foods which produces acrylamides that destroy the important microbes. Eating sterile food (hybridized) can impact our absorption rates as well. All the vegetables in the stores are far different than fresh-picked organic ones because they must be washed regularly due to exposure to mold, toxins, and pollutants. High-sugar low-mineral fruits and refined sugar foods can cause issues because the excessive sugar can damage the intestinal flora. This will be very difficult to repair once the damage is done.

The primarily raw sun food lifestyle exposes you to food choices your body easily recognizes and knows how to utilize. When you move closer to nature and away from the corporate sad diet(even vegans and vegetarians), you instinctively start supporting local organic growers that rarely wash their produce or you can simply start growing your own. The issue of B-12 is, in my opinion, nowhere near the commotion it has caused but definitely needs the proper attention due to the widespread misinformation. If you feel you may have this issue, consult with your physician to verify your levels. I have heard *Dr. Gabriel Cousens* state that the blood test is inaccurate and is leading to misdiagnoses- he feels the urine test is much better. In cases of supplementation, B-12 is one that must be strongly considered if you feel you may need it due to the extreme demineralization of our soil in which our food is grown and the sterilization practices of western medicine. I would recommend everyone at some point use a quality B-12 supplement to restore damaged reserves.

Dairy

"The bigger the lie, the more people will believe it"
Adolf Hitler

In all of the controversies and conflicting information in terms of health and nutrition, I would say none have been more prevalent than the propaganda coming from the milk and dairy industries. At this point in time, the knowledge of conventional dairy being toxic is no secret, or at least one in the know would think. With all the books, lectures, documentaries, and scientific evidence validating the dangers of milk, I am always astonished to see how many people are consuming it every day. The marketing companies have done a remarkable job promoting and ultimately misinforming the public about this substance. The vegan community has completely sworn it off due to it being an animal product and the insanity of factory farming methods. I could easily swear it off as well but the truth is not entirely black and white; not all dairy is the same.

The milk that most people know today is completely different than raw milk, which has been used for thousands of years as nourishment and medicine. In the days of Hippocrates, physicians used raw milk and raw butter as treatment for certain diseases. The vegetarian groups of India cherished the cow as a holy creature. They did not eat cows but milked it to feed their families. Entire nations survived with their main sustenance being raw dairy for their fat and protein source. Raw dairy played a crucial role in times of possible starvation for survival and optimal health. The options back then were also much fewer than they are now. Raw milk was associated with good health throughout the ages right up until the late 1800's when pasteurization was first introduced by Louis Pasteur, a French chemist.

We now know of milk as pasteurized and homogenized. These are two techniques that were most likely intended for good purposes but have gone terribly wrong. Pasteurization is the process in which the liquid, in this case milk, is heated to a specific temperature in order to limit the microbial growth attempting to prevent pathogenic diseases in the consumer. This also prolongs the shelf life of milk and can far exceed that of raw milk. Homogenization is when milk is passed through a small filter at extreme pressures. In doing this the fat of the milk is micronized (made smaller) and dispersed throughout the liquid of the milk in much larger numbers than nature intended.

The combination of pasteurization and homogenization is a clear cut way to weight gain, poor digestion, diabetes, multiple sclerosis, and excessive cholesterol as well as trigger increased hormone production in children from the hormones of the animal and the hormones injected into it. Since pasteurization heats up the milk at very high temperatures, up to 162 degrees, it severely damages the enzymes such as lipase (fats) and protease (proteins) which are required to easily break down and distribute these nutrients. Since homogenization creates high pressure which the milk is forced through, it seems to break up fats, creating a digestive nightmare and causing these fats to not be effectively metabolized, leading to a host of problems as listed above.

Raw milk is easily a much better alternative to the processed version we have grown accustomed to but it should be dealt with a bit of caution as well. We are in turbulent times, agriculturally speaking. Livestock is subject to exposure to chemical sprays, radiation in the air, and carbon monoxide from vehicles that even free ranged animals are breathing in and eating from the vegetation. We must do our due diligence to source the best possible quality. I do believe raw dairy products make it much easier for more and more people to go vegetarian today since everyone's metabolism is different and I believe it is irresponsible to suggest everyone to do the same low-fat vegan diet.

A point of value to note is that some people may benefit from introducing raw fermented cheese into their lifestyle once in awhile because it is a great source of Vitamin K2. This is a very overlooked vitamin that is only now getting the attention it deserves but was actually discovered in 1929 by Danish scientist Dr. Henrick Dam. Vitamin K, which means "koagulation" when referring to blood clotting, has two key components: K1 and K2. Vitamin K1 is widely available in vegetables such as spinach, helping to reduce inflammation and increase bone strength. Although K1 is great, it is much more effective when partnered with K2, which is most abundant in raw fermented butter, fermented natto, and cheese. This was uncovered by Weston Price while studying the health of indigenous cultures. Price referred to K2 as Activator X because it would open the gates in your blood stream to let minerals such as calcium absorb into the bone structure. Price believed that K2 came from wild grasses that free-grazing cows consume and produce in their milk. Someone could eat fresh grass but may not be able to fully digest or absorb what is needed, especially if they are pregnant. Raw grass-fed butter or cheese can be a good option for many people as there is no harm or killing involved, and can allow someone to cover their nutritional bases.

My own personal experience with raw dairy has been a positive one as it has allowed me to transition into a vegetarian and eventually a raw food lifestyle smoothly and with less speed bumps. I would consume it regularly for a short period, then take breaks until I felt it was appropriate to consume periodically. Raw unfiltered milk has a beautiful glow under Kirlian cameras, showing off the life force or enzyme capacity. There must be a good reason raw milk contains enzymes as many people suffering from lactose intolerance are coming from consuming cooked dairy. Make sure raw dairy products agree with you because they are still mucus-forming if consumed too often. I believe they should be used as a periodic tool for those that could benefit from them. It is highly recommended for those who consume raw dairy products (as well as eggs) to source these foods from local farms, or a trusted source that does not participate in any form of animal cruelty or subject the animal to agricultural practices that could lead to contamination in milk products.

I no longer personally support the production or consumption of "cow's milk", either raw or conventional. Although cows on small farms are treated far more ethically then large-scale operations, many(not all of course) of these cows are being milked 365 days of the year. A mother cow's birth cycle is similiar to that of a a humans (nine months). Not only does this add stress onto the mothering animal, it also increases the production of estrogenic hormones which show up in its milk. Historically, indiginous people of all cultures would produce cows milk at very small scale operation for their family, or the immediate community at most. I recommend anyone who consumes raw dairy to switch entirely to goat dairy as it is a far superior health food and is produced at far smaller scales, ensuring quality. When consuming raw milk, cow or goat, it is highly suggested to culture the milk with probiotics due to possible viruses. I would also recommend we all strive to consume dairy products seasonally and with respect since overconsumption leads to formation of industries that partake in the inhumane methods of mass production. This attitude will encourage a relationship between you and your small-scale farmer, guaranteeing the quality of the products you purchase.

(Recommended Book: Not Milk: Robert Cohen)

Cooked food, Factory Farming & the Environment

"In the long term, economic sustainability depends on ecological sustainability"
American Living Oceans (Pew Oceans Report, 2003)

The abusive participation of cooking and killing has led us not only further away from health but far from mother earth as well. A raw vegan/vegetarian lifestyle is not just about cleansing the body or saving the animals, although that is a huge part of it. It is truly about what is most sustainable for our lives as a global community, what would cause the least amount of harm, not only on our personal health, but also on the world as well.

In **The Sunfood Diet Success System**, *David Wolfe* expresses a valid perspective on this subject:

"The cooking of food is by far the biggest waste of resources on planet Earth. Victoras Kulvinskas, in his classic book ***Survival Into the 21st Century****, reports that cooking destroys 85% of the food. When I first realized this, I was staggered. But I did not understand the full implications of this fact. You see, if 85% of the food value is destroyed in cooking, then, also destroyed, is 85% of the time, labor, resources and energy that went into creating the foods. So this idea of eating raw plant food impacts all agriculture, all business, all the economies of the world, all politics."*

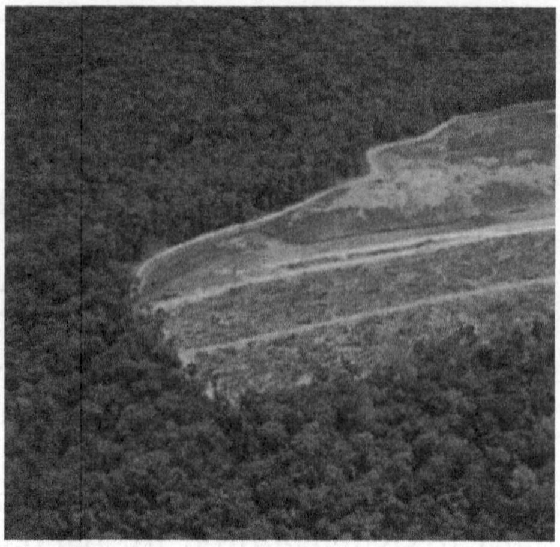

The major deforestation going on is a huge problem for our planet, for all the resources we strip of the earth we handicap our future, and for every tree we remove from nature we dig multiple graves. One of the biggest reasons for cutting down trees is specifically for cooking. Sure, gas stoves and electric ovens are the norm in wealthier countries, but most of the less developed world is still using wood to cook their food. Tropical rain forests are being cleared for cooking food, destroying not only the beauty of the land but the ecological resources that all life requires.

Trees are critically important to their natural ecosystem because they are the distributors of life. Tree roots that are deep in the ground hold soil steady and resist erosion. Trees absorb and store rainwater, reducing run-off and sediment erosion after a storm. This helps the supply of ground water recharge, aids in the prevention of chemicals being moved into the streams, and prevents flooding.

The fallen leaves of trees are excellent compost for the soil. The water deep down in the earth is driven upwards by the roots, providing minerals to the trees which lead directly to the leaves. When the leaves fall they help remineralize the top soil in the earth, giving back to the process. There is a reason the highest mineral content foods in the world are sea vegetables. Trees are often able to dig their roots so far into the soil they bring up all those minerals from the sea water but if there are no leaves to fall then all the minerals fall back down into the ocean and the soil becomes demineralized. The leaves of trees are sustenance for many of the wild life, not to mention the trees themselves are homes for birds, squirrels, and other friends of the Earth.

An area of deep concern is coming from the air we breath and the effects of fossil fuel and bio-mass fuel emissions being spewed into the atmosphere. The black and brown particles called 'soot' that exist in both fossil fuels (diesel, coal, gasoline, jet fuel) and bio-mass fuel (heating and cooking) have been analyzed in their effects on the environment. According to the **Journal of Geophysical Research** in 2009, the combination of the two are the leading cause of global warming second to carbon dioxide. *Mark Jacobson*, director at Stanfords Atmosphere/Energy Program found that soot emissions kill more than 1.5 million people prematurely worldwide each year and afflict millions more with respiratory illness, cardiovascular disease, and asthmatic conditions. This is happening primarily in developing countries where biofuels are used for home heating and cooking.

The dangers of cooking are reaching far beyond just the food now as it is being shown in numerous studies and articles that the soot produced from cooking fires alone could be the most detrimental. It is estimated as many as 400 million stoves fueled by wood or crop residues are used daily for cooking by possibly more than 2 billion people worldwide. Researchers from the University of Illinois, Urban Campaign found out in a field test located in Honduras that the soot from cooking fires, which is darker than those of grassland or forest fires, has a major climate warming effect because they are able to absorb solar energy and heat the atmosphere.

The estimates of wood burning in developing countries produces 800,000 metric tons of soot worldwide each year. In comparison, diesel cars and trucks produce around 890,000 metric tons of soot annually. In addition to the environmental challenges that cooking creates it also causes a strain on the user's health, contributing to respiratory problems, tuberculosis, and eye infections from the smoke according to the research.

"Ralph Waldo Emerson once asked what would we do if the stars only came out once every thousand years. No one would sleep at night, of course. The world would create new religions overnight. We would be ecstatic, delirious, made rapturous by the glory of God. Instead the stars come out every night, and we watch television."

Kathy Freston, The Veganist

I believe the reason the world is in trouble right now is because people are distracting themselves by enhancing problems instead of increasing solutions. The main problem here is the overall lack of knowledge and, in most cases, denial of the obvious. The deeper I travel into researching the key factors of health, the more I identify the same recurring constant that plagues modern society; it is the idea that regularly consuming dead animals in order to become healthy is an intelligent assumption. There is a tremendous amount of misinformation flooding the media from the corporate meat companies who seem to care as much about the health of their customers as they do about the critical state of the planet.

There is an overwhelming bulk of information stating the dangerous conditions that factory farming, slaughterhouses, and widespread commercial fishing poses. All life has an impact on the planet, regardless of how insignificant it may seem. Chaos is created when animals are bunched together in the hundreds to thousands in captivity all over the world.

In her book, **The Veganist**, *Kathy Freston* states, *"It's a little hard to fathom when you think about a small chick hatching from her fragile egg. How can an animal, so seemingly insignificant against the vastness of the earth, give off enough greenhouse gas to change the global climate? The answer is in their sheer numbers. We slaughter around 10 billion land animals a year in this country alone, and 60 billion are slaughtered worldwide. Remember all these animals have to eat- feed mills have to operate, trucks have to tote the feed (and the animals and their carcasses) from here to there. And on and on- producing massive amounts of carbon dioxide (CO2)."*

Commercial farming has huge implications to our water supply. The water that many people are consuming has been influenced in a less than pleasing way from contaminants of large scale farming. According to **FAO (Food & Agriculture Organization of the United States)**, *"Accounting for more than 8 percent of global human water use, mainly for the irrigation of feed crops. Evidence suggests it is the largest sectoral source of water pollutants, principally animal wastes, antibiotics,* *hormones, chemicals from tanneries, fertilizers and pesticides used for feed crops, and sediments from eroded pastures. While global figures are unavailable, it is estimated that in the USA livestock and feed crop agriculture are responsible for 37 percent of pesticide use, 50 percent of antibiotic use, and a third of the nitrogen and phosphorus loads in freshwater resources".*

If the consumption of meat went down considerably then the use of pesticides and chemical fertilizers would drop significantly as well. The use of antibiotics on animals is a response to the chemicals they are exposed to as well as a ravaged environment they live in. The use of growth hormones would have to be reduced or even eliminated because they are given to animals as a direct result to the growing demand for meat. It is said by many that 'almost' all of the soy in the world is being grown to feed animals. Animal agriculture takes up most of all agricultural land and around 30% of the land on planet earth. The combination of factory farming and cooking is easily the biggest cause for the removal of all the worlds forests.

A point that is less announced by vegans, animal rights activists, environmentalists, and health advocates is the destructive effects factory farming has on the workers within the slaughterhouses. The health concerns faced by these individuals should be highly considered as well as the animals, as all life is precious and deserves compassion. It can be hard to extend this concern towards those we hold responsible for the cruel treatment of the animals but, from my perspective, thats exactly why we must do it. When looking at this situation objectively, it becomes apparent that a big percentage of workers are from outside the country, migrating mostly from Mexico or Latin America. This industry is said to employ in the range of 700,000 full-time and part-time workers. I believe most of these individuals are like any common working class citizen, hoping to survive and feed their family despite unbearable working conditions.

"Rather than raise the standards of the industry, many employers have sought to recruit workers who will simply accept less" - "Most of the time we're bargaining just for basic human decency."
Greg Denier, Union Advocate, Los Angelas Times

The top-tier corporations take full advantage of those who feel unable to perform in a new line of work, and therefore breaking any kind of resistance to the inhumane treatment towards humans or animals. As we learned earlier we are deeply influenced by our associations and environment. The atmosphere many endure translates into a emotional numbing which would allow for the tolerance of cruelty in which they are instructed to perform.

The health hazards are so severe that most factory farm workers are advised by their physicians to quit their job as it conflicts with their ability to live. The fear of the unknown is drilled so deep that many would choose to risk long term health and psychological burdens. The attitude and emotional trauma that one would be put through in such surroundings can boggle the rational mind. I look at each human as a pillar of possibilities. I truly believe that if these individuals were given opportunities to find positive alternatives such as ethical farming or proper education then the impact could be tremendous. The consciousness is so low in that industry that it is up to each and every one of us to shine a light for those stuck in the dark to see.

"If slaughterhouses had glass walls, everyone would become a vegetarian"
Sir Paul McCartney

Evolutionary Theory

"The Dogmas of the quiet past are inadequate to the stormy present. The occasion is piled high with difficult, and we must rise with the occasion. As our case is new, so we must think anew and act anew."

Abraham Lincoln

Dietary Evolution Theory

The dietary patterns of any species in nature are based not on philosophies or convenient ideas but what is readily available at that particular time instead. There are no grocery stores or drive-throughs in nature. Only in our concrete cities where we will elaborate complex theories that conform most readily to the story we have constructed in our mind. Many evolutionary theorists believe that humans have "naturally" adapted to certain habits of eating through millions of years, such as incorporating the muscles of animals and cooked food. The behaviors of our ancestors must vary extensively and, at the very root of common sense, we have to know every single conviction we carry about it are highly analyzed assumptions at best, and never solidified as fact. How could we, of modern civilization that is so far removed from anything that resembles the natural world, begin to fathom the great mystery of this ancient planet?

There are vast variabilities all through the human race, which may in part determine one's ability to adapt to certain foods, lifestyles, and climate conditions based on their geographical location. If we look at cultures from all across the world, we find no two identical eating patterns. These patterns are all across the board but, interestingly enough, many different civilizations have enjoyed what we would consider as phenomenal health. This realization alone must fly in the face of promotions that claim a one-way-fits-all approach. It is well assumed that because humans began adopting certain dietary practices, and lived to tell others about it, then we all must have conveniently adapted to it as well.

The factors involved in cultural diversity among ethnic groups is important to consider as it relates to dietary individuality and why some people adapt differently. The up bringing of a culture is predisposed to influences such as belief systems, traditions, values, varying environments, and availability of food. It is easily taken for granted that those of us in the more developed areas of the world have full access to any kind of superfood, herbs, supplements, and information streaming along the global feedback network. It is rarely ever mentioned among different sections of theorists that the biggest marker for human evolution was at the point when communication became world wide. Up until this point, every continent and country was subject to the constraints of their surroundings. It is easy to assume that ancient man lived a certain way, ate a particular diet, and conducted themselves according to the perspective of the theoretical paradigm for the time. The mode of communication has provided us with a wider range of sources from which to gather information and deepen our understanding of those around us.

In the days before automobiles, telephones, grocery stores, computers, airplanes, radio, or trains, cultures have used their ecosystem to teach themselves about life. The oldest thought-out systems of herbalism were developed over thousands of years, through incorporating familiar plants and foods. For instance, the Chinese system of medicine is believed to be over five thousand years old. I am sure they considered their methods to be the best at that time, yet most likely unannounced to them, India developed an effective system similar in age. Each system is unique. They teach different ideas, use all different herbs, and yet both approaches work extremely well. Each set of people has done their best with the tools that have been made available to them. This does not automatically indicate these tools being the best suited for use. It is very possible and very likely that if other options were explored, their genetic results would vary greatly.

It is thought that each ecosystem, based on the unique environmental conditions, has a limited selection of food to procure. The basic idea is that certain foods naturally develop in a given area, therefore the people of that region are better designed to consume that particular food. This kind of argument is used in the defense that cooked and animal-based foods are somehow a natural evolutionary stage in the human timeline. It reflects the belief that whatever we identify to be our ancestors actions, we should also recreate those habitual patterns(such as cooking and killing our food), instead of considering that we may have merely adopted certain living patterns. I find it much more likely that the human race has been freely exposing itself to many various environments that would create the need to adapt. The need to adapt is caused by one of two factors: 1) The climate radically shifts, thus causing a complete change in the biosphere. This could be the catalyst for a quantum leap. 2) The inclusion of a foreign influence, such as poison (virus), new people (disease, cultural reform), and unfamiliar food (cooked food, meat, processed food, sugar, drugs).

The biological set point for humans has not mutated into something else. The original blueprint material before cooking fires has always been raw plant foods; this is what is closest to our genomic material. This does not and will not spontaneously mutate due to the change in direction our species once took. The domestication of humans and animals has influenced genetic mutation more than any other factor. Our inherent code for food/fuel has been lost, and only recently rediscovered through the desperation of adapting to sickness and disease. We will experience illness's and imbalances when we travel too far outside of our natural innate setting.

There has been enzymatic mutations occurring in different cultures responding to the influence of foreign foods, which can be a positive or a negative thing, and either one is not mutually exclusive from another. For example, some groups are able to produce enzymes required to metabolize alcohol whereas some do not. This is the same for raw dairy products. This is easily applied to people who have metabolically adjusted to their cooked food staples. Although this adjustment can be important for changing times, adjustments do not always mean improvements, and sometimes it can create stagnation. It seems to be human nature to make seemingly small alterations to a situation, and coast along that route while being unaware of the consequences far down the road. The incremental choices our ancestors made did not yield results big enough in their lifetime to the point where they would rationally develop any kind of differentiation. The generations following would have been raised into a world already in motion, and they would not have any reference point in which to question their surroundings. There is a tremendous resilience the human being contains. Each cell is extremely intelligent, performing unthinkable tasks to ensure our survival. As amazing of an adaptable species as we are, there is only a certain point where we can alter our biological blueprint until we reach the point of regression.

The truth, as I can best approximate it from my own understanding and holistic vantage point, is that the dietary rigors of our great descendants became irrelevant to the conditions of modern humans. Although we have glimpses of the past through archeological studies, geological records, personal memoirs, and among other resources, I find it difficult to assume we know enough to determine optimal eating habits based entirely on individual findings. The isolation of communities and cultures, as pointed out before, limited a group of people's ability to expand their scope of the world. Prior to open trade and advanced communication, the food sources that were most abundant and accessible would not be questioned. The idea that we could create a completely new lifestyle from what was around us couldn't have existed. We have found that food is not limited to a specific ecosystem. In fact, it would appear that some of the most important foods can be cultivated in a number of natural ecosystems. The practice of world wide farming is an example of this. Many foods that grow predominantly on one side of the globe can reproduce in another, given that the appropriate conditions are available. The famed goji berry that was held at the height of the Chinese herbal system, which was in deep isolation for thousands of years, seems to not only grow in the mountains of China, but can thrive in a diverse assortment of ecological settings. There is no telling where we could be now if ancient man had our availability of information, technology, and resources.

I do find it very important to delve into the history of our lineage to find pieces of ourselves left over by the sands of time. We are ever expanding creatures that benefit from grounding ourselves in ancient wisdom and fueling ourselves with the fruits of the future. It would be advantageous for all of us to not allow the lack of insight from the past to interfere with creating foresight for our future.

Biological Individuality

"Nutrition is for real people. Statistical humans are of little interest."
Roger J. Williams

The theories, ideas, and speculations that we have accustomed ourselves to are largely due to the vast generalizations made by individuals and adopted by institutions. The needs of one may not be sufficient for the needs of many, and the reversal is true for each human being is biologically unique among all others. No two organisms within the same species are entirely identical, let alone the complexity of the human genome. We come into this world and mature through our own process based on factors such as genetic disposition, chemicals we are exposed to from our mothers womb, the environment and atmosphere we grew up in, as well as the culture that shapes our perspective of the world. Each person exists with different experiences, which breed different thinking patterns that ultimately produce much different results. The shape and size of our organs, endocrine glands, heart, muscles, stomach, arteries, and brain are all different among each other. For example, I have two double jointed thumbs while no one else in my family shares this trait; this distinctive characteristic is unique to me.

In 1956, a free thinking biochemist by the name of Roger Williams published a book titled **Biochemical Individuality**. He was the first researcher to be seriously recognized for the concept where nutrition and environmental factors plays a significant role in developing individuality. He was able to effectively point out that although seemingly identical twins share the same genes from the mother, their genetic expression will differ depending in part the nutritional needs of each individual. These needs can be dramatically different from one another as they grow up since the two twins originally developed in different environments in utero. This study was done not very long ago, and unfortunately, it is still under question by traditional medical science whether a developing fetus is a fully conscious being or not, or whether it feels pain or not. It is no surprise to most mothers that all of this and more turns out to be true, which should shed some light on the individuality of human experiences and how that influences the progression of a life. The first face a hospitalized baby will see while coming out of the womb is a man or woman in a white trench coat. The bond between the child and mother nature intended is misinterpreted due to this birthing practice, creating lifelong confusion.

Roger Williams developed a core belief that each of us is built in a highly specific manner in every conceivable way, and this became the foundation for his life's work. He believed that the body can not be averaged, therefore the ideal picture depicting the general human body cannot exist due to the uniquely distinctive characteristics in which we show up in the world. In 1967, Williams wrote: "*It is an inescapable fact that every individual is highly distinctive with respect to the numbers and distribution of nerve endings of all kinds, in eyes, ears, noses, and mouths as well as in all areas of the skin. This has tremendous meaning because our nerve endings are our only source of information from the outside world, if the nerve endings are different in number and are distributed differently this means the information we get is somewhat different for each one of us*". The American Botanist *Albert Francis Blatsly* was quoted by Williams as saying, "*different people live in different worlds so far as their sensory reactions are concerned*".

Moving forward with the understanding of environmental influence on one's individuality leads me to explore the cultural and social implications of dogmatic presuppositions. The 19th century philosopher, *Max Stirner*, played a pivotal literary role in terms of individualistic thinking, breaking away from the constraints of socially imposed "guidelines". Stirner believed strongly that everyone is an individual first and foremost, and is unique in their own way, deeming it unnatural to fit anyone into any kind of fixed ideas. In his 1844 book, **The Ego and Its Own,** Stirner makes the case that all socially regimented institutions rest on empty grounds, such as state, legislation, all systems of education, and religion, including the church that would claim authority over an individual. In the same time period, another prominent philosopher and human rights activist *John Stuart Mill* was spreading his message of individualistic freedom. He was very adamant that each person should be given authority over every aspect of their lives, which he communicates clearly with statements such as, *"it is essential that different persons be allowed to lead different lives"*. It is said that Roger Williams, the German biochemist who is credited for discovering the B vitamin complex, was highly influenced by the works of Stirner and Mill, which would explain his deep fascination into the science of human individuality.

The reason I credit these voices of the past, in terms of social views regarding the freedom to express one's own individualistic nature, is because I clearly see the connection this has on our world view. Roger William's work on biochemical individuality would not have been possible if he was a prisoner to the constrictive thinking of the ideology of the times. Consider his words here: *"The more open space that is created on the planet the more we have put in its place cities which has produced crowding of people. This begs the need for more regulations, rules, and generalizations in which to approach the population"*. This very idea, in my opinion, is the basis for the one-size-fits-all dietary and health approach modern medicine has decided to adopt as a convenient replacement for real remedies.

The words of John Stuart Mill, written down almost two centuries ago, seem very relevant at this point: *"It is true this benefit is not capable of being rendered by everybody alike, there are but few persons in comparison with the whole of mankind, who's experiments if adopted by others would likely to be any improvement on established practice. But these few are the salt of the earth without them human life would become a stagnant pool. And although persons of genius is true are and are always likely to be a small minority, in order to have them it is necessary to preserve the soil in which they grow. Genius can only breath freely in an atmosphere of freedom, persons of genius are more individual than any other people less capable consequently of fitting themselves without hurtful compression into any of the number of small molds in which society provides in order to save its members the trouble of forming their own character"*.

(Recommended Book: Biochemical Individuality: Roger J. Williams)

The Blood Type Theory

The blood type idea, to me, is one that is very fascinating, and opens up a new discussion as to what humans are biologically designed to eat. There is a great deal of controversy surrounding this theory from different circles, some refer to it as "blood type astrology". The core idea is that within each human specific characteristics, such as dietary needs, are intertwined within our genetic code or blood type. Each one of us has been imprinted with a specific blood type that is believed to determine the direction of ones overall quality of health and life span. There seems to be a strong body of research that has created this idea. Although I do not believe it is fully accurate, I do find it to be interesting as it pertains to the "accepted standards of diet". I believe there are multiple factors that go unannounced in the blood type books and research, which must be considered.

There is said to be about 16 identified blood type variations among all people, the most common being O, B, A, & AB. These groups and sub-groups are predicted to identify certain foods that are most easily digestible and familiar for that group. Type O is believed to be the "original" code for human blood types, which has been associated with being hunter/gatherers consuming high levels of protein, of course mostly referring to animal protein. Blood type O's are seen as having the strongest immune system, have the highest capability to metabolize the most variety of foods due to high levels of stomach acid, and can be the most frivolous in our omnivorous culture. Blood type B's are said to metabolize meat in small quantities but seem to do well on diary products. They are noted to be the second longest living group next to O's, both of which have much thinner blood than the rest. It would appear, based on this observation, that the chances of developing disease is lessened. Type AB is said to be the youngest genetic group of the four, and has a wider complexity due to having two dominant traits(A & B). The specifics of this group are mostly assumptions since they only consisting of 2% of the population. What is stated is that AB should eat a mostly plant-based diet, while a little animal protein is acceptable. Blood type A is believed to have been the first mutation of blood type O's in nature. A's are advised to follow through with a vegetarian lifestyle. An overwhelming statistical record shows that more than any other group, the inclusion of animal protein drastically lowers health of A's. Blood type A's seem to have the thickest blood and the lowest amount of stomach acid, which makes saturated animal fat and coagulated proteins very difficult to digest.

"At the dawn of man it is presumed that the original blood type was O and that meat was the primary source of protein. But because of migration to different regions and environments, man had to adjust accordingly. Just as animals have adapted to survive, so has man. Through adaptation the development of the other three blood types emerged. The hunters adapted to vegetarian, or A type. When raw food sources became available, again man adapted, resulting in the B and AB blood types"

The Answer is in your Blood Type, Steven Weissberg & Joseph Christiano

The information regarding blood typing, in my opinion, is important for people to look at and see if there appears to be a correlation since it can be helpful. Beyond that, I strongly feel that this idea is much more specific to those either transitioning into live foods or still eating mostly cooked meals, especially animal products. There is evidence that this type of understanding has worked very well for many people, and it is really not hard to see why that could be. The foods that are being suggested in the blood type diets are whole foods with a strong emphasis on plants, especially for type A and AB. I don't care who the individual is, but if someone introduces more whole foods and plant foods into their lifestyle, then they will be able to produce results. This is merely common sense and should be taken as such.

The one factor I see missing from the discussion is how the needs of someone can change as their lifestyle changes. The problem I have with this kind of idea is that although it promotes individual needs, it also works within a small scope of options that may not be entirely up to date. Our current understanding of the body electrics, higher forms of nutrition, spring water, herbs, and raw foods seems to oppose many of these dietary theories. The best example I find is the common argument that blood type O's require meat for the complete amino acid profile, which we now know thanks to research provided by Max Plank Institute(See Chapter: **The Raw Naked Truth: Meat**) that that idea is not accurate. The great mistake in this argument is that it completely disregards countless examples of vegetarians, vegans, and raw foodists who have outweighed it with their own example. In the book, **The Sunfood Diet Success System**, David Wolfe points out three unique examples of this, including himself, where he himself has been a vegetarian for over 20 years. Dr. Gabrielle Cousens has been a vegetarian for almost 30 years and Dr. Brian Clement has been a vegetarian for over 40 years. Each one of these examples are blood type O's, and are now long term raw foodists. I will also add that each one of these individuals (plus many more) speak of high protein/fat in their own diet, which signals there may be a connection with blood type, while there is zero connection to animal protein.

(Recommended Book: The Answer is in your Blood Type: Steven Weissberg & Joseph Christiano)

The Brain Evolved on Meat

A central debate whether meat is crucial for the human species is the theory that our humanoid ancestors evolved physiologically due to the incorporation of flesh foods. This idea is focused on the thinking that the human brain began to increase in size as a result of ancestral man consuming meat for its caloric density. There is much speculation on whether ancient man would have been able to fulfill the nutritional requirements of a developing brain on mere plants and fruit since the brain needs a sufficient amount of energy in the form of calories. According to some anthropologists, this evolutionary change occurred around 2.3 millions years ago. It is assumed that along this same period, carvings from tools are found in the fossil records, which were not made from a sharp tooth but that of a crafted tool. The idea is that hominids scavenged carcasses, using the tools to extract bone marrow. Researchers theorize that when ancient humans included raw meat from decaying carcass's, their brains expanded, and as a result, became smarter, developing tools, intellect, and superior hunting methods. This theory makes a lot of sense considering that the limitations of food/fuel sources and the brain demands a significant amount of fat for growth and functionality(Specifically DHA). Once again, this idea sounds great in theory but the proponents of it usually are far too swayed with an agenda to debunk the exclusion of meat from ones diet. I personally believe that the original consumption of meat began purely out of survival, and not from any kind of attraction or inherent nutrition needs. The fact is that 40-60% of the fatty tissue in the brain is concentrated from DHA, which would have been mostly abundant in marine sources. If these homo sapiens were consuming fish as a main source of fuel, then this perspective provides more validity.

Another key idea that is almost always left out of the discussion is perhaps food gets far too much credit in the evolution equation. Paleoanthropologist *Harry Jerison* in his 1973 book, **The Evolution of the Brain and Intelligence**, speculates that the brain is first and foremost integrating sensory data of the world around it and responding to that perceived data accordingly. The nervous system is flooded with information about the environmental surroundings as an adaptability mechanism. Jerison states that the human brain would have developed as either a prey or predator. This presents an interesting idea, and perhaps early man became smarter and mentally agile not because of eating animals but out of necessity of avoiding being eaten by larger animals, so the requirement for adaptation creates behavior changes. As the world was shifting into more of an ice age(if the 2.5, 6, or 7 million-year marker is accurate), the overall environment which natives lived would have become instantly altered, including the food supply. Modern day archeologists use fossil records to create an entire picture out of a random finding, assuming this is the true marker or "missing link". The obvious objection to this is that fossil records of any kind can only represent what is thought to be an individual marker for that specific case. This does not factor in evolutionary transitions in periods of rapid change, such as an ice age. Evolution does not just happen as a step by step process, as depicted from the typical stages of our human evolution chart or natural selection as thought of by Darwinian theory. It takes huge quantum leaps, which can be seen by any major social environmental alterations, take the modernization shift from the 1800's or my favorite example, how humans miraculously went from living in isolated caves to building impenetrable pyramids.

"Our historians, anthropologists, and economists begin with a deep-buried assumption that civilizations are meant to progress in one way, as our did: from non-technological and "primitive" to technological and therefore "advanced". If civilization collapses or disappears, it means that environmental or cultural factors kept it from achieving our level of science and rationality, which is seen as a necessary advance over previous form of social organization."

2012 The Return of Quetzalcoatl, Daniel Pinchbeck

The idea that we can find a single object or test fossil, and assume it is some kind of missing link, is not only bogus, but rests comfortable at the height of human arrogance. The assumption that we think we even "know" the quandaries of a world that came before us escapes all reason of sensibility. The human imagination is a master of creating stories that fit perfectly into our own preconceptions, and discounting anything that may oppose it. In my opinion, the biggest assumption being made is that ancient man was somehow less intelligent than we are now. Take the classic Neanderthal caveman portrayal of humans we all were raised with, for instance. This idea was started by a paleontologist, Marcellin Boule, who some believed to carry a prejudice describing "Neanderthals" as dumb witted, brutish, and ape like. This perception was easily adopted and universally accepted by paleoanthropologists thereafter. I find this to be a prime example of a socio-superiority complex that promotes the notion that we are vastly more evolved in our modern day when the actual reality is that we may in fact be much more primitive in our thinking, and our ancestors may have had a much more profoundly conscious outlook on life than we realize. Carnivore theorists love to "remind" us of how the inclusion of meat catapulted the intellect of the entire human species by increasing the physical size of our brain matter. This is not only superficial in nature but we now know it is not the best indicator of intellect. I greatly suspect that our ancestors had tremendously more free time compared to us, allowing them to develop their intellect in ways we would rarely attain. Even our most advanced engineers, along with our modern advancement in technology, admit that it is impossible to replicate the greatest structures, megaliths, and pyramids. If you do not believe in the ancient astronaut theory, which is the idea that we had assistance from beings originating beyond our solar system, then the idea of devolution must be considered. It is impossible to gauge the consciousness of the so-called primitive man, whether they freely chose to eat meat as a temporary survival tool or not. However I do find more and more indications from historical records, current scientific data, as well as my own personal insights, that the inclusion of raw meat, followed by cooking food, was the beginning of an intellectual downslide.

During the turn of the twentieth century, the anatomy of the brain became very popular. Scientists believed that intelligence was linked to the size and density of the brain. Groups of famous individuals, those who have been considered to be highly intelligent, had their brains donated to science for examinations. The results of the findings were far and wide between the studies, disproving this theory. Although many scientists are still divided, isolated regions of the brain have been shown to have enlargements in individuals such as Albert Einstein and Carl Friedrich Gauss, the German mathematician. The most recent research in neuroscience has indicated that brain size is irrelevant to overall intelligence, and the functionality of the brain is more correlated with the activity of neuron connections within the brain. It is now known that every thought, every feeling, and every belief we hold creates a brand new neurological pathway, and this is mostly influenced by stimulus from our environment. The increased activity taking place within the brain would most likely require more calories(nutrients) than what may(or may not) have been available to one set of people in a particular region. Based on that fact, they very likely would have partaken in flesh eating for survival. I do believe that is what people did in extreme situations before it became common place. What I do not believe in is the necessity of meat consumption for the continual evolution in which the human phenotype(genetic expression) is concerned, especially in terms of intellect, innovation, and circumference of world view.

"While ancient homo sapiens certainly exploited large mammals, evidence supporting the importance of meat earlier than 100,000 years ago is scanty. Although early hominids used animal products, we have no evidence that they were dependent on meat as a major part of their diet. While we generally assume that our ancestors would have sought to maximize protein intake through consuming animal flesh, this may be too simplistic a point of view"

The Origins of Human Diet & Medicine, Timothy Johns

I have heard many carnivore advocates in the health field claim that vegetarians or vegans have a much higher risk of mental deficiencies, and eventually will decline in acuity. I often look at statements such as this, and cross reference it with the historical theories propagated by individuals who may be a reflection of their own contradiction. We now know, thanks to scientifically orientated doctors such as George Watson(See Chapter: **Alkalinity**), that the higher rate of acidity in the body, the less our brain is capable of functioning. This is due in part to the lack of oxygen and chlorophyl, and the increase in inflammation resulting in dehydration. This would make it easy to say that anxiety, stress, fear, and irrational thought patterns leading to schizophrenia were much more correlated with heavy meat eating as opposed to the lack thereof. If we take an objective look through history, what is the evidence gathered on such a controversial subject? The obvious truth for me is that nuggets of wisdom have been bestowed upon us for thousands of years from the greatest minds to touch down on this planet thus far. If the continual consumption of meat was a major factor in brain development, then why has our world been shaped and crafted by so many vegetarians?

Historical Records of Most Well Know Vegetarians & Advocates

Name	**Year**	**Professional/Life Focus**
Pythagoras	580-500 Bc	Philosopher, Mathmatician
Plato	428-347 BC	Philosopher, Mathmatician
Plutarch	46-120 BC	Historian, Biographer, "Platonian"
St. Frances of Assisi	1182-1226	Famous Catholic Preacher
Leonardo Da Vinci	1452-1519	Scientist, Artist, Engineer,
Martin Luther	1483-1546	Preist, Theology Professor
Sir Isaac Newton	1642-1727	Physicist, Astronomer, Alchemist,
Voltair	1694-1778	Writer, Historian, Philosopher,
Benjamin Franklin	1706-1790	Scientist, Activist, Inventor, etc.
Ralph Waldo Emerson	1803-1882	Writer, Lecturer, Poet
Henry David Thoreau	1817-1862	Author, Abolitionist, Naturalist
Susan B. Anthony	1820-1906	American Civil Rights Leader
Leo Toistoy	1828-1910	Play Writer, Essayist
Vincent Van Gogh	1853-1890	Famous Impressionist Painter

Name	Year	Professional/Life Focus
George Bernard Shaw	1856-1950	Nobel Prize Winning Author
Henry Ford	1863-1847	Creator of the first Automobile
Mahatma Ghandhi	1869-1948	Social Activist, Visionary
Albert Schweitzer	1875-1965	Theologian, Physician, Philosopher
Albert Einstein	1879-1955	Physicist, Visionary
H.G.Wells	1886-1946	Prolific Writer, Socialist
Nikola Tesla	1856-1943	Free Energy Pioneer, Visionary
Mark Twain	1835-1910	American Author, Poet
Jack LaLanne	1914-2011	Health & Fitness Pioneer
Cesar Chavez	1927-1993	Civil Rights Activist
Bob Marley	1945-1981	Singer-Song Writer, Peace Maker
Friedrich Nietzsche (Periodic Vegetarian)	1844-1900	Philosopher, Author, Revolutionary thinker
Rudolph Steiner	1861-1925	Visionary, philosopher, lecturer, Agriculturist

The Most Natural Diet

The place all of this information seems to lead us is the same place where it began: the iconic question in the nutrition and evolutionary orientated world, "what is man's original and most natural diet?" Every major proponent, practitioner, and personality of every diet, health, and food trend has argued their case, most of the time, while missing what has always been completely obvious. The great debate whether we should be a herbivore, carnivore, frugivore, vegetarian, vegan, or raw foodist rages on into modern times. From what I can tell of human nature at this point in time is that we seem to be inherently omnivores. Humans will naturally eat anything that shows up immediately, finding ways to adapt to their food sources. This idea presents an interesting dilemma for many that believe all humans are designed for one form of fuel, one way or no way. The natural way of approaching dietary lifestyle is through sensory acuity, the ability to taste, touch, and feel what works, and what works for one may not work for another. Naturalistic living involves discernment while unnatural living is dominated by hesitation and doubt. Raw plant food is the most accessible to the most amount of people in nature, and represents 99.9% of the food available on earth. What is most obvious is not usually seen by many. The few that do see it strive to experience the gifts it has to share while the great majority construct theories, ivory glass towers, and institutions in order to entertain easily won debates.

The confusion of the twentieth century regarding nutrition is actually completely natural due to the human condition. The only way to move towards natural living is by moving more and more into our heart and out of the mind step by step. An analytical analysis of how humans once behaved has little to do with where humans are going. The evolution into a plant-based vegetarian diet is the most obvious step towards peace, sustainability, tolerance, economics, and common sense!

Health Begins in the Mouth

Throughout the years, ideas and concepts about health have changed and evolved as new information has come in to overlap the old. We have progressed to incredible heights in our understanding of the human body, and the fundamentals of keeping it in pristine condition. As we move forward in our knowledge, it is always a wise decision to look back at ancient wisdom when we progress too fast for our current pace. When the ideas we are relying on become too complicated for every individual to take action on, it becomes apparent that simplification is needed. We have reached many points in our recent history when the complications of modern living have imposed harsh effects on our state of health, one of those times is right now but its getting better all the time!

In 1894, *Weston Price*, a now famous dentist, had begun to suspect that there was a deep connection between the dental health of people and their dietary lifestyles. Price became very interested in nutrition over the years, and figured that the tooth decay he was witnessing in his patients had a lot to do with food. He wanted to know if cultures outside of the US were dealing with the same health problems that Americans were. Dr. Price set out on a journey across the world to study indigenous people that were still living in their original environment to determine his suspicions, and what he found shocked him. He found that those living on their natural land and eating natural foods had far better teeth health than those on the western diet. He noticed that these people did not suffer from the same illnesses, such as tuberculosis, which was a central epidemic at the time. He noticed that these indigenous cultures had much stronger jaw structures than common westerners, indicating that the health of the mouth is directly linked to the health of the body.

In 1939 Weston Price published his work, **Nutrition and Physical Degeneration**, which chronicled his experience across Switzerland, Polynesia, Africa, and Australia, among others. His discoveries led him to argue that when non-western people would leave their original diet, they would develop the same diseases that western people accumulated. The fact that these illnesses were almost nonexistent in non-western cultures was clear cut evidence of his argument. The western method of commercial food preparation and living methods were believed to be the root cause of all physically degenerative problems facing Americans. He found that as the vitamins and minerals were stripped from the food supply, and being replaced with processed foods containing white sugar and white flour, our teeth and bones degenerated.

The work of Dr. Weston Price is an invaluable body of research regarding most of what I'm talking about in this book. The absolute fact is you are what you eat, and that statement seems to withstand the test of time. The more we move away from nutritionally abundant foods, and attempt to replace them with heavily processed calorically empty food substances, we will experiences problems, without exception!

Teeth Health

The health of our teeth indicates the overall health of our body. If our teeth are decaying, our body will follow right behind. The teeth are constantly being rebuilt and replaced, much like the bones. The teeth are actually living bones feeding off the same mineral compositions for structural integrity. Our teeth are coated with hard enamel, which is the most mineralized shield protecting the dentin(another protective layer) and the pulp, which contains our nerves and blood vessels. The information being delivered to the sensitive nerve fibers in the teeth from our food is giving us a specific education that is either increasing our health or decreasing it. The light density of our food's energy will determine how our bones are being structured. Cooked food weakens mineral absorption while numbing the enzyme activity found in our saliva.

The most important minerals for the bones and teeth are magnesium, calcium, silicon, phosphorus, sulphur, boron, and manganese. Our mouth is fully equipped to repair tooth enamel damage from time to time, but through the extended process of being on an acid forming diet, it gets overwhelmed to the point where we will experience demineralization. The acidic compounds found in soda, candy, hybridized fruit, tap water, artificial foods and ingredients, etc. will eventually cause our bones to leach minerals out of the body, giving us a drastic disadvantage in healing. We must remineralize our teeth by the foods we are eating in order to get everything else back on track.

Vitamin D is very important for the combination of calcium and phosphorus in building strong teeth. Vitamin D (**Triangle of Health: The Sun**) is a hormone that supports us in many ways, and in this case, with the balance of of these two important minerals. The average person has an excess of phosphorus in their diet along with the wrong kinds of calcium (**The Scientific Method: The Calcium Theory**). Phosphorus is used by the body to help filter out the kidneys while assisting in muscle, tissue, and cellular repair. Approximately 85% of the phosphorus in the body is dedicated to our bones and teeth. Phosphorus is an acidic mineral in nature, and must be balanced by good forms of calcium coming from rich organic leafy vegetables. Otherwise, it can lead to tooth and kidney weaknesses. A diet high in cooked and processed foods, animal flesh, eggs, conventional dairy, rice, grains, most nuts, seeds, and potatoes do contribute to an excessive amount of phosphorus, which must be balanced out with green juices, sprouts, and salads.

Massive raw food action can help to work out any physical problem one may have, especially in terms of bone density and teeth health!

It is important to note that many raw foodist's get in trouble with overall mouth health from focusing too much on certain types of food groups such as simple sugars coming from conventionally grown fruits, dried fruits, and nuts without buffering the acidity of these choices with highly mineralized alkaline foods. The over indulgence of high-sugar fruits, in most cases, can degrade the enamel of our teeth in the same way artificial candy bars do over long periods of time. A candy bar is void of all nutrition and full of refined sugar along with a huge storage of empty calories, leaving one full and tired. Fruit with simple sugars are a great source of immediate fuel and antioxidants, but since they lack a sufficient concentration of calories, one must keep eating to sustain energy. The problem this equation poses is that each time you consume fruit, sugar is passing through your mouth, attaching itself to the bacteria in and around the teeth. The difference between the fruit and candy bar is that a piece of fruit has conductive elements, allowing it to actually feed the cells along with the bacteria in the mouth. According to *Dr. Jameth Sheridon*, the bacteria in the mouth can grow at a much faster rate from large quantities of fruit than they will from even smaller quantities of candy(I am in no way advocating candy or refined foods, it only serves as an example). Since certain bacterias thrive on sugar specifically, it is something we must all keep in our awareness as to where we decide to tip the scales.

Whenever sugar or starches enter the mouth, the saliva acts to neutralize the acidic effect they have. A very overlooked aspect of this discussion is that the biggest majority of people have over loaded themselves with cooked, baked, and refined carbohydrates most of their lives, which has depleted the enzymes and antibacterial compounds that are naturally occurring in our saliva under normal conditions. If the defensive mechanisms in our mouth are below optimal function, then the ability to keep conditions neutral will become impossible, which is how tooth decay and gum disease perpetuates. It takes a long time to restructure our body's natural biology after it has been severely thrown off balance. This is exactly why healing facilities, such as The Tree of Life and Hippocrates, have such a focus on organic freshly grown vegetables, sprouts, seaweeds, and super foods while using zero to very minimal amounts of fruits as a way to re-harmonize the entire body. These are the foods that contain integral building blocks for remineralization and bringing back vitality.

Dr. Brian Clement of the Hippocrates Health Institute has stated that the biggest culprit for minerals being removed from the bones and weakening of the cells is not just the sugar in the fruit but the acidity that eating unripened fruit inflicts on the body. Fruit coming from the super market is 100% unripened. In a natural setting fruit only ripens when it falls on it's own accord to the ground, if it is picked prematurely it is not fully developed. Fresh water-soluble fruits with seeds are fantastic for hydration and vitamins, which is important to keep the saliva in our mouth healthy. If you are in the position to do so it would be a great advantage to grow your own fruit trees and let them fully mature before eating them.

The best way to clean the teeth regularly is through eating vegetables, such as celery, which can act as a natural tooth brush. The fibers in celery can seep into the gaps of our teeth, helping to loosen up food particles. Celery is also a good sodium balancer in the mouth because if one eats too much raw foods too fast, they can be hit with potassium burns, this is when our mouth starts getting irritated and burns slightly from too much potassium that is found in most living foods. Foods high in silica, such as radishes, bell peppers, oats, okra, fresh lettuce, nettles, and horsetail, have a powerful effect on the healing of bones. It is recommended by many long-term raw foodists to chew on leaves and fresh grasses. I began doing this, and I believe it has made a distinctive difference. Observing animals in their natural habitat is an interesting experience. I notice my dogs chewing grass all the time, and they are said to have much cleaner mouths than humans do!

Mouth Health

The health of our mouth is the initiating factor in keeping the rest of the body clean and clear of the build ups that can accumulate. When the teeth are strong, the bones are strong, and that will increase the performance of every organ, gland, joint, ligament, and even the brain. If there is toxicity in the mouth, it will leach off into our digestive track. If we have had unnatural contaminants attached to our teeth, the residue can breach through the blood brain barrier, and disrupt our brain's cognition along with our nervous system. We must take extreme care of our oral dentistry as we do with the outside of the body. We do not need to rely on another person to do this either, we have all the tools to be fully self-reliant.

There are a number of things we can implement into our dental health strategy to either bring us back in good shape or take us further away from sustaining vitality longer. Living foods on their own can make a huge difference in one's oral health just by the nutrition, enzymes, hydration, and the chlorophyl content. As we move forward, we discover that traditions of the old and new have given us simple technologies that we can use to determine our own oral care program.

When it comes to brushing our teeth, there are a few things we must alter in relation to the conventional way most people were told to do so. The first thing we have to look at is the toothpaste we are using. All mainstream brands are considered toxic and unfit for use on or in the human body. The main ingredient to look out for is **fluoride,** which is the same additive in rat poisons. It is a known fact that fluoride compounds were added to the drinking water of war prisoners to keep their behavior non-resistant and docile. This chemical has nothing to do with teeth health, but degrade the quality of our teeth over many years of use instead. Fluoride seeps into our digestive track, kidneys, and liver, and has been even shown to contribute greatly to the calcification of the pineal gland in the brain. Other ingredients to pay attention to are sodium lauryl sulfate(skin irritant), triclosan(pesticide), hydrated silica(enamel damager), and anything else you may not understand on the ingredients label.

The truth is, we are becoming much more sophisticated with our hygienic care that amazing products are coming out that are completely natural and have phenomenal results. Nadine Artemis, who created Living Libations, has promoted the use of essential oils as a replacement for standard toothpaste. So much bacteria resides build up in our mouth after eating food and breathing city air that it is more important than ever to pay attention to our oral care program. The use of essential oils is highly beneficial for providing extra protection from tooth enamel erosion, and aiding in the alkalinity of our oral environment. Teeth are bathing in a ocean of saliva that is healthiest at a PH of about 7, which is the same for the best quality spring water. If our saliva is too acidic, then it may contribute to tooth decay, degrading the quality of our overall bone structure. Essential oils have antiseptic and antibacterial properties, improving the quality of saliva, which contains living enzymes and prepares food for digestion. Ingredients to look into for essential oil products are neem, cinnamon, clove, and others.

You can add essential oils to the string of floss when you floss your teeth. Flossing is extremely important to the longevity of our health, removing food particles left over after eating. According to Dr. Mark Merriman, flossing is the single most important thing you can do for you health, and only 18 % of the US population does it. This simple act has been stated to be able to add an upwards of 6 years to ones life if done regularly.

There are other tools and techniques that anyone can easily incorporate into their daily routine to maximize the health of their mouth and teeth. You can add these options in as you go, and by what is easiest. One good habit done each day will yield far better results than struggling to get it all done once in awhile.

Hydrogen Peroxide:

Hydrogen Peroxide therapy has been used as an effective tool for cleaning our oral environment as well as our digestive terrain. Hydrogen peroxide, chemically speaking, contains one extra oxygen atom then water(H2o) making it H2o2. This extra oxygen molecule is used by the body to produce naturally occuring "free-radical-molecules" that help to ward off various forms of bacteria, viruses, and fungal infections. The white-blood-cells(immune system builders) produce hydrogen peroxide using it to oxidize foreign invaders in the body. According to Dr. David G. Williams vitamin C, among other chemical reactions, requires hydrogen peroxide to form in order to fight off infections. He also states that lactobacillus(friendly bacteria) found in the colon and vagina produce hydrogen peroxide naturally as a defense mechanism against infections. Friendly bacteria that reside in our gut are aerobic meaning they thrive in an oxygen rich environment. Pathogeons such as unfriendly bacteria, fungus, parasites, and cancer cells are anerobic indicating that they thrive in an oxygen depleted environment.

This modality is advised here to be used orally as a mouth wash along with brushing your teeth. Make sure you are using 3% food grade hydrogen peroxide for oral use. If you decide to take it internally you will need to dilute it in water. For internal use it has been suggested by many health experts to use 35% food grade hydrogen peroxide diluted in 11 parts per filtered water to 1 part per H2o2. Done orally this is a great way to insure the cleanliness of your oral environment and resist common infections that build in our mouth that make it through our digestive track.

Oil Pulling:

Oil pulling is an age old hygiene system developed in Ayurvedic practices for assisting the bodies natural healing processes. This is a very simple, direct, and inexpensive method to apply to anyones lifestyle. It is suggested to do this procedure on an empty stomach first thing in the morning before drinking water. Begin by pouring one tablespoon of any kind of healthy oil you prefer (sunflower, sesame, walnut, flax, coconut) into your mouth, and swish around without swallowing. Swish the oil around in your mouth like using mouth wash, use your tongue to move it around, coating your gums and teeth.

The idea is to saturate the oil with toxins that use our mouths as a breeding ground to create harmful bacteria. It is instructed by more experienced practitioners to perform this for 15-20 minutes in order to build up a white milk- like substance. When you are done, make sure you do not spit the liquid out into the sink or toilet as oils of all kinds may create a corrosive environment in the pipes, especially coconut oil. When finished, wash out your mouth with fresh salt water, and then you may brush your teeth after.

Tongue Scraping:

Tongue scraping is another technique coming from the Ayurvedic healing system. This has become a popular method of reducing halitosis or better known as "bad breath". When we go to sleep, your body begins its detoxification cycles, which regulate throughout the body. Many of the excess toxins get stored on our tongue. In the morning, you may notice a thick white coating if you stick your tongue out to look. A tongue scraper is easily purchasable in many health food stores or online, it is a metal or copper wire that is used to scrape off the thrush from our tongue. It is suggested that by implementing this practice, we activate our salivary glands, thus increasing our digestion. A build up of bacteria and toxins in the body over time will inhibit our natural digestive ability, making it difficult to process food. This technique can alleviate that issue.

Digestive Health

"Man can survive on one third of his daily food intake. The other two thirds goes to the benefit of the health insurance and medical care industries"

Steve Meyerowitz, Food Combining and Digestion

If health begins in the mouth, then it continues and ends in the gastrointestinal tract, which is the body's digestive system. The body must break down food in order to convert it into units of energy through the process of digestion. The digestive tract is one long tube, starting from the mouth to the anus, where unused waste is excreted. The more efficient our digestion is, the easier our body can extract nutrients from our food. If our GI tract is burdened by food that is hard to process, then valuable nutrition is passed through, and is left over in our stool. In most cases, so much of the nutrients, phytonutrients, and minerals are lost on a cooked diet. Even while on a raw food lifestyle, many people face these problems due to improper food combining, the time in which we eat our food, and the way we eat our food. The art of digestion can be practiced in different ways, just like a great oral protocol, to enhance the results we need to explore multiple approaches.

A belief of mine is that whenever anyone transitions from one lifestyle habit to another, they will carry habitual ways of doing something with them until they can release it from their routine. When moving into living foods, we can take old food habits with us, such as getting most of our calories from starchy carbohydrates or high fatty foods. Those that overeat on foods such as fruits, high fat foods like nuts, raw crackers, avocados, and olives are much better than their cooked counter part, and serve especially well as replacements. As one progresses in their lifestyle, frugality is encouraged so that we do not compound layers on top of each other faster than our body can metabolize it.

When people move into a natural way of eating, a common complaint is that they are having a hard time digesting the fiberous materials. The big long tube I referred to as the digestive tract is one long muscle, and just like any muscle in the body, we begin to lose it if we don't use it. The cooked food diet consists of foods that have become denatured and mushy, requiring little chewing to activate the salivary glands, which produces enzymes for helping to break down and disperse food particles. Someone may need to reacquaint themselves with the sensations of simply chewing live foods. If you practice this in a conscious way every time you eat, your jaw muscles and teeth will become stronger.

If one is too acidic their digestion will be impaired. Eating too much raw fat and protein without enough green vegetables can create powerful stagnation. The most effective remedy for stagnant digestion is vegetable juice, most specifically celery juice for its chloride(salt) content, which goes into producing hydrochloric acid(HCL). A big part of digestion is the necessity of natural salts in the diet. If food is not properly digested, it can sit in the stomach for too long, causing fermentation. This can deplete our HCL over time and hinder our internal organs through the years. Celery, ginger, lemon, parsley, cucumber, and apple juice is a great neutralizer. Vegetable juices flood our body with alkaline minerals and chlorophyl to aid in cleansing. You want to have somewhere around 1-3 real good bowel movements in a normal day to ensure proper digestion. If you feel bloated or backed up, only drink vegetable juice until your rhythms begin to reset normally.

As we eat a meal, it is important to recognize the position that our body is in, such as sitting, laying, or standing up. When we sit down, our organs are compressed, making it more difficult to effectively digest food, laying down is even worse because our body is in a relaxed state with its weight forced on one side. The best position to be in while we eat is standing up straight while our body is in complete alignment, and without compression of the organ system so that our food can assimilate much easier. The standard American family has most likely grown up sitting at the table to eat their meals. Now we can see why many people are fatigued and depleted after a family dinner. It is a good idea to not mix liquids with any solid meals because it interferes with the production of enzymes. A sip of a water may be fine but not a big gulp to wash the food down. If we give enough attention to chewing our food properly, it will be easy for the digestive system to do its job. It is recommended to drink half a cup to a cup of water 20-30 minutes prior to eating a solid meal in order to activate enzymatic function. You can add half a lemon to your water in order to help digestion.

Food combining is important to understand for increasing our digestive health and wellness. Most of us grew up thinking nothing of it but when we deal with raw living foods, we can be impacted faster by poor food combinations. I have to say, after looking at other teachers in the field, and studying myself, the overall message is that everyones body is different, and therefore can break down certain foods differently than others. For example, I have a hard time with different kinds of sweet juicy fruits combined with other fruits, such as a starchy banana, but for others I have seen thrive with that same combination. I personally enjoy and do excellent with a wide variety of vegetables mixed with certain fats, such as coconut oil, olive oil, different nuts, or avocados, where for someone else, adding considerable amounts of quality fats hinders their digestion. You must find where you stand in this equation for yourself because your body carries the experiences and food habits YOU have dealt with, not somebody else.

In terms of food combining, there are some general guide lines that you can play with and use to help you steer clear of problems. Sugars should be consumed before any heavy meal involving protein or fatty-rich foods. Simple sugars, like those that come from most fruits, break down the fastest of all food groups, and feed the bacteria in our body, which causes a fermentation process. If we consume a lot of sugar after a solid meal, this can cause some discomfort while slowing down digestion. In most cases, desert is better off served before a meal or completely on its own. Combining too many fatty-rich foods, such as olives, avocados, coconut butter or oil, and nuts, can cause issues. Healthy fat serves as a transportation vehicle for other nutrients. Most fats are best eaten with a nice salad or by themselves. Fats take longer to break down in the system than all other food groups because one of their big roles in the body is to provide insulation, thus they contain more density. Fats and protein can be combined sparingly since most protein foods have a good amount of certain fats in them. Vegetables and most sweet fruits do not combine very well. Sugarless fruits, such a tomatoes and cucumbers, are great but a fruit such as a pineapple is not a great idea, although a simple apple or berries could work for some people.

When you feel digestive distress due to improper food combining, or simply eating too much, there are a few techniques you can use to help reduce discomfort. Breathing with intention is very helpful to move food along your gastric intestinal system. Sit up, back straight, shoulders up but relaxed, or just stand straight up. Then breath deeply through the nose, focusing from your core while pushing your stomach out. This will expand the belly, creating more space and filling the stomach with air to reduce digestive stagnation. Generally, when people breath, they fill their lungs with air, which can only hold a limited amount. The belly has a much greater capacity for storage as well as stimulating the abdominal muscles. There is an ancient breathing technique called the breath of fire where one sits up straight inhaling in the nose while filling the belly then immediately exhaling through the nose relaxing the belly. This technique is repeated rapidly at one's own pace, either fast or slow.

If you feel the need to help move unprocessed food along, you may perform stomach massages on yourself. This is done in colon hydrotherapy sessions where the practitioner will gently push the organs and colon to help push stagnant particles through. Exercise can help as well, such as light jogging, jumping jacks, biking, or certain types of gym related exercises, or anything that utilizes the entire body, and creates the demand for excessive lung capacity and abdominal integration. I don't recommend a lot of abdominal-specific exercises but more full range movement exercises that involve the stomach instead.

The Sun Food Connection

"Then God said, "I give you every seed-bearing plant on the face of the whole earth and every tree that has fruit with seed in it. They will be yours for food."
Genesis: 1:29

I have spent most of my life as an athlete and, because of this, I was always looking for the extra edge. I began studying nutrition in order to determine how my food choices affected my athleticism. It was soon after discovering raw foods that I found these choices affected everything in my life. Before I dedicated myself to a plant-focused lifestyle I would eat anything because I was burning through all of the calories I consumed and the suggested idea was a young athlete could simply eat a certain amount of calories and burn it off through exercise. I accepted this flawed logic up until the moment I began breaking down prematurely. I began to recognize how the generally accepted concepts of nutrition were not only misinformed and misguided, but they were also very misleading. There are many facets of nutrition we should look at in relation to how our food affects our body so that we may expand our horizons, thus creating brand new possibilities.

This may prove to be the most important and insightful section of the entire book. We are going to explore the nutrition puzzle one piece at a time. Each section is uniquely complex yet, with a little bit of probing, can be simplified and understood so a greater picture of health can be achieved. I suggest the reader use this chapter in particular as a resource and as a way to make immediate choices based on the information presented, picking from the vast options on the sun food menu.

Calories

"One can thrive on half the normal intake of food as long as we consume high electron-rich nutrients"
Dr. David Jubb

In the nutrition puzzle, the base of our intake is in the form of calories. The general idea of nutrition is strictly focused on caloric intake, which would constitute as mainly macronutrients consisting of carbohydrates, fats, and proteins. This has been the main way of gaging nutrition in the diet/weight loss field. In light of nutrition science, coupled with ancient wisdom, we are crossing over into a new field of in-depth understanding.

Just like in all of the areas of nutrition there is a major difference between cooked nutrients and raw nutrients as well as cooked calories and raw calories. The sources we choose to get our main calories from should be strategically investigated depending on your own personal metabolism. The way you process certain types of food is unique to you and should be carefully studied. I personally thrive on protein and plant fats as a dominant source of calories on top of a wide range of green leafy vegetables. I enjoy a vast assortment soaked nuts and seeds which make for a great source of calories. I love olives, avocados, and coconuts as a regular source of quality fats. One third of my caloric intake, on average, may be coming from carbohydrates such as fresh water-soluble fruits depending on the season. It is important to state that vegetables are not prominent sources of calories; they are great for cleansing, mineralizing, chlorophyll, and fiber to maintain a balanced lifestyle but they are not ideal as a main source of calories. However, green leafy vegetables are still an important foundation of 'nutrition'. We will explore the difference as this subject progresses. (See Section: **Raw Philosophy, My Personal Diet**)

It is important to make the distinction between what people "think" they need in terms of caloric requirements and what the body "actually" needs to thrive. I have noticed very significant differences in my eating habits, needing less and less even as a dedicated athlete. When the body is properly fueled and hydrated it seems to require less frequent portions. You can relate this idea to a car: if you fill up your car with quality fuel and the machine is in perfect working condition it can more efficiently use the fuel, spacing it out longer as opposed to a car that is using low-quality fuel. A car using low-quality fuel will burn through it much faster and require more frequent trips to the gas station.

The idea that someone needs 3000 to 4000 (or more) calories per day is preposterous, and does not apply if one were living in a natural environment. This concept only makes sense when we are surrounded by food products in a "civilized" society. Cooked calories are devoid of so much of the nutrients that the body has trouble absorbing the full spectrum and, in many cases, people eat far too much and disrupt proper digestion. This causes people to put on a lot of body fat while rarely getting any nourishment. Most people on diets are counting calories without understanding that calories make little difference when looking at the quality of what you're eating. If you eat high quality food your body will not require constant feeding because it is being nourished at the cellular level. The vast majority of people are merely feeding the bacteria and microbes that reside in their gut but their cells are starving, causing them to gain weight and create dis-ease in the body.

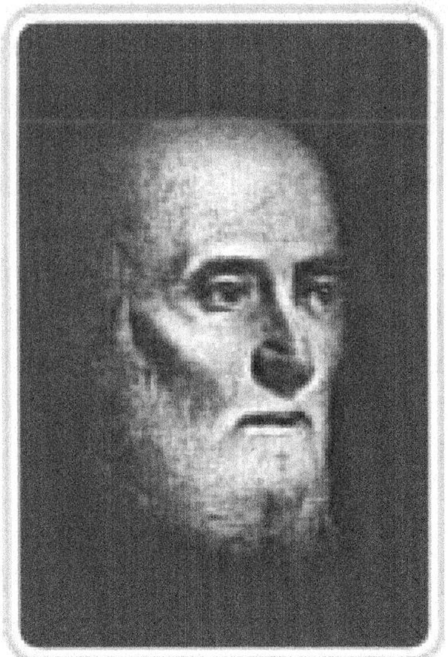

The phrase *"the less you eat the longer you live"* most likely was inspired by Luigi Cornaro, an Italian nobleman of the 1500's. Luigi became violently ill at the age of 35 and, on the recommendation by his doctors, began removing alcohol and rich heavy foods from his diet. He became remarkably healthier from this change. He decided to reduce his entire food intake to 12 ounces of solid food a day, split into two meals per day, and drank pure grape juice. He lived to be 102, retaining all of his faculties until the end of life, passing away peacefully in his sleep. The quality of food available in Luigi's time was far below what is at our grasp now. By living simply and not burdening the body with harsh requirements Luigi was able to live healthily to 102. Imagine what is possible if we can adopt a similar philosophy with the options we have today. When someone moves from a heavily cooked and meat-based diet to the raw organic plant-based diet they are essentially on an optimal calorie restriction program without the restriction.

"Eat food, not too much, mostly plants."
Michael Pollen, The Omnivores Dilemma

The idea of moving towards calorie restriction can be extremely beneficial for those who are seeking weight loss, improving an illness, or maintaining a balanced lifestyle. The area where people can run into trouble is eliminating individual macronutrient groups for long stretches of time. In the short term, this can be very beneficial and help assist in detoxification. However, in the long term, one should focus on creating harmony with all food groups in order to promote maximum results.

Over the years of reviewing all kinds of diet programs, ranging from low carb, low fat, low protein, and anything of a restrictive nature, there is one question that arises in my consciousness: each one of these programs is sold as a solution to a problem, correct? Yes, correct. However, once the problem is solved, the exact measurements used to it are no longer viable as a step by step plan to move forward even though the core principles may remain the same. The methods must change in order to produce further results. An idea that I have been promoting is not so much about dropping the amount of certain foods as it is about finding your own perfect ratio in which you find harmony with what you choose to eat. This idea has been around for thousands of years. The longest living people in the world do not necessarily eat perfect but, from what I can tell, they spread the ratio out wide and only eat when hungry. Biochemist *Barry Sears* presents a valuable approach to dietary lifestyle in his book **The Zone Diet**, which is entirely focused on creating the perfect ratio relevant to the reader's metabolism. Sears was originally involved in cancer therapy where he found that patients would experience major results when their hormones became balanced as a result of creating balanced eating habits. With this concept Sears formulated the idea of being in the "dietary zone". He criticizes low-carb diet approaches, claiming they completely miss the bigger picture where balance is created through moderation as oppose to complete restriction. I have to agree with Dr. Sears' idea and say this is one of the more sensible ideas in the diet field.

Find out for yourself if you do not already know what your metabolic preference is towards macronutrients. This is an important aid in helping you find out what types of foods might be more appropriate for you. Although this is never exact, it can steer your nutritional program in a way that agrees with you. You can do a personal version of what is called a glucose tolerance test in order to see how you respond to different raw foods and what macronutrient ratio works best. Pick your favorite fruit to eat in the morning, and only eat that until you become satiated. Then see how you feel an hour later. If you feel you need to keep eating to stay in balance then you will want to incorporate other food groups. If you feel like your energy levels are where they should be, then that may be the right fit for you. Do this with foods you enjoy that fit into the protein, carbohydrate, and fat categories over a few weeks as your body adjusts. I always recommend we drink at least 1 liter of clear water first thing in the morning and only begin eating when you are truly hungry.

Carbohydrates (Sugars)

Carbohydrates can be broken down simply in two words: carbon and hydrogen- a long-chain of carbon with hydrogen/oxygen bonds linked to it. This the main storage of quick-release energy in the body. The term carbohydrate is generally associated with cooked starches such as bread, pasta, cereals, pancakes, and processed sugars such as candy, chocolate, and different types of jams. The term "carbo-loading" in the sports nutrition world usually refers to an athlete taking in a huge amount of cooked and/or processed carbohydrates in order to create depths of energy reserves for an upcoming event. The main sources of carbohydrates in the sun food menu would be fresh fruits eaten as close to the time they were ripely picked in their natural form. ALso, raw wild honey is a phenomenal carbohydrate source which is being used by many more athletes nowadays.

Sugar is a very important nutrient for the complete picture of energy production. The brain requires glucose to supply energy for steady concentration as the brain cannot store glucose separately so it must get it from food sources. Glucose in the body can get used up very fast when we experience mental fatigue or heavy stress. The amount of processed and cooked carbohydrates eaten seriously contributes to the rise in all blood sugar related problems we encounter in our world. It is important to consume the right kinds of sugars for optimal health because the wrong sugars (refined sugar) will cause counterproductive effects in your body and begin to leech alkaline minerals from your bones, causing poor bone density, frail skin conditions, over acidic conditions, and possibly neurological disorders.

The mineral content of fruit is important because large amounts of sugar without the balance of biologically active minerals in the body can create blood sugar problems over time. This is easily seen with the overconsumption of processed substances like candy, cooked chocolate, pastries, spaghetti, and soda (not even food, combination of chemicals and artificial sugar). According to *Dr. Joseph Mercola (Mercola.com),* a tablespoon of sugar in the blood will bring our blood sugar levels to a fatal level. Healthy levels are about a tea spoon on average. If excessive amounts of sugar is released into the blood stream it will signal alkaline minerals such as magnesium, silica, and calcium (bone minerals) to act as a buffer or defense against the acidity from the overload of sugar. Following this response, these alkaline minerals become lost through constant urination that sugar stimulation can cause. You may require more natural sugar (glucose) if you are very active. If you are not very active, then you may not require as much natural sugar, and should pay more attention to the quantity of sugar you are consuming (yes, even natural sugars).

There has been some controversy over carbohydrates in recent years, with claims indicating that these macronutrients are bad for us. This type of promotion has caused a lot of fad diets to flood the market such as the no-carb diet, or low-carb diet, and other diets of this nature. Based on the information above, carbohydrates are extremely important, but thedohydrates that exist.

There are simple sugars and complex long-chain sugars, both of which are important but play different roles. The carbohydrates can also be known as a *saccarides,* which is the greek word known for sugar. The simple sugars that you find in fruit (fructose, glucose), table sugar (sucrose), and the sugar naturally occurring in milk (lactose) are known as *disaccharides* or *monosaccharides*. These are short-chain sugars that act as immediate fuel for energy because they act in the blood instantly. These sugars should be eaten with special attention to energy increase or decreases within your body. Usually a decrease will come from consuming too many simple sugars in one sitting.

There are complex sugars are known as polysaccharides. These are long-chain units of sugars that link together similar to a chain pulling a large object behind it. These complex carbohydrates act as a more sustainable form of fuel that takes longer to digest, and, as a result, these sugars take more time to release into the blood stream like a time release capsule. Monosaccharides are the most basic form of sugar, mono-meaning "one". Disaccharides contain two molecular bonds. The next tier of saccharides are called oligosaccharides, which are slightly more complex sugar molecules found in mothers breast milk and in plants. Polysaccharides are extensively more complex and are able to carry out far more functions than any other class of sugars. Where sugars found in mothers breast milk may contain six monosaccharide bonds, polysaccharides may contain hundreds to even thousands of bonds! Polysaccharides are a great discovery in the nutrition field because these macromolecules do much more than allow one to sustain energy longer. They have powerful effects on our immune system by acting as a barrier between our cell wall and the outside environment, protecting us from pathogenic invasions such as bacteria, viruses, fungal growths, and toxins. You can find polysaccharides in goji berries, noni fruit, bee pollen, raw honey, oats, and properly grown green vegetables like wild grasses, medicinal mushrooms, sea vegetables, and aloe vera.

The eight essential sugars known as glyconutrients:

- Mannose (aids in production of "cytokines", increases cellular communication, anti-inflammatory, lowers blood sugar levels)
- Fucose (abundant in human breast milk, helps aid our immune system)
- Glucose (stimulates memory, used for fast energy, glucose must be balanced by other glyconutrients otherwise blood sugar levels can become too high)
- Galactose (increases calcium absorption, anti-inflammatory, known to trigger long term brain function)
- Xylose (antibacterial, antifungal, aids digestion, increases cellular communication)
- N-Acetylgalactosamine (more research is being done, has been shown to increases cellular intelligence)

- N-Acetylglucosamine (the joint and cartilage supplement "glucosamine" is derived from this polysaccharide, anti-inflammatory, increases brain cognition, has been shown to aid in the prevention of known diseases)
- N-Acetyneuraminic Acid (abundant in breast milk, aids in brain cognition and learning ability, aids the immune system, has been shown to have positive results on high blood cholesterol levels)

(Recommended Book: Sugars that Heal, Emil I. Mondoa, Mindy Kitei)

Sweeteners

The topic of sweeteners has been under high scrutiny in the health food community for many years. There is a collection of conflicting information regarding which sweeteners are considered healthy and which should be avoided at all costs. This is one of those areas that can become subject to general assumptions and oversimplification among health leaders. Sweet foods have been a staple in the human diet all throughout recorded history. The desire for a sweet stimulation through our taste buds is a natural desire. One of the great misunderstandings in nutrition is discernment between how indigenous cultures thrived on certain food classes and how modern day humans sustain themselves on food. For example, honey has been the favorite sweetener of all tribal people who had access to it. It is the world's most natural sweetener, and is possible the densest source of calories found in nature. In the natural world availability to this food was limited, and therefore they could only consume it in moderate quantities per person. In our abundant culture, we have unbelievable access to honey and could literally eat it in large amounts every day if we chose to. The extreme tendency of modern day behavior, dietarily speaking, is to latch onto certain substances that excite our taste buds. The overall abundance causes many people to become attached to this experience since there is virtually no shortage of it in their life and, in this case, sweet-tasting foods.

Dating back to the 15th century, the original "drug" of choice in Europe that many of us would consider "substance abuse" was refined sugar. This reality has not changed in the last 500 years. Although the form in which refined sugars enter ours lives have dramatically altered, the substance abuse has skyrocketed beyond comprehension. The amount of soda, artificial energy drinks, packaged sweeteners, beer, and synthetic juices have flooded the food market and has made its way into every sector of society. The original soft drink was formulated from mineral water from natural springs with lemon and sweetened with honey. The modern day sweeteners of choice such as high fructose corn syrup(crystalline fructose), aspartame, and sucralose (splenda), among many others, are extremely deceptive in their marketing, allowing someone to believe that these are healthy choices when in reality they are socially accepted drugs with catastrophic repercussions. These chemical sweeteners can be found in all forms of processed foods, breads, baked goods, pasteurized dairy products, all processed drinks, frozen foods, breath mints, gum, and all forms of candies. These sweet additives have long term detriments. For example, aspartame has been claimed to damage the frontal lobes of our brain, resulting in a complexity of life long neurological disorders. Common substances consumed, such as "diet" soda, is one of the biggest offenders to health on the planet. There is nothing nutritive about this chemical formulated liquid. These kind of drinks contain a chemical compound known as "excitotoxins" that over stimulate nerve cells, eventually exploding these cells in our brain. This is one more reason why 100% of processed/artificial food should be completely removed from our diet.

In the ongoing discussions regarding the appropriate usage of natural-based sweeteners, there appears to be a large body of information missing. There is no definitive answer as to whether sweeteners are good or bad- it relies heavily on the constitution and physical condition of the individual consuming them. I think sweeteners are fantastic and are a critical bridge for most people coming from a western diet. In the overall picture of identifying the different forms that we experience taste it is my belief that we actually must lessen the amount of sweets in our regular diet. We have pushed the sweet button to its most extreme conclusions not once or twice, but most likely every day for the majority of our lives. This has caused most individuals to lose all sense of the wide variety of other tastes that are integral for the full spectrum of nutrition and food intuition. There is a time and place for everything in the natural world, and sweet is only one sliver. There is also bitter, astringent, salty, spicy, and sour. The incorporation of all these incredible tastes brings a new revelation to the relationship we have with our food and condiments. It also greatly enhances the subtle taste of sweet foods and sweeteners because our taste buds become reactivated and less desensitized from only having one taste fraction in the diet.

The strong tendency to gravitate towards only sweet foods can and, in more common cases, will likely lead to fungal growths such as candida and any variety of cancerous growths. In the average daily diet people, over the age of 35-40 are playing the blood sugar game which determines how that persons energy levels may remain steady or fluctuate throughout the day. Unbeknownst to the average American, the chronic consumption of heavy meat, cheese, and cooked carbohydrate dishes are used indirectly as a way to balance blood sugar levels. The dense meat and gluey thick nature of conventional animal products acts to absorb the rush of sugar coming from artificial dessert and soda products.

We have learned in the healing field that the receptors for insulin pick up sugar and deliver it right to our cancer cells. Each one of us contains what are known as "cancer cells". However, this does not mean we have what is known in the medical world as "cancer". The proliferation and abuse of these cells is the cause of cancerous growths. According to recent cancer research, cancer cells may contain anywhere from six to thirteen times the insulin receptor sites as normal healthy cells in our body. This appears to be one of the key reasons why some individuals can handle sugar consumption while many others cannot. When someone is consuming foods from the standard american menu the symptoms and signals of sugar overdose can be extremely subtle due to the shielding of dense animal foods. When someone embarks on a healing diet of plant rich foods they remove that dense shields, forcing them to get much more in touch with their body and becoming much more sensitive where, in the past, the same behavior may have passed by them without a moments warning.

For those who are looking to lessen the glycemic load in their diet there are many great options available to play with:

- Stevia: This herb originates from the Andes mountains and has a false sugar taste. Stevia contains no sugar. This is one of the most popular sweeteners for those with sugar sensitivities and low-glycemic diets. Stevia is available in the whole herb, concentrated liquids, and powders.
- Goji Berry Soaked in Water: This is when we soak dried goji berries in water and strain them out, preferably one day later. The subtle sweet sugars will disperse along with some of the medicinal properties, creating a great base for any smoothie or an afternoon beverage.
- Lucuma: This is a Peruvian fruit that has been cherished for it's incredible aroma and creamy taste. The powdered version is available to use as a sweetener and creamer. The best ways to use Lucuma powder are in chocolates, smoothies, and raw pies.
- Mesquite: The leguminous plant from northern Mexico known as the mesquite pod makes for an excellent sweetener for drinks, chocolates, teas, and raw confections. The bean pods are grounded down into a powder and can be used in addition to other sweeteners for a more rounded out flavor.
- Yacon Root Syrup: The sweet syrup of the yacon plant is an extracted agent that can be used as a low-glycemic sweetener. In Bolivia, the root of the yacon plant is consumed by diabetics to help even blood sugar and alleviate digestive disturbances. Yacon root syrup contains somewhere between 30%-50% oligofructose or oligofructan which have been shown to not increase blood glucose levels.

Fats

The best source of healthy fats come directly from nature, and raw plant fats are the best aid in helping to promote beauty as they help make the skin glow and the hair thicker. Plant fats contain oils that our body requires for not only our outward appearance but also for digestive health and increased brain function. The foods that contain the most nourishing fats are coconuts, avocados, raw seeds, raw soaked nuts, durian fruit, cacao (raw chocolate), and olives. You can find cold-pressed oils such as hemp seed oil, avocodo oil, extra virgin olive oil, algae oil, and flax seed oil which make excellent salad dressings as opposed to cooked or processed oils.

Good quality fats in our diet are mandatory for health, brain development, and long life. Fatty tissue in the brain act as insulation for nerve cells called the myelin sheath. If this sheath is damaged or removed we develop neurological disorders, reducing our ability to think clearly. The brain is made up of more than 60% fat according to *Dr. Udo Erasmus*, author of **Fats that Heal, Fats that Kill**. The body uses good fats to act as a shock absorber for our organs, tissues, glands, and all of our cells. Raw plant fats also act as a much more sustainable source of energy than just simple carbohydrates alone. Fats slow down the release of sugar into the body so combining a piece of fruit and a fat source such as an avocado, coconut or durian fruit would work synergistically, allowing you to have extended periods of energy. Many vitamins are primarily fat-soluble, meaning they require quality fats in order to be digested, and absorbed into the body. These vitamins are A, D, E, and K.

The brain is being run primarily on electrical impulses from proteins (peptides), electrolytes (potassium, sodium, magnesium, calcium), glucose, and water. The fatty insulation surrounding the nerves is crucial for helping direct the electrical currents to where they need to go.

Saturated Fats, Monounsaturated Fats, & Polyunsaturated Fats:

There are different ways in which fatty acid formations(hydrogen atoms bonded with carbon atoms and glycerol) express themselves. A **saturated fat** is when these carbon atoms are saturated in hydrogen. Saturated fat has been a source of scrutiny for some time but, like all forms of fuel (food), it depends on the form in which it is ingested. Consuming raw sources of saturated fat has numerous health benefits that aid in the fine tuning and lubrication of the body. According to the research it has been shown to help the liver alleviate fatty deposits that store toxic compounds. Most of the body's toxins are built up in excess fat storage. This is also why the saying "eat more fat in order to lose fat" is true. Saturated fats can also have positive effects on respiratory and lung functions. The air spaces of the lungs are thinly coated with a layer of *surfactant,* and the fat content of this material is 100% saturated fat. Many people are warned to stay away from saturated fats and, because of this, they tend to replace it with vegetable oils or trans-fats which provide no benefit from the raw materials they actually need. Babies that are withheld from their mothers breast milk may suffer from premature physical problems and an underdeveloped brain since approximately 40% of mothers natural milk is saturated fat. The best source of saturated fat is going to come from coconuts and coconut products and organic butters such as raw organic dairy and cacao butter.

By definition, an unsaturated fat is a fatty acid that contains at least one double bond (carbon atoms) within the fat chain. A **monounsaturated(MUF)** fat has one double bond, a **polyunsaturated(PUF)** fat has two double bonds or more. The difference between the unsaturated fats and fully saturated fats is that hydrogen atoms are burned in order to create energy when double bonds exist within the fatty acid chain. The cells require hydrogen to create energy or else oxidation occurs. The large consumption of fats (especially PUF) in cooked form, especially cooking oils, could explain why so many people are focused on antioxidants which is really actually an attempt to replenish damaged cells that are not being effectively hydrated.

MUF can help lower bad cholesterol levels and increase the good cholesterol(LDL). Walnuts, almonds, pistachios, avocados, and olives are high in MUF. PUF are extremely beneficial only in their raw untampered form. If heated, exposed to light, or processed PUF have the greatest risk of going rancid, becoming very detrimental to health. The omega fatty acid family comes from polyunsaturated fats which I explain below. The foods highest in PUF's are walnuts, sunflower seeds, sesame seeds, unsalted peanuts contain PUF's. I always recommend raw jungle peanuts over conventional peanuts due to the aflatoxins and mold contamination of conventional peanuts on the market.

Cooked, Rancid, and Trans Fats

The difference between cooked fats and raw plant fats is very steep, causing much confusion among those looking to increase their health. Many believe that fats will make them fat. This is only true in relation to cooked fats or an overconsumption of unsprouted nuts depending on your metabolism. As we know, when you cook something it alters the molecular structure of the food. When we deal with food such as **animal fats**, **rancid fats** from oils, and **trans fats**, this is specifically where people run into problems. Whenever an *unsaturated fat* is introduced to heat it converts into a trans fat (Elaidic Acid), which results in becoming partial hydrogenated (hydrogen) instead of a complete hydrogen bond being created, completing a *saturated fat.* In the case of cooking unsaturated fat or trans fat, it can create a chemical response due to it not normally occurring in nature. The body does not know how to break it down into adequate nutrition. Trans fats have been linked to an increase in blood cholesterol while lowering the good cholesterol(HDL) that helps form hormones. This increases the risk of certain heart diseases, which is the leading cause of death among men and women. The foods that contain trans fats are mostly crackers, cookies, cakes, pastries, fried foods, doughnuts, french fries, and margarine. Food labels that claim to have no trans fat can be misleading and still contain traces. This is why a food practice high in raw organic and fresh food is ideal because there are no hidden surprises.

All oils should be stored in a dark spaces, away from frequent exposures to light like the sun or artificial florescent lighting. All oils should be kept at low temperatures and inside a dark ambler glass jar to avoid oxidation. Oils can become rancid very fast from being oxidized from light, high temperatures (heat or cooking), and oxygen.

(Recommended Book: Fats that Heal, Fats that Kill, Udo Urasmus)

Avocados:

One of the main things I suggest people do is to start eating avocados when coming off a conventional diet high in cooked and animal foods. These foods are very important in the sun food lifestyle as a transitionary food or a staple in the long term. Avocados make transitioning into raw foods much easier because they are a soft fatty fruit which provides excellent calories without the heaviness of cooked foods.

Avocados are likely the favorite food of most raw foodists worldwide. Everyone I have talked to has had a deep relationship with this fruit at some point in their journey, including myself. Some plant foods can come into one's life and leave for a short time, only to reconnect further down the road, making the bond even stronger than before. For me, avocados is such a food. I believe this special fruit has the power to open one up to the world of raw plant foods by acting as a replacement for the dense meat and standard cheese products many have become addicted to and are struggling with. Raw plants alone, such as a salad, are not always enough for many people, especially when transitioning. Adding 1 or 2 ripe avocados can be the best strategy in completely changing the eating experience.

The smooth soft texture and important oils make this a great brain food. Around 75% of the avocado is mostly monounsaturated fats! This fruit is very high in many B vitamins and has a great deal of potassium, far exceeding the traditional banana. High consumption of avocados has been shown to dramatically lower blood cholesterol levels. This is also an obvious result of lowering meat consumption plus adding in superior nutrition such as the famed avocado!

Olives:

The long standing ancient fruit has been mentioned all throughout history. The Athenians claimed the olive has its origins in Athens. Greek mythology talks about Athena winning patronship of Athens from Poseidon, the god of the sea, with the gift of olives. Another legend of Athens states when the Persians burnt down the city and the olive trees were destroyed. On the very day they burnt down they grew back to the height of two cubits. The Quran mentions olives multiple times in interesting ways, quoting the Prophet Muhammed, "Take oil of olive and massage with it- it is a blessed tree". The famous Greek physician Hippocrates is said to have recommended olive oil to heal health aversions such as ulcers and muscle cramping.

The olive truly is a special fruit bearing its mysteries of health, vigor, glow, and longevity to all who embrace it.

The olive leaves and the oil that is pressed from it has been linked to a long healthy life by nearly all the centurions who I have personally studied and met. Those later in their years with the energy of their youth usually lower their consumption in total calories and focus on a few staples. Such staples are olives and olive oil more than anything else that seem to come up. This is a fruit extremely high in minerals such as calcium, iron, magnesium, zinc, copper, potassium, and selenium. Like the avocado, it is high in B vitamins along with vitamin A (beta-carotene), vitamin E(alpha-tocopherol) and K. Olives are made up of important fats called oleic acid or omega-9 fatty acids, a monounsaturated fat. This plays an important role in cellular health, adding an extra buffer to the cell wall. This helps shield the mitochondria and DNA within our cells from oxidation along with the reinforced antioxidants olives contain.

Using cold-pressed extra virgin olive oil in a dark amber glass is the only way I suggest due to the light sensitivity of all unsaturated oils. Cooking degrades all oils and is advised to use as minimally as possible if cooking is still in the equation. Instead of cooking with it try using the oil as a organic salad dressing. You should be considerate of how you combine fats. Refrain from too much avocado or nuts if you consume a lot of olives and olive oil. Play with different raw plant fats and rotate them so your body can get used to it and filter them easier. Luckily, with raw plants, even if you over consume them or combine them inappropriately you will not suffer the consequences of deep fatigue that cooked or fried foods can impose.

I personally prefer to eat Peruvian sun-dried olives because most others in jars are pasteurized and soaked in unnatural compounds (ferrous gluconate) to darken them or preserve them longer. Naturally ripened olives are perishable so it is advised to seek out black olives that are water-cured in a salt solution and/or sun-dried.

Durian:

Perhaps one of the most outrageous and addicting food experiences a sun food enthusiast can indulge in is the durian fruit. One would hardly suspect durian was a food at all from its appearance as the outer layering is covered in a tough protective spiked husk. Underneath is a soft bulb shaped fruit with a custard-like consistency. This is truly the dessert nature had always intended. The durian can give off a foul odor that can become abrasive or even offensive to some if they are not accustomed to it. I did an event called the Raw Chocolate and Durian Festival in California where I was approached by many concerned people asking if there was a gas leak in the building. After investigating the situation for almost an hour, I found out the strong smell was lingering from a durian that was cut wide open and placed on the stage. To the untrained nose, this fruit can reject even the strongest individual. To a seasoned sun food superhero, this is the most enticing of smells. I have actually noticed after surrendering to this pungent odor the smell has seemed to weaken or in some instances go away all together.

Durian is known by some as the king of all fruits. It is unlike any fruit in the entire world for its fat and protein content. Durian is highly concentrated in the **serotonergic**(serotonin pre-cursor) amino acid Tryptophan. Many natives in countries where durian is widely available say when one consumes too much of this fruit it can cause euphoric or even intoxicating behavior. This can be likely caused by the tryptophan. Durian not only is a great source of protein and a good source of raw fats but also contains a large amount of carbohydrates as well. This fruit has a high amount of dietary fiber, which makes this a great laxative and digestive aid(I know this from experience!). In its raw state it contains a good quantity of vitamin C, most B vitamins and essential minerals such as potassium, manganese, copper, magnesium, and iron.

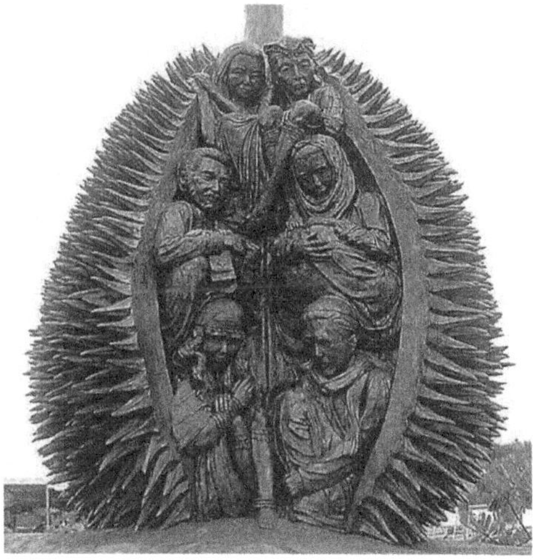

As we currently know, Durian has been consumed for at least 600 years but most likely much longer. The king of all fruits is native to Indonesia, and Malaysia but is now highly popular in the Philippines, Bali, and most frequently cultivated in Thailand. Anyone can purchase frozen durian in its original shell at most traditional asian grocery markets in your local area. When you have your first durian fruit use a butcher knife edge to cut in the middle, similar to how you may cut a coconut. Take a moment before you dive in to calm your mind and spirit knowing this is truly a rare experience most people you come in contact with will never experience (unless of course you share it with them).

Coconuts:

One of the most important foods in the world without a doubt must be the coconut. This is a food that not only tastes amazing, can hydrate and replenish someone living in the hottest climates, but can also literally save someone's life in critical care. Coconut is a fan favorite among raw food advocates and all other foodies alike. The oily meat is so nutritious that it is widely used for skin care and cosmetics for providing excellent benefits. The water of the coconut is a gift from the heavens itself, containing the most plentiful amount of electrolytes (electrically conductive free ions-"minerals") which is balanced by proteins, fiber, and vitamins. One could survive in tropical climates where coconuts are native for extended periods time from this one food and I strongly believe many cultures that coveted the coconut actual did resort of this.

In the Philippines, the coconut tree is often referred to as the "tree of life". It is known as "The tree that supplies all that is known to live" in Sanskrit. In Sri Lanka history there is a poem called The Mahavamsa dating back to 589 A.D. which gives early mention of the first planting of coconuts. Interestingly enough, there is a Coconut Research Institute of Sri Lanka who's mission and vision is to generate technologies to create knowledge and limit the challenges in the coconut industry in order to increase sustainability of this food source.

Coconut water is truly amazing in its health preserving and anti-aging qualities. The trace minerals in coconut water are bound by free ions of electrolytes aiding our nervous system, thus making this an ionic mineral source. This means these minerals are much more conductive in our body than ordinary food sources and definitely most mineral supplements. The water is almost identical to that of human blood plasma, which is said to consist of 55% of our blood. The other 45% of our blood is hemoglobin which can come from chlorophyll. In wartime, specifically the Vietnam War, they would use the coconut's water as a blood plasma substitute, gathering coconuts up in preparation for a big battle. In developing countries there has been many cases where they have used coconut water as an intravenous hydration fluid.

The above information could be a great indication on why many cultures such as Polynesians, Hawaiians, and Filipinos have excellent health and skin eventhough they eat many fried and fatty foods in their diets. The blood is literally being replenished, providing hydration to the cells which transfers over to all parts of the body. What an outstanding food!

Along with a great source of important saturated fat coconuts also contain Medium Chained Fatty Acids which are fatty acids inside Medium-Chain Triglycerides(MCTs). This form of saturated fat requires much less effort to digest and uses less enzymes than saturated fats coming from cholesterol-soaked meat products. Coconut oil is comprised of around 60-66% MCTs, making it highly absorbable and easy to store in the body for usable and easily accessible energy reserves.

MCFA's help promote weight loss by metabolizing in the body completely different than the LCFA(Long Chain Fatty Acids) in animal foods. LCFA's take a much longer time to process in the gastrointestinal tract (GI Track), requiring powerful enzymatic support along with salts from the bile to break them down and use as nutrients for the body. This has been correlated with excessive body fat production over time, and most directly related to the overconsumption of cooked/oxidized unsaturated fatty acids.

Dr. Ray Peat who has been a champion for the benefits of coconut products explains that farmers tried using cheap coconut oil to fatten their pigs in the 1940's. The farmers were looking to fatten up the animals to increase their weight for greater profits. Opposite of intentions, the farmers ended up with lean, more active, and hungrier pigs. This resulted in the use of corn and soy to slow down the thyroid of the animals and cause them to gain excessive weight instead. Coconut products seem to be hormonal precursors, activating hormone production such as the thyroid gland hormone that controls how quickly the body uses energy, creates proteins, moderates metabolism, and assists in the regulation of all other hormones. The thyroid is considered the shield gland of the body existing in the neck, protecting us from physical dis-ease. If the shield is deactivated or suppressed we begin to experience health issues such as potential weight gain. In the case where someone may have hyperthyroidism(extremely increased activity) or hypothyroidism (extremely decreased activity), coconuts and coconut oil may be the best thing to jump start the healing process.

(Recommended books: The Coconut Miracle, Bruce Fife)

Omega Fatty Acids

There has been a lot of discussion about omega fatty acids and how important they are to the development of overall health. There are 3 categories to be aware of: Omega-3, Omega-6, and Omega-9, all of which have their role to play for abundant health. The sources in which we get our omega fatty acids has been widely debated and many of the non-vegetarian proponents believe you must consume fish oils in order to get the best form of omega-3's. According to Dr. Udo Erasmus, that is not completely accurate as he has stated *"Whats interesting is that fish don't actually make fish oils, the oils are made from the food they are consuming which are algaes from deep in the sea"*. This is important for everyone to know because if one is purchasing a conventional fish(farmed fish) that is raised by humans in order to get their omega fatty acids they will be at much greater risk of becoming deficient since fish are incapable of producing the oils themselves. The massive charge by fishing operations claiming fish oil is a requirement to health in many cases could be linked to the idea that most of the fish could be completely fished out of the ocean by 2040 if the same trends continue, which it most likely will.

It is important to pay special attention to the amount of omega-3's in relation to the omega-6 fatty acids we are consuming on a regular basis. A problem many raw foodists (and everyone else) can run into is the overconsumption of nuts, seeds, and also avocados because these are all dominantly omega-6 containing foods. Inflammation is an issue that arises commonly from such a practice because omega-6 fats are inflammatory by nature. The ideal ratio of omega-3 to omega-6 is 2:1 while most people consume a 20:1 ratio of omega-6 to omega-3's, completely the opposite of an ideal situation. Most people are consuming heavy amounts of omega-6 fatty acids from animal fats, cooked and rancid cooking oils, and trans fats from fried foods. Omega-3 and Omega-6 fats both share the same pathway into the body so we end up crowding out the one fat or the other when consuming too much of either, resulting in potential deficiencies.

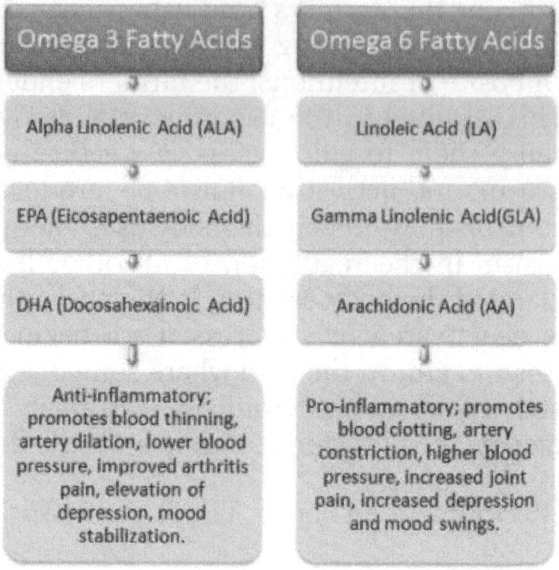

The discovery of omega-3 fatty acids came in the 1970's when researchers studied the Greenland Inuit people inhabiting the Arctic regions of Canada, Denmark, Russia, and Alaska. They noticed that these people consumed a large amount of fat, primarily from seafood, and rarely had any cardiovascular disease. This is important information because many believe a high-fat diet is harmful. In reality, a high-fat diet may be the best source of fuel for brain power, muscle building, and long term energy of all macronutrient sources when consumed in the correct raw form.

The short chain essential fatty acids LA (linolenic acid) and ALA (alpha-linolenic acid) in plant foods such as flax seed, chia seeds, and hemp seeds may convert into long-chain omega 3 fatty acids when a body is clean and contains a good amount of magnesium, zinc, vitamin B6. B3, and vitamin C according to Dr. Erasmus's research. When we combine these forms of omega-3 with coconut oil we increase the rate of conversion into its destination forms. Beyond just having good genetics, our lifestyle is the determining factor in our omega-3 conversion within the body. This conversion could be up to 5% whereas it can be much greater in women due to the demands of pregnancy. Studies have shown and confirmed that the conversion rate is dramatically slowed down based on standardized food consumption.

The long chain fatty acids at the other end of the conversion are EPA (Eicosapentaenoic acid) and DHA (Docosahexaenoic acid). EPA is specific to the brain, having positive effects on depression symptoms and those with suicidal behavior. EPA is the precursor for DHA. DHA is key for our eye health, sperm production, and a major portion of our brain function. Without enough DHA in the body we can fall into nervous system problems and has been linked to Alzhiemer's disease. DHA constitutes at least 40% of polyunsaturated fat content in the brain and 60% in the retina of the eyes according to the research. At least half of our neurons cell membrane is strictly DHA.

The concentration of DHA in a healthy mothers breast milk has been stated to be anywhere from 0.07% to more than 1.0% of total essential fatty acid content. This is more evidence that the choice to skip breast feeding is a very dangerous choice for the wellbeing of a newborn. If a woman is pregnant or wanting to become pregnant, she should look into taking supplemental DHA from a high quality algae source such as Marine Phytoplankton(See Section: **Super Foods**) which contains significant levels of EPA. Dr. *Gabrielle Cousens* has also stated that Blue Green Alga(E3 Live) and algae oils contains significant amounts of the long-chain fatty acid EPA. According to Dr. Cousens, studies show when you take E3 Live your DHA levels do improve.

There is an ongoing discussion whether vegans or vegetarians can get adequate amounts of the required DHA they need to be in complete balance. I am not qualified (nor is anyone else) to tell you that you should stay away from all animal products; only you are. Therefore if you feel the need to add in an animal source I suggest looking into Krill Oil or the highest grade Fish oil you can find to mitigate the potential of toxic exposure. If you do use these products they should be done in a periodic fashion as to provide the nourishment needed without getting into over usage as we would strive to remove ourselves from as much negative karmic behavior as possible (if this concept pertains to your individual philosophy).

Dr. Udo Urasmus has been quoted as saying *"Those needing DHA the least are Vegans who are on raw diets because they are going fresh, whole, raw, and organic. They are closest in line with nature and our life made a genetic program to only live in line with nature, not live out of line with nature.*

Protein

The word protein is broken down in greek terms as pro-tee-un or proteios which means "primary". This is important to understand when identifying protein sources. Plant foods contain "primary-protein", animal foods contain secondary protein which is non-essential and by definition inferior.

Protein in the field of nutrition is probably the most misunderstood and misinformed topic being debated over all others. In the sports and fitness world it would always be stated by coaches and trainers that you must have animal protein to build muscle and repair torn tissue fibers. The issue is so forced upon athletes and those interested in health that the supplement companies are constantly coming out with new products such as whey protein, soy protein, and isolated amino acids to flood the shelves. The vast array of those products are coming from contaminated sources, are completely artificial, and have absolutely nothing to do with health. Whole live foods contain not only the most recognizable forms of protein for the body but organic and properly grown plants also have the highest quality amino acid profiles that can be digested and used as building blocks so that our body is not overly stressed by having to break down food for over extended periods of time.

I always find it fascinating how the strongest and longest living animals in nature seem to be herbivores. Gorillas are a popular example, being enormously strong, fast, and powerful while getting the majority of their sustenance from plants. Elephants are the largest mammals on earth. They spend most of their time eating which they require 330-375 pounds of food on a daily basis to meet their caloric needs. They their sustenance entirely from grass, leaves, twigs, roots, fruits, flowers, and vegetables- that is amazing!

I have seen in the raw vegan community that a lot of people will recommend nuts as a main source of protein. I have found out from my own experience that vastly over eating nuts that most nuts are actually a fat-dominant food. This is actually why most people binge on nuts while transitioning into a live foods lifestyle. If you soak and sprout nuts the enzyme inhibitors will deactivate and release the viable amino acids. The conception that flesh foods are mostly protein is not entirely accurate either. It turns out that what people are getting in terms of satisfaction from meat is mostly fat, not quality protein. This clearly explains why there is a disconnect in terms of what protein is and where the best sources come from.

Protein is essentially a strung together set of amino acids that all have their own individual function. The essential components to an amino acid are hydrogen, carbon, nitrogen, and oxygen. Amino acids are critical to the development of the entire human body and form together to create what we understand as protein. There is said to be 22 amino acids which are standard in the body, 20 of which are locked in our genetic code and 8 of these are what is called "essential amino acids". Essential amino acids are essential because they are not produced naturally by the body, and therefore must taken from food sources. Amino acids all have their own unique properties and roles they play in the body. Just like all nutrients that come from whole foods, amino acids work best in synergy with each other so it is crucial to get the forms which are going to be from raw sources. The essential amino acids that are required to activate the supporting cast are as follows:

- Isoleucine (aids in endurance, tissue and muscle repair, boosting energy levels)
- Leucine (aids in the regulation of blood sugar in the liver)
- Lysine (promotes the immune system, antiviral properties)
- Methionine (sulfur-containing amino acid, potent antioxidant, aids in cell and nerve function)
- Phenyalanine (aids in blood sugar regulation, mood enhancer, tyrosine-neurotransmitter precursor)
- Threonine (aids in complete protein balance, promotes liver, immune system, central nervous system, muscle tissue and collagen(skin) health)
- Tryptophan (mood enhancer, 5-HTP-serotonin precursor, mental relaxant)
- Valine (enhances energy, mental focus, central nervous system, helps supply muscle tissue with glucose storage, preventing muscle breakdown)

Protein is essential for the complete formation and performance of the human body. Approximately 70% of the body's dry matter weight consists of proteins. Everything is being influenced by the quality of protein and how absorbable it is. We need protein for building muscle and tissue formation and for proper brain cognition. Protein helps make minerals activate more efficiently, producing balanced hormones. We cannot disregard the need for quality proteins. The popular vegetarian theme that says we do not need all the amino acids to thrive is not accurate and can lead to further deficiencies. It can get you by for a short period of time but, after a while, the depletion of essential amino acids and your own personal protein needs will contribute in deficiencies such as physical break downs, mental and mood imbalances, hormonal disorders, and other possible issues that can arise.

What's interesting is that I believe the reason many vegetarians/vegans have defended their position that protein is overrated is strongly based on the push by the carnivorous sectors of the health community stating how critical animal protein is for human development, and claims that vegetarians will end up protein deficient. They point to the fact that many people, including athletes lose body weight and become skinnier on a meatless diet. Protein deficiencies do not always show up as muscular or endurance weakness's- they generally show up as neurological imbalances. Protein deficiency is the long standing myth surrounding the vegetarian centered lifestyle which turns out to be false in terms of athletics. Vegetarians are becoming noticeable superior in their athletic performance. Record breaking vegan and raw food athletes are emerging all across the podiums, spanning through all professional sports and olympic circuits. (See Section: **Peak Performance, Athletic Performance**)

Hemp Seeds:

It is beyond most peoples imagination that one single seed can produce so many innovations of the future while being one of the best sources of nutrition for the human body. The hemp plant has received a lot of bad press due to smear tactics in the early 1900's, leading to the government-enforced ban on the plant, claiming it was a drug all the while ignoring the legalization of life-damaging substances such as coffee, liquor, and pharmaceuticals (all proven to have dangerous side effects). The word hemp is often confused with its more commonly known associate, marijuana, which both are classified as *Cannabis Sativa*, and are derived from the same genus. The hemp plant contains extremely low amounts of THC(tetrahydrocannabinol), the psychoactive compound in the marijuana plant. It would take unreasonable quantities of ingesting hemp to feel any effects but the powers that be have withheld the importance of this plant from the public. Now so much information has surfaced that it has become widely available for all to benefit from it.

The health benefits of this food are so tremendous. It is a complete protein source that has the potential to aid in nutritional needs worldwide. The main source of protein people are turning to are from cooked, denatured, hormonally altered, and ultimately unsustainable formations of animal byproducts that hinder not only our health, but our karmic connection to the earth. Hemp seeds contain perhaps the perfect ratio of amino acids in the form of globular edestin and albumin. Of the total protein profile in hemp seeds, 65% is globulin and 35% is albumin. Edestin is the protein closest to our blood plasma which is albumin. Hemp seeds are most likely the closest protein source to the human biology and therefore should be an abundant percentage of our nutrition strategy. Globulin, like albumin, is a part of our natural blood plasma, performing many catalytic functions involving hormones, enzymes, antibodies, hemoglobin, and fibrogin which are all constructed out of the protein Edestin. Globular proteinsm, such as edestin, are major carriers of information in the body to travel through the blood stream, initiating various chemical-reactions such as neurotransmitters in the brain and white blood cells(immune system). Hemp seeds also contains the essential fatty acid ALA and sulfur-bearing amino acids that decrease inflammation in the body.

"Hemp seeds contain all the essential amino acids and essential fatty acids necessary to maintain healthy human life. No other single plant source has the essential amino acids in such an easily digestible form, or has the essential fatty acids in as perfect a ratio to meet human nutritional needs".

David Wolfe, Super Foods

Chia Seeds:

Salvia Hispanica, otherwise known as Chia, has been a staple in the Meso-American diet dating as far back as the Aztec civilization. Cacao and chia were their main sources of nutrition. Just as they used cacao beans as a form of currency they would do the same with chia seeds because it was such a prized food. The Aztec warriors and runners are said to have completely sustained themselves through a full day on as little as a tablespoon of chia seeds. This food was so important to the Aztec culture that when the Spaniards conquered the land, they completely banned chia from cultivation to strip the people of their sustenance and identity. In *Christopher McDougal's i*nspiring book, **Born to Run**, he brings to light that one of the greatest long distance runners (barefoot runners) alive were an indigenous tribe in Northern Mexico who's main source of food was derived from chia seeds.

Chia seeds are not only a great source of omega-3 fatty acids, but also important minerals such as phosphorus, calcium, manganese, copper, zinc, and iron. They are also a complete protein source. In the plant world, foods with a full spectrum of amino acids are not as rare as people may think but certain foods do get special mention based on their own unique properties and characteristics they contain. For athletes, chia seeds are a perfect source of long sustaining fuel and bioavailable protein, especially for endurance sports. When chia seeds are soaked in water they become gelatinized, allowing them to absorb the water content and the seeds to expand. The seed's ability to absorb water makes for a perfect hydration tool while running, playing basketball, cycling, swimming, or any other high-intensity activity. I have done many tests on myself to see how hard I could push myself with the least amount of food or even water needed to perform optimally. I have seen that my water and food requirements are greatly lowered as I exercise when I consume gelatinized chia seeds and goji berries earlier in the day. I once rode my bike 20 miles on a hot summer day(101 degrees), most of which was at high intensity and I felt no ill effects as I did not eat or drink anything for hours during or after. I do not recommend anyone do that without years of prior athletic experience but I do suspect that the ancient people would use chia seeds in a drink to sustain their daily activity with little to no other nourishment in times of lack.

Enzymes

The discovery of enzymes may, in fact, be the most important finding in human nutrition. It represents the prime difference between cooked food and raw food.

Enzymes are of the utmost importance to the basic function of the human body and overall longevity. When we are born, we are given a deposit of enzymatic value that is stored in our enzyme bank account. Throughout the time of our lives we are spending these enzymes as we conduct our lives, much like the way we spend money. If we have the live-fast-die-young mentality then that is exactly what we can expect. If we are more conservative, taking our time, and heeding more caution, then we can more efficiently make use of this limited storage. It may seem like you have a lot at first If you have a million dollars in your bank account, but if you spend each day without ever putting anything back in you will eventually become depleted. This is exactly what most people do with their health- the game ends right there when the enzyme load reaches zero.

"Humans eating an enzyme-less diet use up a tremendous amount of their enzyme potential and lavish secretions of the pancreas and other digestive organs. The result is a shortened lifespan of sixty-five years or less as compared to 100 or more years. Also resulting will be illness and a lowered resistance to stresses of all types both physiological and environmental."

Dr. Edward Howell, Enzyme Nutrition

Enzymes are considered catalysts in the body that allow the activity of all other functions to take place. In many ways, your enzymes are like the workforce which uses the raw building materials you have for their appropriate use. If you have the right tools but no workers then the tools are still inefficient on their own. The tools in this case are vitamins, minerals, and other nutrients that the body must disperse where needed. Enzymes help break down nutrients such as proteins into amino acids, carbohydrates in their respective forms of sugars and starches, and fats into absorbable fatty acids. Lactose in dairy cannot be broken down properly without the enzymatic aid that is lost through the heating process of pasteurization. This is why raw organic dairy is always a far better choice then conventional dairy.

The importance of raw organic living foods is found in their ability to partially break down in the body on their own. Enzymes are being utilized and manufactured in different areas of the body such as the pancreas, brain, heart, kidneys, muscles, and lungs. Whenever we eat cooked or denatured food that has been stripped of its own enzyme account it forces our body to compete for enzyme availability. When the digestive track requires this kind of assistance to break down food matter it handicaps other bodily functions and reduces the limited enzyme account you began with. According to *Dr. Edward Howell*, who has been considered the lead authority worldwide in enzyme research, the depletion of enzymes in the body leads to premature aging and age-related afflictions such as various cancers, heart disease, diabetes, and other chronic conditions. In the alternative healing field, researchers are finding the use of pancreatic enzymes, such as trypsin, to be very effective for dissolving blood clots and can be used for breaking down the active protein casein found in cow's milk, a known contributor to cardiovascular disease.

There are three distinct categories of enzymes to be aware of: metabolic enzymes, digestive enzymes, and food enzymes. Metabolic enzymes are the main factors that work behind the scenes to initiate all major functions within the human body. According the Dr. Edward Howell, our organs, tissues, and cells are run specifically by our metabolic enzyme cascade and the depletion of these enzymes, in particular, is the root cause of every major dysfunction within the health of mankind. Digestive enzymes are activated by the alimentary organs to help digest carbohydrates, fats, and proteins. Food enzymes are encapsulated within all raw and living foods that are either eaten from the ground or prepared/dehydrated in most cases under 118 degrees Fahrenheit(47.8 degrees Celsius). According to the research, generally, when food is cooked between the temperatures of 120-170 fahrenheit, indispensable nutrients and enzymes are lost.

Cooked and processed foods are void of food enzymes which, over time, will influence digestive disturbances, leading to the depletion of our valuable metabolic enzyme storages. To put this fact into perspective, it has been calculated that it takes exactly 12 metabolic enzymes to create one digestive enzyme in order to break down foods that do not contain their own inherit enzyme. This is exactly why when most people following a standard western diet reach 50 years old they are "over the hill"- the body begins to break down, debilitation sets in, and we lose all sense of our digestion due to increased constipation, and lack of daily bowel movements. This is easily turned around and does not have to be the reality for you if you do not want it to be; there is a better way.

In the ground breaking documentary, **Simply Raw: Reversing Diabetes in 30 days**, the lives of six diabetic patients were chronicled and placed under the care of world-renowned raw food and holistic physician Dr. *Gabrielle Cousens* who runs the Tree of Life Rejuvenation Center(See Chapter: **Symptoms of Society, Diabetes**). They were all restricted from eating cooked foods and animal products of all kinds while introduced to a living food cuisines. Within only 2 weeks, everyone that stayed on the program dropped their insulin in half or completely dropped off of insulin. This example leads me to believe that Dr. Howells perspective on the importance of living food enzymes must be greatly considered.

Many nutrition and health researchers suggest that enzymes are burnt up by stomach acids, thus dispelling the validity of a raw food approach due to it's high enzyme cascade. This is an inaccurate suggestion as it appears these protein molecules cannot be broken down by hydrochloric acid. It is known in the science of raw food nutrition that digestive enzymes survive in our intestines, where they can be effectively absorbed into our bodily tissues, aiding in the break down of old food residues left over from a primarily cooked and animal-based diet.

I would like to quote Dr. Edward Howell in an interview he participated in responding to the claim that all enzymes are destroyed once they hit the stomach:

"When you eat food, acid secretion is minimal for at least thirty minutes. As the food goes down the esophagus, it drops into the top portion of the stomach. This is called the cardiac section, since it's closer to the heart.

The rest of the stomach remains flat and closed while the cardiac section opens up to accommodate the food. During the time the food sits in the upper section, little acid or enzymes are secreted by the body. The enzymes in the food itself go about digesting the food. The more of this self-digestion that occurs, the less work the body has to do later.

When this 30 to 45 minute period is over, the bottom section of the stomach opens up and the body starts secreting acid and enzymes. Even at this point, the food enzymes are not inactivated until the acid level becomes prohibitive. You see, food enzymes can tolerate chemical environments many times more acid than neutral."

Just eating raw foods for most people is not entirely sufficient for re-populating the body's enzyme availability since the vast consumption of cooked and processed foods have greatly hindered this function. Enzyme supplements are a great addition to the equation. They must be plant based, containing the basic enzymes for complete digestive assistance such as protease (protein), lipase (fats), amylase (carbs, sugars, starches), bromelain (from pineapples- break down protein), and papain (from papaya juice- also aids in protein break down). HCL(hydrochloric acid) can be a very effective as a supplement if your HCL levels are too low, sometimes a result of too much alkalinity in the diet without sufficient acids in the stomach. Citrus fruits such as lemon, limes, oranges, and grapefruits can be very effective for this, especially when pressed for a concentrated juice you make yourself.

Possibly the most important reason for live foods and enzyme supplementation is the fact that the transmutation of minerals from one form to another is made possible through liver enzymes. As we age the severe break down of our physical functions and mental acuity may be linked to this fact. For instance, the over abundance of calcium formations in the body causes the aging process to be accelerated.(See Chapter: **The Scientific Method: Calcification**)

It is also important to know that most seeds and nuts contain what is called enzyme inhibitors known as phytic acid(phytates). These inhibitors are locked inside the seed to protect it from prematurely sprouting and dying. Seeds and nuts require sufficient moisture to properly sprout in a way that you are able to receive the nourishment from it. You can soak nuts or seeds in a bowl of fresh spring or filtered water overnight and use it the next day. Cooking can also be used to ward off enzyme inhibitors but, consequently, it also destroys the enzymes so therefore this is never a preferable route. All food, in one way or another, contain inside of them a toxic component that is only offset by the sufficient synthesis of enzymes. Wheatgrass, for example, contains high amount of cyanic acid or cyanide which is known as a poison but healthy cells contain an enzyme known as beta-aromatase neutralizes this toxin and allows it to pass through the urine.

There is a vast amount of information on enzymes in the form of books, online videos, and research studies that continue to evolve. It is my belief that this subject will be at the forefront of all health-related conversations among the scientific community of the future as we progress in our nutritional understanding.

(Recommended Book: Enzyme Nutrition: Dr. Edward Howell)

Chlorophyll

The green pigment that is found in all plants and algae's is called chlorophyll. It gives leaves their color and is needed for photosynthesis to occur, a process that allows plants to absorb light from the sun and convert it into a viable energy source. Chlorophyll is almost identical to hemoglobin (human blood) except the central atom in our blood is iron whereas it is magnesium in plants. Chlorophyll is nature's greatest blood cleanser and blood builder. You can tell in plants when their chlorophyll content has decayed. In leaves, for example, the green display is replaced by an orange, red, or brownish color that is from injury or oxidation. When our bodies are lacking in chlorophyll we are much more susceptible to oxidative stress responses(free-radical production) in the body, increasing the aging process.

The color green is synonymous with vitality, energy, and life. It is the color-coded symbol of nature and where there is a flourishing arrangement of this sign there is life force present. Chlorophyll builds the body from the inside out. When the inside is clean then you can assume it is also green. The vibration of green energy in nature is clearly one of peace and ease. Animals that are focused on vegetation have a dominantly alkaline state, exude ease and relaxation whereas the animals that are carnivorous having an acidic state are more defensive and aggressive. Neither is wrong nor right but it is an important distinction that needs to be drawn as it also applies directly to human beings in society.

Green leafy vegetables are important for their alkaline mineral content which promotes balanced blood-sugar, stress reduction, clear thoughts, and muscle relaxation. Many people getting into raw foods will over eat nuts and avocados initially which are heavy foods containing more acid-building minerals such as phosphorous, sulfur, chlorine, etc. Those suffering from anemia can help alleviate this condition with more fresh organically grown green vegetables and herbs. Herbs are highly alkaline and have strong medicinal properties. I enjoy a wide variety of greens and herbs such as parsley, cilantro, watercress, basil, and sometimes dandelion mixed with all the other goodies.

Besides the leafy green vegetables we are more accustomed to in our health food stores or local farmers markets, one of the best sources of chlorophyll is in fresh grass like wheatgrass or wild grasses. Grass is rich in many different compounds such as protein, omega-3 fatty acids and CLA (conjugated linoleic acid). According to *Kim Evans*, author of **Cleaning Up! The Ultimate Body Cleanse**, one key reason many vegans and vegetarians are unable to keep up their lifestyle with no meat or dairy products is because they do not get enough CLA which is found in animal products primarily because the animals are consuming large amounts of grass. Healthy grasses

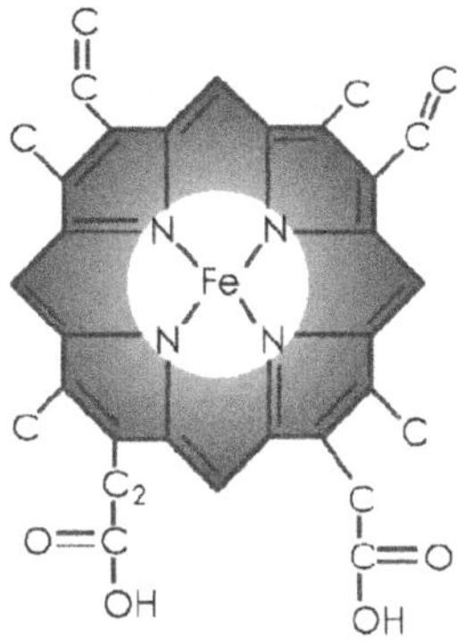

Human Blood Hemoglobin

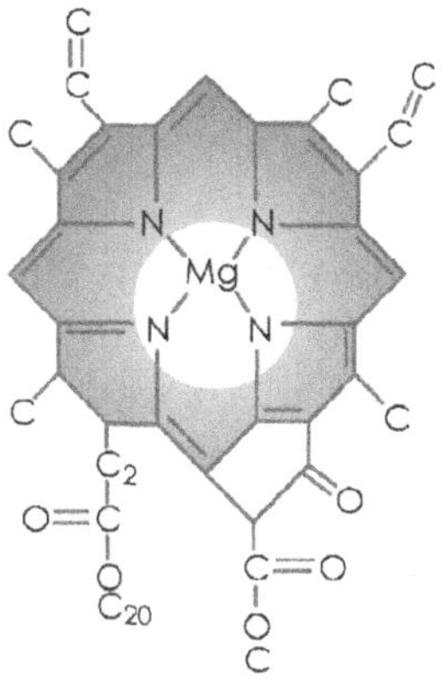

Plant Chlorophyll

that are kept away from outside smog and pollution are one of the best ways to fuel your body, brain, and blood with chlorophyll. It is extremely difficult for the human stomach to break down a hand full of grass like a horse or zebra would. The solution to this is to go to the juicer. If you can incorporate a wild grass juice (or vegetable juice) into your life once a day it will cause profound shifts in your metabolism, clarity of mind, as well as encourage a more enchanted perspective of life.

Wheatgrass juicing has become extremely popular and for great reasons. It is widely available in many health food stores and raw food juice bars. I would encourage anyone to pour down as much wheatgrass juice shots as your palette can handle! You can add wheatgrass shots into your normal green juice as a daily discipline and notice the magic that develops inside your body.

The most basic and simple advice I can give would be to consume as much foods that contain alkaline minerals and high water content. Water is a conductive substance that forms an inner environment, allowing for the stimulation of minerals in our body. If we are lacking adequate water then dehydration sets in, and we actually begin to lose minerals in our body at an accelerated pace. This causes increased fatigue, joint/bone deterioration, skin blemishes, and aging, which is essentially physical oxidation. Chlorophyll is one of natures most potent antioxidants which can be broken down into liquid-oxygen.

The beginning of any dis-ease is the complete lack of oxygen, all relief whether physical, emotional, or spiritual begins through the reintroduction of oxygen.

Chlorella, a green algae usually found in a powder or tablet form, is known to be the highest chlorophyll containing food in the world and is easily mixed into a green juice, super food smoothie, or added into chlorophyll shots. Chlorella can be somewhat of a warming food so you can also substitute it with Spirulina (cooling food high in green pigments) during the summertime. See more information on this algae below on the Section: **Super Foods**.

Flowers

Flowers may be the most under recognized piece of natural nutrition yet they are an indispensable factor in the beautification of the human garden. We admire the unique shapes, arrangements, and colors of these plants in many ways. They can symbolize the feelings of passion and appreciation from a loved one as well as providing intense visual stimulation from one who is tuned into natural magic. One may reach glimpses of bliss or euphoria by inhaling the lingering scent of a mature flower. A lifestyle focused on beauty and attraction would be easily complimented by the inclusion of these subtle yet powerful botanicals.

The term flower power that was heavily announced in the 60's was a notion of peace among all people and living in accordance with mother nature. This was a beautiful concept in speech. However, the problem in those days was the people were eating all the wrong food which ultimately drove this movement into the ground. People were ingesting burgers and soda while being distracted by alcohol and smoking marijuana bushes. Instead of talking about flower power they should have been consuming the flowers. Perhaps then they would have been much more tuned into what nature has been attempting to move towards all this time.

It is not commonly suggested by many to eat a wide variety of flowers like it is to eat vegetables and fruits. The nutrition that we can derive from flowers is unique as these plants are concentrated in minerals, micro-nutrients, vitamins as well as special bioflavonoids(powerful antioxidants). Flowers are the source of one of natures most favored foods, honey. The nectar and pollen of flowers contained within this treasured food is extremely nutritious. The traditional use of flowers for culinary purposes dates back thousands of years in such cultures as the Romans, Chinese, and Greeks, among many others. Flower petals can be added to salads for a simple and colorful dish. Those interested or involved in raw food cuisine can create spectacular entrees, adding a bit of their own brand of "flower power".

Not all flowers are considered edible so I suggest looking into a good reference book on the subject. The use of pesticide and herbicide sprays has reached into much of the botanical wild life so caution is advised. Do not consume flowers in closed quarters such as nurseries, schools, florists, houses, or on the side of the road due to car exhaust. You can look into growing them yourself in your own backyard and/or purchase them at your local health food store.

A brief list of Flowers you can explore:

- Dandelion (Linolenic fatty Acids, anti-bacterial, antioxidant, liver protection, diuretic, pectin- "helps remove toxins & heavy metals", vitamin c, has been used as an anti-tumor alternative as well as an anti-plaque by dental researchers, recommended for menstrual cycle regulation)
- Hibiscus (Vitamin C, Iron, Calcium, Niacin, potent antioxidant, recommended to balance cholesterol levels and lower blood pressure)
- Chamomile (anti-inflammatory, aids in digestion, stress reduction, and nerve repair)

Salt

Salt seems to be the subject of confusion and controversy born out of the inaccurate suggestions to leave it out of one's diet. The conflict stems from the lack of differentiation between iodized table salt which acts as a processed food preservative and the natural life sustaining salt that has aided civilizations throughout world history. The simple fact is that we require salt to function appropriately. The complete absence of natural salts like celtic sea salt or even himalayan salt can lead to drawbacks in ones ability to sustain energy, focus, produce digestive acids, hold onto weight, achieving proper mineralization, and retain water. This category of nutrition must not be overlooked by those who are serious about activating their highest health goals.

The problem many face is that almost all commercially processed foods contain the the wrong kind of salt. These commercial salts are chemically cleaned, stripping it of all the essential minerals and trace elements our body needs. The poor quality salts we want to avoid, such as table salt (white salt), are heavily refined and concentrated forms of sodium chloride which makes salt similar to artificial and refined sugar; it is white poison. In 1924, a preservation agent known as potassium iodide was added to table salt assuming it would help prevent thyroid disorders that are thought to be caused by an iodine deficiency. Dextrose(main ingredient in corn syrup) is used in refined salt to prevent potassium iodine from chemically breaking down into iodine and evaporating away. Other known chemical preservatives and bonding agents in table salt are calcium silicate, ferric ammonium citrate, silicon dioxide, sodium ferrocyanide, magensium silicate, magnesium carbonate, propylene glycol, calcium phosphate among many others. Every single allegation made towards salt is based on the effects of chemically-enriched table salt.

Refined salt is a likely contributor of hypertension, mood disorders, adrenal exhaustion, brain fog, thyroid disorders, and immune system failure. Naturally occurring sea salt, according to Dr. Brownstein, can aid in the reversal of each of these ailments.

Salt resides as a cornerstone for sustaining youthful strength and pursuing longevity. The english word salary is derived from salarium which where wafers of salt that were given to Roman soldiers as part of their wages. It is documented that in medieval Europe salt was used as a popular remedy for chronic headaches. The headache-relieving effects of sodium have been well known in earlier times as well. Sodium helps to regulate blood pressure and pH balance. Dehydration largely has to do with the body's inability to hold onto water. Natural salts help our cells absorb water properly and thus hydrating us at a much more effective rate then filtered water on it's own. Sodium is a physiological requirement for the functionality of our physical faculties. The element potassium, abundant in raw plant foods, works on the "intercellular fluid"(inside the cell), while the sodium works on the "extracellular fluid", creating a necessary balance. According to Dr. A. True Ott, sodium combines with potassium as a chemical pump to move hydrogen and oxygen molecules in and out of the cell, resulting in healthy energy production. Raw foodists generally get plentiful amounts of potassium but can be lacking in sodium if they have left salt alone for too long, resulting in difficulties retaining healthy weight.

The purpose of adding in heavy amounts of salt is misused by most as a way of adding flavor to their food, this is an inaccurate focus of salt, yet works extremely well nonetheless. Salt is the ideal mineral supplement which embodies what is called "the mineral matrix". This is the complete formation of every known and most likely unknown element present in nature. Salt should always be consumed in its natural form, never cooked because cooked salt is completely not absorbable in the body, creating intercellular disturbances we often see plaguing people on high-cooked diets.

Understanding salt's role as a conductor in our bodies is key because salt is not merely of a molecular makeup; it holds electrical charges which respond to the nervous system in the body. Salt holds the frequency of the earth and of the ocean which, in turn, increases our own frequency, allowing us to be more alert, focused, hydrated, and has been shown to reduce muscle cramps when good quality salts were missing from the diet. Salt has been used as a healing therapy for Dysautonomia (autonomic dysfunction) which is a disease affecting the nervous system. Common symptoms of this are regular fatigue, adrenal fatigue, excessive thirst, dizziness or light-headedness, panic attacks or anxiety, hypertension, numbness or nerve pains. A common response is also intense salt cravings, which indicates again that there is a sodium deficiency occurring. The reason many people crave meat is purely because they are feeding on the salt in the blood to help balance their own constitution. Without the juiciness of the blood and salt, a piece of meat would be no more appetizing than a dry piece of rubber.

"Without the elements of potassium and sodium found in salt, we could neither think nor act"
Dr. Barbara Hendel, Peter Ferreira-Water & Salt: The Essence of Life

Electrolytes play a crucial role in our health on numerous levels. Salt contains the ionic mineral elements that make up the electrolytes sodium, potassium, calcium, and magnesium among many others. Electrolytes help the functioning of our entire cellular wall, allowing for all other physiological performances to become possible. Our ability to rehydrate ourselves is greatly dependent on electrolyte replenishment which also helps balance our blood pH levels. Every level of the human experience is being affected by electrolytical influence. This is not to be confused with the kind claimed to be found in popular sports drinks. As a long time athlete, I personally have a bottle of spring water with a dash of salt and feel much more rejuvenated and focused than I did on those inferior substitutes.

When someone is cleansing on a living foods diet, it is generally suggested to get off all salt completely due to the overaccumulation of refined salts in the body. Living foods contains a massive amount of potassium and it floods the body as the salt is absent. Eventually we do want to bring natural salts back in to help balance the two elements.

(Recommended Book: Water & Salt: The Essence of Life: Dr. Barbara Hendel, Peter Ferreira)

Fermented Foods

The traditional practice of fermented foods is an integral part of raw food nutrition. There most likely has never been a point in history where people have needed this more than right now. We are living in a society that is very "anti-bacteria", believing all bacteria is harmful and should be removed from our foods. Fermented foods help assist beneficial bacteria for optimum digestion as well as protection from invasive organisms. The increase in over sanitation with chemicals to somehow shield us has actually contributed to lowering our natural defense mechanisms and opened us up by breaking us down. *Sally Fallon*, author of **Nourishing Traditions**, asks this question in regard to the upheaval of new viruses, intestinal complications, parasites, and frequent health problems:

""Could it be that by abandoning the ancient practice of lacto-fermentation, and insisting on a diet in which everything has been pasteurized, we have compromised the health of our intestinal flora and made ourselves vulnerable to legions of pathogenic microorganisims?" Like the $2.97 gallon jars of dill pickles Vlasic sells at a loss at Walmart, are we undermining our health and even economic well-being by our insistence on "more, faster and cheaper?"

The lacto-fermentation that Sally Fallon refers to in this quote is the process in which lactic acid is increased in raw foods as a preservation method. What this does is not only help food last longer in a raw state but it also increases enzymes and good bacteria which allows the food to strengthen ones digestion, especially if they are having stomach problems. All throughout history, cultures would use salt, water, and different spices to soak in a jar or crock pot over a certain duration. As we can tell from looking back in history, people had much stronger teeth, bones, and digestive power than the general public does now. The most well known examples of common fermented foods are kimchi and sauerkraut, which is basically fermented cabbage sometimes mixed with cucumbers, cauliflower, garlic, salt, and spices.

It has been shown that we have at least two brains in our body. There is one in our head, which seems to govern our lives, but often overlooked is the brain in our stomach called *the edenteric nervous system*. It appears that most of what is being processed in the brain is being signaled from our gut and is immediately transmitted to the other receptors in the body. This gives a completely new understanding to the law of "you are what you eat" since the foods we put into our bodies are literally controlling some of the most important facets of the human experience. This includes our immune system and our neurotransmitter functions such as serotonin and melatonin release. This also explains how food directly influences our emotional state- the energy and information of a certain food is meant to educate our cells to perform certain tasks within the body. *Dr. Michael Gershon*, a lead researcher on the topic, states that "*nearly every substance that helps run and control the brain has turned up in the gut*". Gershon also goes on to saying that "*details of how the edentric nervous system mirrors the central nervous system have been emerging in recent years.*"

"95% of the serotonin in your body is produced and stored in your intestinal tract."

Dr. John Douillard

The reason why the above information is so critical to understand is because when we have a depletion of good bacteria or 'microflora' in our gut and intestinal wall, along with the introduction of antibiotics, refined sugar, excessive sugar consumption, factory farmed meat, and genetically modified foods, we lose our ability to defend against the foreign agents that are introduced. Fermented foods are predigested in the culturing process which will help break down in the body. The addition of healthy bacteria from fermented foods actually work to consume the bad bacteria that is damaging to the central nervous system that we now know is occupied in the stomach.

I was first introduced to the idea and information on probiotics, fermented foods, and bacterial science by *Donna Gates*, who has created one of the most popular dietary protocols focused on this principle called **The Body Ecology Diet.** To dig in deeper on the topic you can look into her book.

Super Foods

This is probably my favorite piece of nutrition to talk about because of the remarkable effects super foods have had in my life. Based on countless research studies, years of history dating back further than any common foods we grew up with, and the extremely unique qualities the foods that belong in this category possess, I personally believe this is the future of food and medicine as a joining of the two integrates pieces of peak performance nutrition.

The term "Super Food" has been used to describe unique foods that exceed the nutritional qualities of more commonplace foods. A super food is a nutritional tool that, in many cases, acts like a supplement but is 100% food. Foods in this unique category are truly special because they create a bridge for people to cross over into raw foods easily. Most food choices act as bulk, merely calories with its active alkaloids(plant medicines) stripped out due to hybridization and extreme processing methods. The reason Americans spend over $100 on supplements each month is because the food they are eating does not contain the minerals, antioxidants, vitamins, alkaloids and adaptogenic qualities they desperately need in this time of extreme pressure and stress.

Super foods can be a huge aid in detoxification for those that are eliminating toxins from the body. Due to the lack of the mineral quality of most dietary regimens people are on, people are suffering from demineralization. This is important to know especially when cleansing because, in many cases, their bodies are relying completely on the fatty content of conventional foods for sustenance. When this sustenance reserve is taken away without its appropriate replacement, the body may sometimes turn on itself for sustaining nourishment.

In the health field, the deep-rooted information in food is rarely talked about or even considered. All food receives its information from the soil it came from and the hands that touched it before it came to you. Excessively cooked foods contain information that is distorted and lost, confusing the body. The immune system is constantly working to decipher the message but, over time, it becomes lost in translation. I never had this insight until I started eating super foods and made it a complete lifestyle. Now I literally am gifted deep insights daily when I least expect it. Super foods are the superior human activation tool that has presented itself in this time of unlimited possibilities. As the research on food gets deeper and analytical data continues to present new information, it seems the potential for growth on all levels continues to expand where the potential for sickness decreases.

The true value of forming a lifestyle centered around super foods, whatever that looks like for you, is that they will help alleviate the obstruction we have caused ourselves in the past from the dietary programs we have been on (or lack thereof). Super foods then begin to allow us to access deeper regions of our genetics which, in turn, allow us to activate increased physical performance, mental acuity, and elevated feelings of euphoria, helping to remove all issues of mood disorders and creating harmony within our golden temple. They also begin to set up a health and vitality account in our centralized banking structure that exists within our own structured lifestyles. We actually can consume foods that will cause us to reap incredible results five to ten years down the line. This is opposite to the regular approach of eating foods that cause us to lose equity in the overall value of our longevity.

(Recommended Book: Super Foods by David Wolfe)

Goji Berries:

The legend surrounding the Goji Berry, otherwise known in the Chinese herbal system as Lycium or Lyceum(latin binomial term dating back to "Plato's school of learning"), is vast and nothing short of intriguing. It has been associated with robustness, vitality, and slowing down the aging process. There are many stories to articulate the healing power of this plant throughout its long history. One of these stories speaks of a water well that was dug near a Buddhist temple sometime during the Tang Dyansty (800 A.D.). This well became surrounded by goji vines which found their way into the water. People would come to this well to pray and drink the water they believed was extremely rejuvenating. There has been a deep link between long healthy life and the regular consumption of this fruit, especially in a tea form similar to how the people in the story consumed it. In the Chinese herbal system, Goji Berry(Lycium) is considered the number #1 tonic herb dating back over 5,000 years in history. The ancient Chinese herbal alchemists considered the goji to be the key herb to introduce someone to their expansive herbal emporium. This food/herb was believed to be the tool that could teach someone about all other herbs in this system. It's the most revered "gateway medicine" ever discovered.

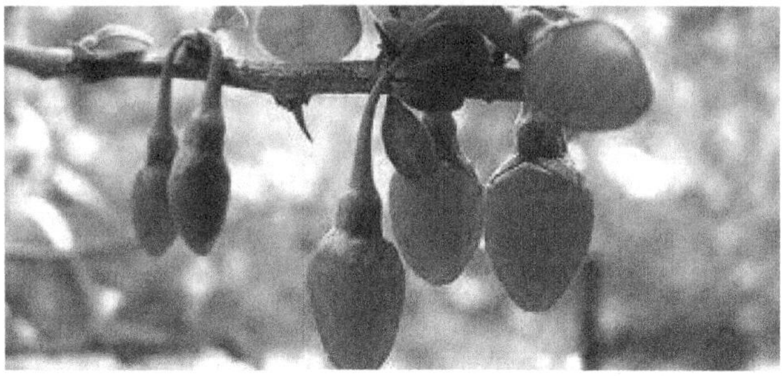

The nutrient properties of this fruit are nothing short of astounding, signifying what a true super food is. It is a complete protein, containing 18 amino acids. The only other fruit in the world that is also a complete protein is the mulberry. This is important because those on conventional diets are lacking in "quality protein". Most children are severely undernourished and are very resistant to most "health food" selections. Goji berries become a great champion in the health world for the simple fact that you can hand a kid a bag of goji and they will eat it- there is no opposition because it tastes good!

Goji berry is known as a great aid in eye health for its wide range of carotenoids such as beta-carotene(strongly colored pigment), zeaxanthin (is inside the eye retina, provides pigments of color), lutein(found in the eye retina, antioxidant), lycopene (antioxidant), cryptoxanthin (stimulates DNA repair of damaged cells), and xanthophyll (oxygenated carotenoids). It has been shown that people consuming a diet rich in carotenoids occurring in natural foods are much healthier and have a far lower rate of chronic illnesses than those who do not. Studies also confirm my own intuitive belief that supplementing with these isolated constituents does not increase the effects simply because they must work synergistically with one another in the way nature intended. This berry can help strengthen the capillaries in the eyes and promote much greater resistance to eye problems many face later as they age, such as cataracts. The theory in the Chinese system of medicine believes that the health of the liver expands the health of the eyes and goji berry is certainly a liver-enhancing food and herbal remedy.

The ancient fruit contains important unsaturated fats including essential fats such as linoleic acid and alpha-linolenic acid. This gives us the brain oils we need for cognitive function and improving cardiovascular health. Goji berries are one of the most mineral-rich fruits on the planet as it contains calcium, potassium, iron, zinc, phosphorous, selenium which help bring balance for many who experience sugar sensitivities where they cannot handle heavy sugar-containing fruits. Goji Berries contain Vitamin B2(Riboflavin), which is essential for metabolizing fats, proteins, and carbohydrates where the goji berry interestingly has a complimentary combination of all these macronutrients.

Something I believe that makes Goji Berries especially important is the polysaccharides they contain. This automatically puts this berry on top of all other fruits that do not contain these long-chain slow-burning essential sugars. These are considered essential to the structural development of the human body for many reason which you can refer back to the section on **Sugar**.

As we accelerate the aging process through non-thought out food selections and environmental pollution exposure, we see a vast decrease in the production of our vital hormones. Goji berries contain a compound known as sesquiterpenoids which help the body produce a central anti-aging hormone which aids in the protection of our longevity. This unique fruit is the only food that has been scientifically verified to actively increase our natural production of human growth hormone (HGH) through a secretion by the pineal and pituitary gland. This may prove to be the most beneficial function of this berry, helping to explain why it has been associated with longevity for thousands of years. HGH is naturally produced by our pituitary gland when we are children to fuel childhood growth, muscle/tissue growth, bone density, and organ function through life. The secretions made by the pituitary gland tend to lessen as we age, especially due to improper lifestyle, which contributes to the break down of our physical and mental faculties.

In the Eastern world, Goji berries have been revered for their ability to help those in their late years to regain sexual virility, decreasing infertility that we are seeing more and more of in current times. In the interesting book, **Adaptogens** by *David Winston* & *Steven Maimes*, Winston and Maimes cite a Chinese study on infertility that was done on 42 men who were having very low sperm counts. These men were given 1/2 ounce of goji berries a day. After two months, thirty three patients had returned to normal levels of fertility and, according this study, all of them were able to father children!

When selecting goji berries be aware that many brands contain pesticides and/or red dye to present a bright red color to the berries. Goji berries have become very popular in the health community. For this reason, many companies have looked to capitalize on this growing trend, cutting corners to supply inferior products. I personally only select Heaven Mountain Goji Berries by Dragon Herbs for consumption. These berries are sun dried and vacuum packed immediately to retain moisture and nutritional quality. If you are dealing with goji berries that are dehydrated then you can soak them in water for a few hours to re-enliven them.

(Recommended Books: Adaptogens: David Winston & Steven Maimes)

Maca:

Maca is the great root vegetable in the radish family that is indigenous to the Andes Mountains of Bolivia and Peru. This plant has a long history as a human food some say dating back as far as 4,000 BC (possibly 1,200 BC) as a fully domesticated crop. Throughout history this plant has been famous for its fertility-enhancement qualities. There are many stories in its lore about those later in their years who have been able to father or mother children when they previously could not due to infertility. The Incan warriors were said to have eaten large amounts of maca root before battles to increase strength and energy. There was a point in its history during great political change that maca was almost made extinct and the knowledge of it was lost until the late 1900's when it resurfaced. Maca has become a subject of great interest due to its legend and chemical composition that make it stand out as a medicine, a super food, and an adaptogenic aid in our modern society.

The harsh stress of an industrial environment has forced us to adapt in unnatural circumstances. The state of our health will naturally shape itself in relation to the most consistent influences of the environment we surround ourselves by. Since we are disconnected from the natural pulsations of the earth we are deficient in electrical-fuel to support our stress defense shield (thyroid), our immune system (white-blood-cells), and our endocrine system. Maca performs in the body like an herb but is consumed as a food that helps us adapt to the stressers of the world physically, mentally, and emotionally. Maca is something everyone needs to know about for the simple fact that this food is known to help regulate hormonal imbalances. There is a tremendous percentage of people who experience hormonal fluctuations coming from poor nutrition coupled with toxins adversely affecting biological homeostasis(balance point).

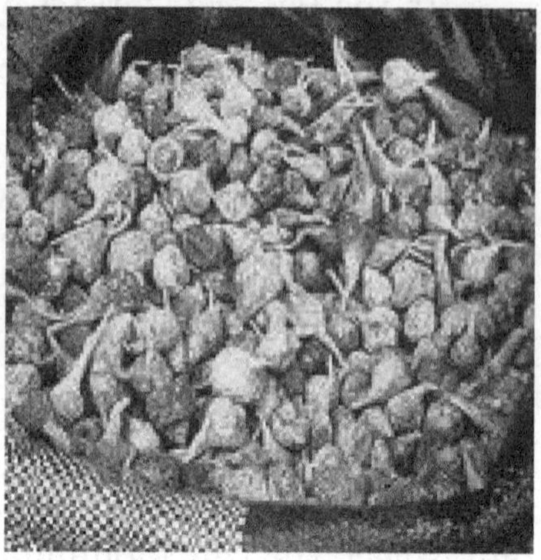

New information that has come out in recent years has shown that maca has positive effects on the hypothalamus, the small almond-sized gland in the brain that controls numerous biological functions such as linking the nervous system to the endocrine system by way of the pituitary gland. Super foods such as cacao, maca, goji berries, blue-green algae, spirulina, coconut products, and marine phytoplankton are feeding our glands because our nervous system can send out signals to the rest of the body through the nourishment of the brain, activating specific hormones. Since the endocrine system is directly affected by the functionality of the hypothalamus, the hormonal symphony of the endocrine system becomes secreted in the brain such as TRH(Thryotropin-releasing hormone) for stimulating the hormone(TSH) for thyroid production. The hypothalamic and endocrine combination regulates emotional behavior and may be the reason for so many years of anecdotal studies of sexual virility which does not just increases sexual performance but also acts as a hormonal trigger, giving one their "power" back, and taking a seemingly docile individual and transforming them into an empowered citizen of the planet.

Maca's nutritional profile has also been linked to its ability to alleviate sexual dysfunction. It contains a unique chemical called p-methoxybenzyl isothuocyanate which is correlated with its aphrodisiac qualities. A 12-week long double-blind clinical study performed by the department of urology in Morgagni-Pierantoni Hospital in Forli, Italy examined the effects of 50 caucasian men who were all affected by mild erectile dysfunction. The group was separated randomly by those taking a dry powder extract of maca root and those merely taking a placebo. The study found both the groups had significant improvements but those who took the maca extract had noticeably higher results in their physical health and all around well being.

Maca was extensively studied by *Dr. Gloria Chacon De Popovici* who was born in Peru in the 1940's. Her studies on this power plant lasted for 40 years, leading her to write a book titled **The Importance of the Lepidium Peruvianum Chacon(Maca) in the Nutrition and Health of the Human and Animal 2000 Years Before and After Christ in the Twenty First Century**. Her work on maca has led her to amazing findings and health benefits that have restored this plant from almost becoming extinct. NASA approached Dr. Popovici about the implementing maca into their nutritional supplement program because they found through testing that animals lost their reproductive ability when in space so, as a result, NASA astronauts began taking maca to reverse this condition.

Marine Phytoplankton:

Marine Phytoplankton is one of the most important food substances for the future of human nutrition. It is considered to be the basis for all living organism on the planet. In the vastness of the sea there are tiny microscopic single-celled algae called phytoplankton. They are filled largely with chlorophyll, giving them a strong green pigmentation and increasing oxygen in the muscles of those who consume it. Phytoplankton account for up to half of the photosynthetic activity on our planet, resulting in the production of a great deal of the earth's oxygen present in the atmosphere. All animals and plants in one way or another depend on this bacteria or algae as it is a direct link to all of our food supply. The animals, such as bears, that catch fish are consuming phytoplankton as well because that is the food of fish that the bear consumes. The tiny oceanic shrimp called krill are also consuming phytoplankton as well which is where they get their unique health properties. Whales who have the largest nervous system in the world consume krill. As phytoplankton moves through the food chain it influences every form of life from start to finish.

Marine-based foods are essential for complete nutrition because an over reliance on land-based foods may lead to deficiencies in trace minerals and micronutrients that are abundant in sea vegetation such as seaweeds and algae. Phytoplankton is an incredible source of brain nourishment as it contains the long chain omega-3 fatty acids EPA and DHA, which are most commonly sourced from fish. However, due to heavy metal contamination and the over fishing in the oceans, fish sources are not advised. As a powerful vegan source of nutrition this is a great aid for brain fuel which most of the population is becoming increasingly absent in. Refer back to the section on **Omega Fatty Acids.**

The beauty of a food like this is in its ability to directly feed the cells of our body with out the interferences of digestion. The process of digesting our food many times gets in the way of assimilating key nutrients, and therefore we do not always absorb what is needed. Food is a stimulant(cooked food always) in most cases, increasing our blood sugar levels significantly. When the food is void of nutrition we experience energy spikes and energy reductions contributing to an over-stimulated adrenal gland. In order to digest food our body must use enough energy to do so. The harder it is for a food to break down, the more energy must be used to disperse the proteins, sugars, oils, etc. to their destination. Initially, the body has to identify the food and then convert it into useable forms of energy. Phytoplankton does this immediately without conversion, meaning it does not waste physical energy and actually creates deposits in our energy savings account within our cells. These cellular energy currencies are referred to as nucleotides(ATP, ADP, GTP) which literally will bypass the mitochondria (energy storehouse for our cells) so the energy packets are delivered right away to the cell whereas most foods must pass through the mitochondria like a processing factory for the rest of the body to receive nourishment.

Marine Phytoplankton contains possibly the most complete package of nutrition of any food known in one source. It is a complete protein source containing every essential amino acid not present in the body originally and every non-essential(but important) amino acid said to be over 60% protein by weight and 100% bioavailable. These characteristics are virtually unheard of in the nutrition world. Phytoplankton has every known mineral that the human body requires and perhaps every mineral constituents we do not even know of yet. This is not surprising considering its origins is deep within the ocean where the abundance of minerals reside. According to *David Wolfe* in **Super**

Foods, Marine Phytoplankton contains massive amounts of B vitamins such as B1, B2, B3, B5, B6, and B12, along with vitamin A, C, and D.

Because of Marine Phytoplankton's concentrated liquid form it is easily used by anyone of any age especially children that are being raised with inferior building blocks to begin the construction of their lives. Those that are older can truly benefit from this food by regaining what was lost by certain degenerative dis-eases or conditions by filling in the holes that may have gone empty for a lifetime. This is truly a substance that must be considered in every health program!

(Recommended Book: The Longevity Now Program by David Wolfe)

Aloe Vera

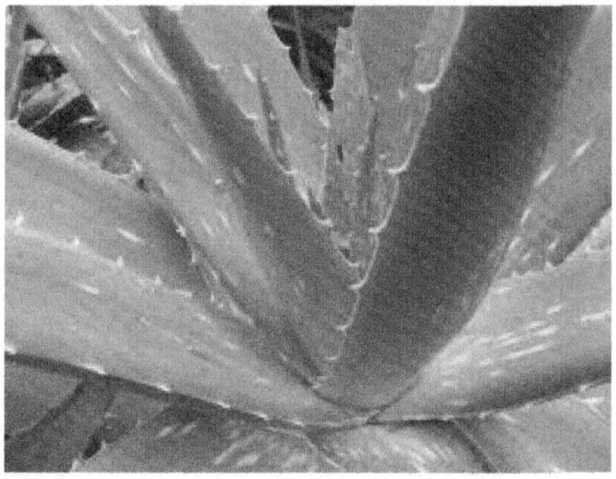

Aloe Vera is one of the great survival plants in the world. Said to originate to fruition in Africa, it now flourishes across the global landscape in temperate and tropical climates. This plant has been passed down through the centuries for its unique healing properties. The Egyptians are the first people in recorded history to utilize Aloe. It is rumored that the two Egyptian queens, Nefertiti and Cleopatra, used Aloe Vera frequently as part of their beautification routine. This plant was highly revered by the Egyptians as well as other cultures. The Mahometans viewed Aloe Vera as a religious icon, hanging it in the doorway believing that it would protect them from negative spirits. The people would create a mixture of aloe and myrrh for embalming upon the death of a Pharaoh. People were allowed to enter the funeral of the esteemed king so long as they brought at least one pound of aloe vera. The lure of this plant has only escaped a small portion of the planet. Aristotle is said to have convinced Alexander the Great to conquer the land of Socotra (now Yemen) for their aloe vera plantations. In the times of the Crusades, the Knights of Templar concocted a drink made out of palm wine, hemp, and aloe pulp. They called this "the elixir of Jerusalem", believing this would add considerable years to their lives. Arab traders had brought aloe to India and Persia by around 600 BC. The Arabs figured out how to separate the gel from the outer shell. They called this plant the "desert lily" for it's inner and outer uses.

The history of aloe vera continues to span far across continents, making it's way to Great Rome, China, Spain, Portugal, Holland, France, and Britain. Every stretch of land that has had its hands on aloe began to revere it and incorporate it into their own healing systems. Christopher Columbus discovered aloe vera on his second voyage to America reporting, *"Four vegetables are indispensable for the well being of man: wheat, the grape, olive, and aloe. The first nourishes him, the second raises his spirt, the third brings him harmony, and the fourth cures him."*

Aloe vera exhibits an extraordinary array of plentiful and highly unique properties that make this a true super food in every way. The plant displays a husky green armor where inside of each one of these sturdy leaves lies a mucilaginous gel. The aloe leaves must be filleted off in order to consume this potent medicinal food. Aloe can be used topically and internally. It is suggested in this book to use it both ways. It is not widely recommended here to use many of the store-bought aloe vera concentrates or drinks as many are filled with preservatives and do not even remotely contain the medicinal qualities this plant is known for. The soft gel is highly concentrated with the long-chain sugars known as polysaccharides, providing satiation, long-term energy production, anti-inflammatory properties, and informing our immune system with highly advanced "biological-data" in which to perform better. The white blood cells that make up our immune system operate more efficiently on certain types of nutrients such as these bitter polysaccharide sugars. These rare sugars help modulate our immunity, which helps fight back all forms of infection such as fungal, viral, and nano-bacterial(calcification). Viral infections, in particular, are a major concern in the world at large. They are even smaller than bacterial organisms and require a viable host to survive. They invade our cells and, once in the body, begin to replicate virus cells in place of what was once a healthy cell. Aloe vera is a powerful ally in the deconstruction of these virus-producing organisms by restoring the delicate balance of our inner terrain.

The glyconutrients (polysaccharides) in aloe vera help to boost the immune system by producing antioxidants that help identify and eliminate free-radicals in the body. Antioxidants such as vitamin C and E are present in aloe along with increasing the production of the glutathione synthetase enzyme in the liver. Glutathione is a powerful antioxidant that is important for the development of our white blood cells as well as preventing damage to other cellular capabilities that hinder as oxidation occurs. Every area in the body can be affected by the increased production of glutathione such as the liver, amino acid transport, enzyme activation, protein synthesis, and critical metabolic reactions that influence DNA repair.

Research studies done at the Medical Plant Information Centre, Mahidol University in Bangok showed that aloe vera juice on its own could have significant effects on diabetic patients by lowering blood glucose and triglyceride levels. A study was conducted with two groups out of 72 patients with diabetes mellitus. One group took one tablespoon of aloe juice(not even the whole gel) twice a day and the other was administered a placebo. Their results showed that after two weeks, the fasting blood glucose levels of the patients who drank the aloe juice was generously reduced and continued to improve as the study progressed.

In the book, **Sugars that Heal**, *Emil I. Mondoa, M.D., Mindy Kitei* attests to a case where Aloe Vera was used to help stabilize a cancer condition where traditional medical treatment was ineffective.

"In a 1998 study conducted in Milan, Italy, twenty-six patients with advanced solid tumors (including cancers of the breast, gastrointestinal tract, brain, and lung) who hadn't responded to traditional therapy were treated daily with 20 milligrams of melatonin, which has been shown to induce some benefits in untreatable metastatic

cancer patients. Another twenty-four patients received 20 milligrams of melatonin daily plus a tincture (alcohol-based liquid) of Aloe vera, 1 milliliter twice a day. A partial response was achieved in two of the twenty-four patients treated with melatonin plus aloe, whereas none of the patients treated with melatonin alone improved. In addition, the cancer stabilized in fourteen of the aloe patients, compared with only seven of the melatonin patients."

This plant is best known for it's topical uses along with it's astounding digestion-enhancing properties. Aloe aids the body in calming the digestive system and can be helpful for many digestive disturbances such as ulcers and irritable bowel syndrome. Our internal surface structure is lined up with epithelial cells that are responsible for connective tissue maintenance where aloe vera supports the replication of these cells. When our inner environment is clean and functioning optimally then our outer environment begins to show it. The topical application can be remarkable for sunburns, scars, psoriasis, open wounds, and fire burns. I remember staying under the sun for too long during a festival. My skin showed sign of severely sunburn by the next day. I filleted a aloe leaf and stuck the gel on my forehead, smearing it all over my face for the day. Two days later my sunburn was gone. It is suggested to hold the gel on a specified location for hours to an entire day, depending on the severity of the wound, for best results.

Noni Fruit:

Perhaps the most exotic, intriguing, and bioactive fruit on earth is the Morinda Citrifolia or better known as the Noni Fruit. This fruit has a very unattractive pungent odor as it ripens. This quality has gained noni the reputation as the cheese fruit or even vomit fruit because of its powerful taste- definitely not something for the weary individual. Noni is one of those special plants that seems to grow wildly in harsh terrains such as volcanic ash beds, lava-strewn coasts, and all over the tropics. I personally believe that an environment in which a plant grows has profound influence on its genetic make up, exactly the same way a baby develops inside a mothers stomach. Noni is always in season and always producing fruit which suggests that is was intended as supreme nutrition for human consumption. Cacao, coconuts, and goji berries are also unique in their year-round growing cycle. If you have these four foods together then you have something special! The amount of nourishment you would receive in one day would be more than most would get in a month, let alone a lifetime.

The chemical and nutrient composition of noni is very interesting. Noni is possibly the best source of polysaccharides of any food in nature along with aloe vera. As mentioned previously, these essential sugars have a powerful effect on our immune system, helping us repel foreign invaders in the body. This fruit is a great source of minerals such as magnesium, potassium, selenium, iron, zinc, copper, and sulfur. The juice of the noni fruit is said to be an excellent source of vitamin C.

There have been a lot of research studies done over many years to determine the effectiveness of this fruit in healing with many interesting discoveries discovered along the way. According to the research, noni appears to reduce tumor growths by activating the immune system. It is considered to be one of the best aids in digestive wellness being a natural antiseptic and helps against certain types of harmful bacteria. The noni fruit has been shown to work at the cellular level, increasing cell rejuvenation and functionality.

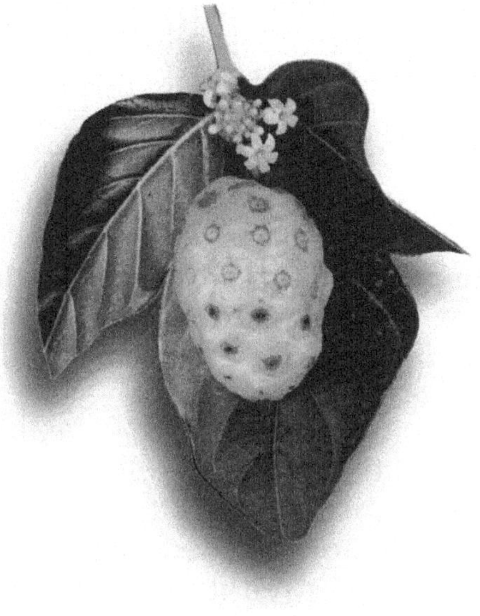

Dr Ralph Heinicke did research studies in Hawaii on the psychologically active compounds that are contained in the fruit. He spent 45 years doing research on the alkaloid Xeronine inside Noni which seems to be the key constituent for improving cellular health. His belief is that the juice of noni actually increases the ability to regenerate damaged cells and also is the reason for the psychological responses that many report after drinking noni juice.

Spirulina:

The famed algae of South America, spirulina is one of the premier foods of the future. Given the research, the historical usage, and bioavailability of pure nutrition, spirulina is one of those leaders in the field. I have become a big fan of this food for my own lifestyle and can see how it dramatically can alter the health of anyone in any situation. The most current reemergence of this ocean algae was in 1964 when Belgian botanist Jean Leonard brought it to the modern world. Before that nobody really knew anything about it. Usage of spirulina as a food staple dates back further than the early 1500's when Hernando Cortez came to the Aztec nation. In Mexico City, Spirulina was the main protein source consumed for hundreds of years and, because of the knowledge we have gained, we are seeing the wisdom of the past.

Spirulina is most likely the best source of protein of any food in the natural world being 50-60% bioavailable, containing every single amino acid in a raw form. What makes Spirulina such a superior protein source to any dense food is that it can be put into a glass of water and immediately transported into the blood stream. It is rich in fatty acids and omega fatty acids such as Alpha-linolenic acid (ALA), Gamma-linolenic acid (GLA), Linolenic acid (LA), Stearidonic acid (SDA), Eicosapentaenoic acid(EPA), Docosahexaenoic acid (DHA), and Arachidonic acid (AA). Spirulina contains a great combination of B vitamins that play a big role in metabolism. They work best in synergy with one another coming from a centralizing food source, such as spirulina.

There is a massive amount of pigments that reside within spirulina, giving it a deep green pigmentation. Pigments in foods such as spirulina all have their own properties which, in this case, they all come together to create a superior nutrition source. Pigmentation in spirulina is related to eye health and nervous system function. Some of the pigments in spirulina are Beta-Carotene (eye retina health), Zeaxanthin (eye retina), Chlorophyll (Blood Health), and Xanthophyll (Eye Protection), among many others.

One of special interest is phycocyanin, the blue pigment that seems to have a powerful effect on multiple areas of health. In the book **Healing with Whole Foods** by *Paul Pitchford* clearly states the benefit:

"Important to note in the area of prevention, spirulina is richly supplied with the blue pigment phycocyanin, a biliprotein which has been shown to inhibit cancer-colony formation. Predominant blue pigmentation in food is rare. The blue color tends to promote astringency, a drawing together. The chemical reality of spirulina's blue color is demonstrated by its effect in the brain. Here phycocyanin helps draw together amino acids for neurotransmitter formation, which increases mental capacity."

Research studies have indicated that spirulina has the ability to block the replication of HIV T-cells in humans. It has been shown to help malnourished children with or without HIV to increase weight gain and improve anemic conditions. A study done in 2007 showed that spirulina actually improved antioxidant potential of patients who were given it for 16 weeks. The blood plasma of these patients showed that the antioxidant levels had increased. There is no doubt that this will be one of the most important food sources, along with other micro algae like chlorella, marine phytoplankton, and blue green algae, as we go into the future.

"Best food for the future"

The United Nations World Food Conference of 1974 speaking of Spirulina.

Adaptogenic Herbs

The term adaptogen refers mainly to herbs that have restorative effects on the body in times of stress, anxiety, and fatigue. This can also be referred to as tonic herbs, a class of herbs that can be consumed regularly like food. Tonic herbs are different from other herbs where certain herbs, such as garlic and echinacea, are only to be consumed periodically. In the current circumstances of daily life tonic herbs or adaptogenic herbs have never been more needed to help us cope with the stresses of modern living. Adaptogens can be used intelligently as tools for increasing immune function, hormonal regulation, decreasing inflammation, strengthening the heart, increasing brain health, aiding the endocrine system, and dramatically increasing sports performance.

"All plants contain adaptogenic/tonic compounds, because plants have to contend with a good deal of stress themselves"
James Duke, PHD, Scientist & Ethnobotnist

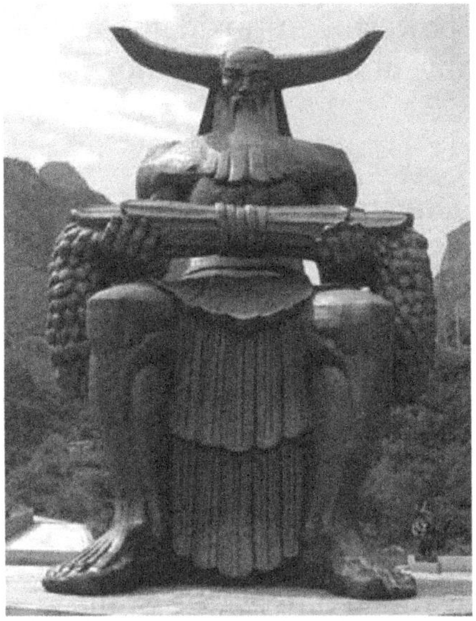

The popular theory of nutrition is a broken system that is lacking the most important piece- the plant medicine. The standard American diet may in fact be the single greatest contradiction in our world and offers no solution within the parameters of socially accepted thinking. The strict raw vegan approach offers great solutions but remains problematic if the herbalism piece is left out. Standard fruits and vegetables, organic included, are not enough to create a complete picture of nutrition. The bitter alkaloids(plant medicines) have been removed through the process of hybridization. In many cases, the plants that endure the harshest terrains become very strong and therefore can be of much better use than domesticated plants. These plants are considered wild foods or wild herbs.

In the natural flow of life we are changing much like the weather during the transition of seasons. We will always require different means of nourishment and healing in our journey. This is exactly why there is so much dis-ease in our world today. People are reaching for pills, which are all synthesized from plant sources originally. Companies attempt to extract what they believe to be the active ingredient in the herb and highly concentrating it. Eventually that is what shows up in the pharmaceutical industry. The reason why this never works is because the body does not know what to do with that one ingredient in a chemical form. It is the combination of all the ingredients that make it work, exactly like a finely dialed-in team of experts. In the ethical way of practicing herbalism there is a theme which states "Non-Interference with Nature" and "Do No Harm"- this is what herbalism is really about.

The use of herbs as physical treatments have most likely been used far beyond our recorded history. Botanical remedies are definitely the oldest form of medicine with the longest and most effective track record without question. It is said Emperor Shen Nong, somewhere around 2700 B.C. in ancient China, wrote the definitive work on Chinese herbalism titled Shennong Bencao Jing, listing 365 medicinal plants and their appropriate uses. In India the traditional healing system is known as Ayurveda which translates to Life(ayus) Knowledge(veda). This system has been in use some say past 2000 B.C. where the earliest used plant was turmeric. The first major writing in Ayurveda is the Charaka Samhita by Charaka. The usage of herbs in health has been uncontested and it is my feeling that this same usage in the modern form is the future. The result of this will likely be an appropriate synthesis between scientific innovation and ancient wisdom.

The reason tonic herbalism is coming into play so profoundly in this time is because we must flood our bodies with adaptogenic substances as we are forced to adapt to our stressful surroundings, allowing us to adapt and thrive in stress-filled conditions. The idea we want to adopt for maximum efficiency is incorporating the best herbs we know of from all of the ancient systems; this will be the future of medicine. These plants have rare compounds that are shared by many adaptogens such as polysaccharides, alkaloids, saponins, flavonoids, triterpenes, and other powerful antioxidants which contain intelligence that can work on our health in ways conventional food cannot.

"The Top 5 Chinese Herbs"

- Reishi Mushroom- known as the spirit mushroom, activates the intelligence of our immune system, adaptogen, anti-stress herb, polyssacharides.
- Gynostemma- one of the most revered herbs in Chinese lore. Increases energy & clarity, powerful adaptogen, brings in balance, calms the nervous system, anti-stress herb.
- Ho Shou Wu- one of the most powerful adaptogenic substance in Chinese history. Enhances the cardiovascular system and the immune system, boosts sexual health, improves clarity and brings balance.
- Cordyceps- this mushroom-herb was historically consumed only by the Chinese emperor and was no allowed possession by the commoner under penalty of death. Increases stamina, restores physical energy, anti-stress herb, increases brain health, improves sexual virility.
- Ginseng- this herb is legendary in Chinese medicinal history. Increases alertness, natural energy, stamina, and regulates blood sugar levels. Contains special phytochemicals known as "sapponins" that improve our immune system.

"The Top 5 Ayurvedic Herbs"

- Ashwaganda- referred to as the Indian Ginseng. Relieves stress from the body, antibacterial and antimicrobial herb, stimulates the immune system, helps speed the healing process, can increase the efficacy of the thyroid gland.
- Mucuna Pruriens- See Section: Leaving Behind Excess, The Adrenal Glands.
- Tribulis- renowned for its capacity to increase sexual function. Significantly increases testosterone levels as well as acting as a diuretic and cooling agent.
- Shilajit- the name means destroyer of weakness. Contains up to 85 known minerals, high concentrations of humic and fulvic acid which help with cellular nourishment and detoxification.)
- Turmeric- famous for its anti-inflammatory and antioxidant benefits which work to support our immune system and helps to lower bad cholesterol. Research is also showing anti-fungal and anti-bacterial compounds.

(Recommended Book: Ancient Wisdom of Chinese Tonic Herbs: Ron Teegarden)

Supplementation

Supplements are all about designing your own personal insurance policy which can be likened to insuring your business. In the natural food community there is sometimes a big debate and even controversial arguments in regards to if we need to be taking supplements. The general assumption is that we can always get all that we need from locally-grown foods. Significant tests have been done to show even the highest quality organic foods being grown today are at least 5 times less nutritious than they were 50 years ago due to extreme soil demineralization. The introduction of whole food concentrates such as super foods, green powders, dried herbs, and raw organic protein powders have given many people a much better road to travel. Whole food concentrates are natural foods that have been low temperature dried and converted into a powdered form. These are not the same as isolated mineral or vitamin supplements that exclude one constituent while leaving out the other essential co-factors. With the concentration of organic minerals and trace minerals, vitamins, phytonutrients, antioxidants, amino acids, and complimenting nutrients, we can receive much more with much less. Here is the way I look at: this is my main source of bulk nutrition. Whole raw organic plant foods (fruits, vegetables, nuts, seeds) are great for our macronutrient needs and should remain at the foundation of most peoples intake to keep in balance.

When searching for supplements that may be of benefit to you it is important to first understand the drawbacks of the supplement industry and tread lightly at first. The standardized supplement industry is a heavy cash cow that produces what can be deemed as "counterfeit nutrients". In many ways the more "intelligent" man becomes the more mediocre the results he produces. In terms of supplements, this statement is spot on and is explained further below in the section on minerals. In order to explain this let me share a few examples of how a good idea(nutrient supplements) can be taken far out of rational context.

Vitamin C is a powerful tool for the beautification of our skin by helping the body produce collagen for the repair and growth of important bodily tissue such as cartilage, ligaments, tendons, and blood vessels. It helps with the healing process of cuts, burns, and wounds as well as being a powerful antioxidant. In extreme cases of vitamin C deficiency an onset of scurvy(skin blots, bleeding/spongy gums) is very common, especially for those who do not consume fresh vegetables or fruits often. The nutrient known as Vitamin C in supplemental form has been labeled "ascorbic acid". This is a false identity because ascorbic acid is the "chemical-name" for vitamin C and does not produce the result that true vitamin C does. Ascorbic acid will not produce the same results of completely alleviate scurvy as real vitamin C does. According to Dr. Robert Marshal, every time someone ingests 500 milligrams of purely isolated ascorbic acid they develop 50 milligrams of skeletal calcium (calcification). The natural forms of vitamin C are heavily present in organically grown citrus fruit. Beyond that, the whole food concentrates of choice are camu camu, amla berry, and acerola cherry.

Vitamin E is the given term that refers to a group of eight chemical forms(four tocotrienols and four tocopherols) that are fat-soluble and contain significant antioxidant properties. This classification of chemical compounds was discovered in 1922. Ever since then it has been long discussed which form of vitamin E is most beneficial. Tocopherol has been long considered the true form of vitamin E. We now have realized this is not the entire story and has created supplemental issues. A researcher by the name of Dr. Barry Tan discovered the value of tocotrienols in contrast to the isolated tocopherols when he was on a mission to find active compounds found specifically in plants. Dr. Tan explains that he witnessed the ripening and opening of the annatto plant where the seed had no “protective-flesh” whereas fruit has a fleshy layer surrounding the seed. He thought to himself, if there is no flesh to protect the seed then what is protecting the seed from the inside? He came to discover through analysis that the annatto plant contained high vitamin E compounds but to his amazement there was no tocopherol content- it was 100% tocotrienol(delta & gamma). Dr. Tan simply explains the distinction of these two vitamin E compounds in relation to their protective features. He says tocopherol is like a common police officer who remains within their limited protective reach of a town. Tocotrienols he explains is like a state trooper who can branch out through the entire state (body) and provide extraordinary assistance in protecting from outside influences. Dr. Barry Tan cites a UC Berkeley study that was conducted in the 1970s where it was shown that tocotrienols has 50 times the efficacy in protecting our cells then tocopherols by spinning around the cell 50 times faster. He states that the molecular size of tocopherol is vastly larger then it’s counterpart, meaning that tocotrienol performs in the body with greater dexterity and can reach out through the body much more effectively.

Vitamin E (tocotrienols) has been shown to be extremely effective in two primary areas of cardiovascular health: cholesterol and inflammation. According to Dr. Tan, when tocopherol in isolated form is disproportionate to tocotrienol it can block the absorption of tocotrienol, thus acting as a catalyst for excessive cholesterol in the liver and increasing blood pressure. When our blood becomes too thick it sticks onto the cell wall, causing a stagnation and blockage of oxygen through our blood stream. Tocotrienols can work to loosen the clustered red blood cells and help in allowing the blood to move much smoother, similar to an untampered river. Vitamin E’s role as a super antioxidant has been shown to prevent protein oxidation and lipid (fat) peroxidation after physically straining exercise. Foods that contain the correct source of vitamin E are anatto, palm seed, and rice. Palm oil has been shown to be a very good supplementary source of vitamin E. The whole raw food concentrate comes from rice bran which is a great addition to smoothies and raw chocolate creations.

While we aspire to get all of our nutrition from whole raw foods in ideal circumstances we also aspire to have optimal heath at all times. Investigate the source and quality of any supplements you may choose to incorporate into your lifestyle.

(Recommended Books: Supplements Exposed! by Dr.Brian Clement, Supplement Your Prescription by Dr. Hyla Cass)

Supplementing for Pregnancy:

In regards to pregnancy, considering all bases is not only necessary but could easily be considered neglectful not to. The physical needs of the pregnant mother changes dramatically and must be addressed with intelligence and sophistication. Extremely religious views on diet and health have absolutely no place in this equation. A person may live however he or she chooses but to bring a new life into the world requires a wide scope of options, nutritionally speaking. However this picture looks for you, consider each option carefully. This is in no way a complete list but merely food for thought. The use of the word supplement in terms of ingredients stated below is meant to be derived from whole foods specifically. If this cannot be done then we move onto high-grade supplemental products. If you, your spouse, or someone you are close to is pregnant look into the chapter **The Karmic Perspective: Sacred Birth.**

I am very much opposed to the low fat idea in dietary literature regarding pregnancy and for women in general. Woman are designed by the creator to carry more body fat than men. The "thin is in, fat is out" mentality has negative effects on the health of future mother(women in general) and could result in severe deficiencies or even miscarriage of the baby. A general body fat percentage for a healthy woman approaching pregnancy may be 18-20% or in many cases generously higher. This does not mean it will be obvious on the outside as many lean and toned individuals(mostly women) have much more body fat than one would assume.

Below is a brief but concise list of essential elements for a birthing mother to apply, all of which have been elaborated on in greater detail throughout the book.

- EFA (Essential Fatty Acids) Non-Vegan/Vegetarians: Krill Oil, Vegans/Vegetarians: Marine Phytoplankton, Flax Oil, Hemp Oil, & Algae Oil
- B Vitamins- B3, B5, B6. B9, B12 (most important), B17
- Vitamin D (hormone), Vitamin C, Vitamin A, Vitamin E, Vitamin K2 (See Chapter: **The Raw Naked Truth: Dairy**)
- Essential Amino Acids (Tryptophan, Cystine, Tyrosine, Phenylalanine may require supplementation in some cases)
- Essential Sugars (Polysaccharides)
- Neurotransmitter Modulating Agents (See chapter: **The Chocolate Revolution: Magic of Cacao** & **Symptoms of Society: Drug Addictions**)
- Minerals (Magnesium, Iron, Iodine, Phosphorus, Silica, Sulfur, Chromium, Selenium, Zinc)
- Enzymes (Organic Plant Based)
- Immune System Protecters (Medicinal Mushrooms, Herbs, Antioxidants, Super Foods, Bee Products)
- The Triangle of Life (Highest Quality Water Possible, Barefoot connection to earth, & Exposure to Sun Light)

Minerals

The mineral make up of a healthy, intelligent, and balanced human being is vital to the sustainability of these qualities. Due to the aggressive farming and wild life depletion practices of the agricultural industry, the mineral compounds in the soil have risen to the surface, beginning from the advent of agriculture, and have been swept away into the oceans. Our food-plants can take carbon monoxide from the air using the sun's energy through photosynthesis to manufacture carbon-based compounds such as cellulose, vitamins, amino acids, and fatty acids. However, what they cannot manufacture on their own are minerals. There are over 90 known required minerals for the optimization of our physical and mental capabilities. The body's electrical system run primarily on the utilization of minerals as every aspect of our nutrition needs the assistance of full-spectrum minerals and trace minerals to activate their assimilation and efficacy in the human body. Minerals are identical to a tuning fork or even a radio station, allowing us to tune into higher thoughts, vibrations, and life experiences. If we are lacking in proper ionic plant-based minerals we are incapable of adjusting the dial of our power grid that lights up our mind and body. The wide range of deficiencies people suffer from can, and in most cases will begin to reverse as the body becomes remineralized. Patients who lose blood are administered intravenous saline solution (salt water/sodium chloride) to prevent and remedy dehydration. Patients who experience a heart attack are given minerals before doctors apply an electric charge through electronic paddles. The electric current would not effectively charge into the body to revive them without proper mineralization. The heart conducts electricity which is being run on minerals.

It is said by some that you can fool someone that only has 4 minerals in their diet but it is impossible to fool someone who has 90 minerals. My friend Hoi Sauce believes that salt is the perfect "lie detector" substance.

"95% of all Americans, regardless of age, have mineral deficiency".
US Dept. of Agriculture, 1975

When exploring mineral supplementation it is important to understand what form and sourcing of minerals conduct electrical transfers in the body. Plant-based minerals are essential because these are "ionic form minerals". Ionic refers to an element/mineral having a positive or negative charge. Mineral supplements that are merely "elemental-minerals" based strictly on the scientifically-accepted "Periodic Table of Elements" are insufficient for absorption in the human body. Ionic minerals help to produce greater equilibrium and facilitate biological changes necessary for the nutrients in our food to go where needed. Angstrom-sized minerals are the most effective form in which to supplement as these are micronized plant-based minerals that can immediately be distributed throughout the body when taken sublingually(under the tongue).

If one strives to obtain their full spectrum mineral requirements from a whole raw food source primarily then I would recommend low-heat-air-dried grass powders and seaweeds as these are the two most mineral concentrated food categories in the human diet.

Zinc: One of the most unique and exceptional elements for health is zinc. Zinc is perhaps one of the greatest antioxidants for the body. A process known as galvanization is used in the routine of coating iron, aluminum, and steel with thin layers of zinc to evade corrosion. This mineral is used to keep steel from environmental rusting. When activated in ionic form it can do the same thing for the human body. Zinc strongly influences the prevention of virus and bacterial production. Zinc can quickly penetrate the bodily fluids, especially our saliva, creating a greater level of sanitation in the mouth, protecting against harmful bacterial replications that form acids that tear away at our tooth enamel. Zinc is essential in aiding the male reproductive system and producing healthy sperm levels. As well as greater results in healthy libido, zinc also has been shown to effectively promote healthy hormone and brain functions. Zinc is also involved in every function of insulin metabolism, helping to prevent insulin resistance in diabetics.

Magnesium: The most deficient mineral in the western diet appears to be the most needed for its capacity to address a multitude of health aversions. Magnesium is the primary mineral responsible for over 320 enzymatic reactions in the human body. Magnesium may, in fact, be the greatest supporter of physiological activities including heart health, brain function, bone density, nervous system maintenance, peristalsis(bowel movements), muscle relaxation, alleviation of menstrual cramping, as well as increasing alkalinity. Experts in the field of brain health and nutrition agree that there is a profound correlation with ADD (attention deficit disorder) symptoms and frequent magnesium deficiencies. A specific enzyme, delta-6-desaturase uses magnesium to help convert omega-3 ALA into omega-3 DHA for proper brain function. A chronic magnesium depletion can, and most likely will, lead to muscular tension. Magnesium aids in increased flexibility and physical strength. Magnesium is abundant in chlorophyll-rich foods as it is the central molecule in chlorophyll. The number one source of magnesium in nature is raw cacao beans(raw chocolate beans) which contain magnesium in therapeutic doses.

Sulfur: The healthy maintenance of our tissue fibers, ligaments, muscle tendons, and joints are heavily reliant on sulfur. Nervous system conditions such as palsy, multiple sclerosis, and parkinson's disease are due in part by the break down of the thin protective material that coats our nerve fibers known as the myelin sheath. Once these layers are edged off of our nerve fibers, the nervous system begins to become oxidized from acid-producing oils, foods, false sugars, radiation, EMFs, and other known toxins. Sulfur is critical for collagen synthesis which builds our skin, hair, and nail cells. Sulfur aids an effective liver and helps to scavenge free-radical production in the body. See MSM below to find additional information on this mineral.

Iodine: This mineral is becoming increasingly more important as pollution and radiation become prevalent in our world. Airborne pollutants, pesticide sprays, radioactive compounds, and plastics influence the shutting down of our irreplaceable thyroid gland. The two thyroid hormones thyroxine and triiodotyronine contain significant levels of iodine which is used to produce hormone functionality. Iodine deficiencies can show up as goiters which is an enlargement of the thyroid gland. The mental and physical growth stunting condition known as cretinism is due to untreated deficiencies in the thyroid hormones resulting usually in hypothyroidism, which is generally due to a maternal thyroid disorder. Iodine has been identified as the single mineral responsible for the prevention of this condition. Iodine also plays a role in other areas of the body such as the eyes, gastric mucosa, the mammary glands, the cervix, and salivary glands acting as an antioxidant for these portions of the body. This mineral assists in enzyme reactions and helps to regulate the cellular functioning in energy production.

Vanadium: This trace mineral has been found to be extremely effective in treating those with diabetes and insulin sensitivities. It helps with the absorption of blood sugar transport into the muscular system as well as reducing elevated cholesterol levels. According to *Dr. Gabriel Cousens* in his book, **There is a Cure for Diabetes** he states, *"Clinical trials have found a significant decrease in insulin requirements in patients with insulin dependent diabetes after vanadyl sulfate therapy."*

Germanium: This element in its inorganic form has been used as a semi-conductor for electronic equipment. This mineral is still being analyzed and tested for its efficacy as an organic supplement. It has been said to stimulate the body's production of interferon, which is a naturally occurring anti-cancer agent. The Nobel Prize winning biologist Dr. Otto Warburg states that germanium increases the delivery of oxygen to the cells, slowing down cancer growth. The primary issue behind cancer growth is the lack of oxygen. Germanium has been found in plants such as garlic, comfrey, aloe vera, and ginseng.

Silver: The element of silver is one of the most prized mineral/metals we know of in our world. Silver is the most thermal-conductive(heat transferable) metal and is said to be the highest electrical conduit of any known element. Ionic silver displays toxic effects to many forms of bacteria, fungal infections, and viruses. The potent germicidal effects of silver can defend against microbial production. Silver is the original antibiotic. In World War I silver compounds were utilized to prevent the onset of dangerous infections. This was as era prior to the invention of conventional antibiotics. Silver coins were once placed in milk bottles to further the freshness of the milk. The people of ancient Rome and Greece both used silver for several purposes, such as the treatment of deep wounds and skin burns. It was also used to disinfect water and food for long term storage. If the immune system has been compromised then regions of the body, such as our spinal fluid, will be extremely vulnerable to bacterial infections, which can cause the back issues many suffer from. Ionic silver can aid this by creating a secondary immune system to support the regions of the body that our primary defense shield may not detect. It is rumored that the introduction of silver utensils began with the intent from Europeans to infuse silver particles with their food as to improve their health. These particular Europeans were known as the "blue-bloods".

Selenium: The mineral selenium is widely found in raw brazil nuts, giving this food a high standing among the nut category. Selenium is a powerful antioxidant and immune system booster. It is suggested by many studies that the human immune system requires selenium for the development of our white blood cells which defend against infections and illness. Selenium seems to protect the cells from free-radical damage from a deficient diet and environmental toxins. In *A. True Ott's* book, **Wellness Secrets for Life**, he states *"when scientists in Arizona gave one group of men and women 200 mcg. selenium daily for seven years, and another identical group a placebo or 'dummy' pills, they made an interesting discovery. The group that took selenium were 42% less likely to develop cancer than the group that took the placebo"*. Selenium plays a role in the production of proteins that are involved in healthy sperm. Male infertility has been associated in part with low selenium levels as well as other vital elements such as zinc. It has been established that activities such as smoking, excessive alcohol, and taking birth control pills can reduce the availability of selenium in the blood.

Copper: Copper is said to be the third most abundant trace mineral in the human body following zinc and iron. It is found in every tissue in the body but most heavily concentrated in the liver. In the 1870's copper was found to play a major role in the body's metabolism because it assists critical enzyme function. Copper helps to manufacture melanin, which is our original hair pigment as well as improving skin tone. The mineral iron requires copper for proper transportation and utilization in the blood. Many iron deficiencies symptoms such as Anaemia could be in fact a copper deficiency. Copper seems to be an essential element for the production of the thyroid hormone thyroxine as well as helping to build the myelin sheath that protect our nerves. The super-antioxidant superoxide dismutase (SOD) is an enzyme that relies on copper to activate free-radical protection which can take place during the normal metabolic process, especially if our immune system has been damaged in any way. According to the literature, when copper is not present in the body, SOD production is greatly reduced and oxidative stress becomes more pervasive. Zinc in combination with copper helps to influence the production of SOD. Copper also acts as a co-factor in manufacturing elastic fibers in the arteries and brain, as well as helping the structural proteins that build bone and connective-tissue.

Copper is unique among most minerals as it is said to be mostly absorbed in the stomach. This means that in order to utilize copper one must make sure their hydrochloric acid levels are at a normal range, otherwise copper deficiency will be much more likely. Another word of mention is that zinc and copper both compete along the same passageway into the small intestine and one may block the other out if zinc supplementation is heavily consumed. Both of these minerals can be done in intervals of each other, or make sure to consume high zinc- containing foods (pumpkin seeds, cacao, sesame seeds, watermelon seeds, garlic) and allow copper supplementation to take greater effect.

Chromium: This mineral is the most popular elemental-form mineral in metallurgy for coating steel because of it's unsurpassed durability and effectiveness to resist corrosion. Chromium is vitally important to the balance and regulation of blood sugar. Blood sugar imbalances that can result in hypoglycemia are generally linked to a chromium deficiency. This mineral, especially in combination with vanadium, signals enzyme reactions that are involved in the body's tolerance of glucose. Low levels of chromium often result in low blood sugar, pre-diabetes, and diabetes itself if carried out for too long. Laboratory studies have been conducted in animals, one showing a 33% increase in lifespan after supplementing with chromium. Chromium is also pulled out of our tissues as a result of a fast food/processed food diet.

MSM: *Methyl-sulfonyl-methane(MSM)* is an organic form of sulfur that was originally discovered from *DMSO (Dimethylsulfoxide),* a water-soluble compound that has great effects on detoxification and breaking up bad calcium formations in the body. It has been known that sulfur-rich foods such as beats, red onions, eggs, and radishes are very good for the skin because sulfur strengthens collagen repair. If someone has, over years of time, become affected by calcification then eating raw foods alone may not be enough to strip out these negative bacteria forming organisms from the body. (**See Section: The Scientific Method, The Calcium Theory**)

Calcium-forming Organisms (CFO) like to attach themselves to stagnant or creaky areas of the body constructing their own haven to set up shop. MSM helps to lubricate our joints, repair tissue damage, improve skin, nail, and hair damage and make our overall body run better. If our body is running optimally then these CFO's have no where to set up shop because the terrain they are most comfortable in is not available and therefore they are easily removed. All joint and bone problems seem to have a calcification problem attached to it, MSM can literally save someone's life and strip away many chronic issues one may have been struggling with for years. Those that have been affected by mercury amalgam fillings in the mouth can use MSM in their personal detoxification strategy. The mercury fillings in ones teeth are extremely close to the brain which, over time, will leach off and de-sheathing the protective layers surrounding our nervous system, leading to a series of neurological problems. Sulfur is a powerful remedy against mercury toxicity and should be used every day in such cases.

In the book **The Miracle of MSM** the authors Stanley W. Jacob, Ronald M. Lawrence, and Martin Zucker cite a particular medical study out of many that shows the importance of sulfur in bone health and osteoarthritic conditions.

"The journal of Bone and Joint Surgery and the journal of the Southern Medical Association during the 1930s, which described the use of intravenous and intramuscular injections of sulfur for arthritis. These studies found the cystine content of fingernails to be 25 percent lower in arthritics. Cystine is a sulfur amino acid that helps build hard tissue such as fingernails and hair. In one of these older studies, when a group of 100 arthritics were given a solution of sulfur intravenously, pain was relieved in many cases and the cystine fingernail test returned to normal."

MSM is not only a great sulfur-bearing compound but the untold story behind it is that it is a methyl group donor as well. Scientific research is now finding in many cases of cancer, such as breast cancer and reproductive cancer, that when certain hormones(Estrogen, Progesterone, Testosterone) are out of balance then there are methylation isssues. The methyl groups are used by our body in order to detoxify chemicals, heavy metals, bad estrogens (non-methylated estrogens), and pesticides. We have been so heavily exposed to these mentioned substances that it has inhibited the bodies ability to produce methyl compounds, especially if our estrogen levels become too high. Methylation affects our hormones, it affects our enzyme and protein efficiency, and greatly influences our genetic expression where non-methylation in our DNA can lead to certain genes being deactivated. It can also have a great effect in the embryonic state of a fetus as its developing in the mothers womb.

MSM can be a powerful tool in anyone's arsenal. The foods that we eat are profoundly important but, when you can back it up with organic compounds that do the deep work then it makes everything else much more effective. MSM can be taken in a pill or powder form, or in a skin lotion. I recommend taking a plant-based MSM supplement if you have the option.

B Vitamins:

B-complex vitamins are essential in any health program for the support of our metabolism, nervous system, immune system, brain development, as well as cellular growth, aiding in muscular tone, skin and hair health among other functions as well. B vitamins are water-soluble nutrients that work together in the same way amino acids do for proper protein utilization. The old idea was that vitamin B was a single vitamin, such as vitamin C. We now know B vitamins are a wide array of nutrients that work best consumed together and each have a specific function in our body.

B1- Thiamine is important for our metabolism, helping our body create energy from the food. The nerves of our cells require thiamine for adequate performance, especially in the brain. Those that have abused alcohol have been reported to have severe thiamine deficiencies which is also linked to a poor diet. Impaired thiamine utilization ultimately causes a magnesium deficiency and storages of thiamine in the liver is reduced.

B2- Riboflavin plays an important role in the body's ability to metabolize key nutrients such as fats, proteins, and carbohydrates. Vitamin B2 helps create oxygen from nutrients for the cellular process of storing and catalyzing energy. Riboflavin deficiencies sometimes show up as cracked and redness on the lips, cracks around the mouth and sore throat, dry skin, damage to the mucous membrane, and sensitive blood-shot eyes. Riboflavin is also subject to oxidation from light.

B3- Niacin has a deep connection with the addictive behavior of cigarette smoking. Niacin is almost chemically identical to the nicotinic acid and niacinamide which is almost identical to nicotine (stimulant compound in cigarettes). Nicotine binds to nicotinic acid receptor sites in the brain, causing the dopamine (pleasure, relaxed) response one feels from smoking. Vitamin B3 can be used to help alleviate such conditions so look into niacin flushes for help with this. Niacin helps open up the blood vessels, improving blood flow to all points of the body and brain, inducing relaxation and well being. Jungle Peanuts have been reported to be the best source of niacin in nature and are aflatoxin-free(conventional peanuts are contaminated).

B5- Pantothenic Acid is a water-soluble vitamin that was discovered in 1919 by biochemist Roger J. Williams(See Chapter: **Evolutionary Theories, Biochemical Individuality**). B5 helps metabolize and synthesize fats, proteins, and carbohydrates as well as a range of other biological roles essential to life. Pantothenic acid deficiency is rare due to its abundance in most food sources. Raw foods that contain the most pantothenic acid appear to be avocados, broccoli, and royal jelly to name a few.

B6- Pyridoxine is needed for healthy neurotransmitter function such as serotonin, dopamine, norepinephrine, and epinephrine. B6 has a major part in enzyme function which stimulates the conversion of the neurotransmitter pre-cursor 5-hydroxytryptophan (5-HTP) into levodopa (L-Dopa). Vitamin B6 has been used in efforts to reduce parkinson's disease because of the dopamine pathway helping to restore the nervous system and brain health. B6 deficiencies have been associated with depression, arthritis, and inflammation.

B9- Folic Acid is important for the health and reproductive ability of our cells, especially for infancy and pregnancy. B9 is required for the maintenance of our DNA structure and protecting us from cellular damage. Folic Acid helps the synthesis of proteins in the body to construct adequate building material. It has been shown to have positive effects on the mineral density of bones and improving bone marrow health.

B12- Cobalamin is of much concern in all circles of health and has been subject to controversy. There is in depth details on Vitamin B12 in the chapter **The Raw Naked Truth**.

B17- Laetrile, otherwise known as Amygdalin, is a 4-component nutrient consisting of two parts glucose(sugar), 1 part cyanide, and 1 part benzaldehyde. Laetrile has been a subject of harsh controversy by the Food and Drug Administration (FDA) in the numerous claims and testimonials of its ability to alleviate the effects of different forms of cancer. The FDA does not approve B17 and, because of this, most people have never heard of it. The "reason" for the scrutiny of laetrile is because it contains cyanide which is considered extremely toxic. Cyanide in its pure free-floating form is very toxic but when it is locked up with other molecular components it becomes an essential nutrient similar to vitamin B12(Cobalamin) which is also known as cyanocabalmin, the cyano being the prefix indicating a cyanide-like compound.

Edward Griffin, author of **World without Cancer,** states that many foods, such as almonds, once had high quantities of amygdalin but have been bred to release it of its healing quality in order to produce a much sweeter, less bitter product. He strongly suggests that as we moved away from bitter foods, and more towards sweet processed foods, the rates of cancer increased dramatically, which is exactly what we have seen in the last 80 years. The amygdalin or B17 supplement is nothing more than an apricot seed extract, making it a whole food supplement.

Vitamin D:

The importance of getting enough vitamin D in our body has been on the forefront of many health discussion in recent years. There has been a tremendous bulk of information that has risen to the surface regarding this topic. We know Vitamin D is completely unique among all other vitamins, mainly because it is not a vitamin at all. Rather it is hormone that has a relation to virtually all major body functions. When the skin is openly exposed to the Ultra Violet Ray Bands(UVB) of the sun, vitamin D is transported into the blood stream, making its way to the liver where it must be converted into the *prohormone calcifediol.* Through a set of physiological conversion steps this hormone precursor is able to synthesize into a biologically active form of vitamin D called D3 (not to be confused with D2). The most significant aspect of vitamin D is the fact that it has tremendous influence on our genetic expression. According to the research, the vitamin D receptor belongs to a certain class of proteins (nuclear receptors) found in the cells responsible for working with the steroid and thyroid hormones as well as other molecules in the gene pool. Vitamin D's influence throughout the body is dependent on how well it is absorbed and ultimately synthesized that determines its enormous benefits.

There have been many debates on whether you can receive all that you require from the sun alone. The sun is the natural source of how vitamin D is produced within the body. My personal belief is that most people can utilize all they need from natural exposure from the sun but, due to multiple factors, it is becoming increasingly harder to do this. Researchers over the years have found common similarities between conditions such as cancer, flu, and autism in relation to vitamin D deficiencies. There seems to be increases in these ailments in areas further away from the equator and in winter where there is far less sunlight. Studies are showing autism births are occurring mostly in March when winter is ending. This is when vitamin D levels would be lowest due to minimal exposure to the sun's UVB. Dr. John Cannell, a leading researcher on vitamin D, believes that the leading cause for autism is intimately linked to deficiencies of this master hormone. Dr. Cannell's belief is considered a "theory" but it is one that holds a substantial weight behind it which I documented in the Resource section (**Scientific Research Studies & Valuable Articles: Vitamin D**). The rates in autism began to rise right around the time that the public was warned to stay out of the sun, coincidently vitamin D deficiencies rose at that same time as well in the early 1980's. We now know, without any doubt, that the sun is our best friend and the false marketing we were force fed for years has been leading us astray. This is a literal quote from the American Academy of Dermatology: ***"Appalling that anyone in good conscience could make the claim that intentional sun exposure- for any length of time- is beneficial".***

Vitamin D deficiencies have been associated with psoriasis, eczema, anxiety, insomnia, loss of hearing, muscle pain, arthritis, rickets, auto-immune disease, pregnancy complications, and there is much talk linking this epidemic with diabetes type-1. Kids today are growing up very sheltered and indoors for far too much time, inhibiting their ability to produce healthy vitamin D levels. This idea, coupled with the fact kids are not being active outside like we all used to be, is likely a large factor in children being diagnosed with diabetes type-1. The link between the sun and exercise is critical because obesity has been shown to decrease the vitamin D absorption rate and also increases one's requirement for the activation of this important hormone. This factor extends probably even more into the adult population because the exposure to the sun is minimal from busy careers, families, and obligations. The more dances around the sun we take(aging), the harder it can be to produce vitamin D3. When we do spend time in the sun the common trend is to put on any kind of sun screen which impairs the skins ability to make vitamin D3(See Section: **Triangle of life, The Sun**). Vitamin D3 can also be washed off of the skin if we immediately shower after sun exposure. I suggest people wait at least 45 minutes to an hour before showering after sun exposure. I noticed that after years of running in the sun I would always enjoy laying out while the sweat rolled off my body. This gives the body down time to relax and the oils to seep into the pores of the skin.

The unique role vitamin D plays in outstanding vitality cannot be overlooked and is becoming extremely well known in mainstream circles. I truly believe that the reason rare individuals such as inediets (See Section: **Deconstructing the Diet, Breatharianism**) are able to sustain such a lifestyle is greatly due to spending so much time in the sun. It is very important for those living in cities to have our vitamin D levels checked through appropriate blood testing. I would love to insist that spending more time under the sun will work for everyone but the fact is over 90% of the western population is believed to be severely deficient. Therefore proper supplementation is advised to cover all bases as it is pointless to take chances with ones health if it can be avoided. I highly recommend the reader look into Dr. Joseph Mercola's work online on this subject as he has perhaps the most detailed and up-to-date information regarding vitamin D.

The BeeGan Ethics

Life is the flower for which love is the honey.
Victor Hugo

For so work the honey-bees, creatures that by a rule in nature teach the act of order to a peopled kingdom.
William Shakespeare

In nature all things are perfect; there is an order that cannot be dictated by human hands. All things must work together with respect for what the other brings, which is the proper way for the inhabitants of nature and humans to live together. The importance of bees in our world is underrated on many different levels. The bees are important for certain ecosystems as a major pollinator of flowers. Bees crosspollinate from the flower to other plants. The flower contains the sexual reproductive pollen of nature, and it is delivered to other plants by bees in order to help them fully develop. Pollination of food crops, such as blueberries, strawberries, cucumbers, melons, and many other crops, is good to know due to the misuse of pesticides and other environmental attributes like nearby suburban developments putting pressure on the health of this wild life. The organic bee keepers are doing a phenomenal service, and I believe we should do whatever we can to support their efforts in keeping ethical bee farms up and running.

The general vegan ethic has been on the fence with bee products since they are derived from a living animal. This is an idea that many are becoming more relaxed about considering, in most cases, the bees are not being harmed. In fact, the bee farmers I have met and heard from seem to have a deep relationship with their bees, much like a family pet. As we become much more sophisticated in not only our health approaches as well as our moral approaches, many are seeing the sense in lowering the walls that certain rigid doctrines can create. I am completely in agreement with the vegan ethic as far as harming bees along with all creatures but I also know that the benefits of bee products for humans are far too important to simply ignore. A quote I heard from Gabrielle Cousens opened my mind which is *"A human out of balance is far more impactful on the environment than the life of a fish"*. I have seen that some people do better with some animal products in their diet occasionally whether it may be raw dairy, bee products, or the deer antler extract (traditional adrenal tonic in Chinese herbalism). These are all things that can be procured without harming the animal. I believe this is the partnership aspect we have with certain creatures in this world. We work with these animals, feeding them, and taking care of them. In return, these animals give us a portion of their truly unique sustenance.

The use of bee products has spanned across the frontiers of recorded history. It may be possible that no other animal has had more of an intimate connection with the human species than bees. The magic of honey during ancient times seems to be shrouded in a bit of mystery and the attraction to it must have been instinctive to indiginous peoples as it surely has been for wild animals. Despite the opinions of many "experts", we truly know very little of early man's true eating habits. We do have good evidence that one of the staples of many cultures was the use of honey and pollen. Countless biblical references have been presented such as Proverbs 25:16: "*Hast thou found honey? Eat so much as its sufficient for thee*". The book of Ezekiel shows true in Ezekiel 16:13: "*Thou didst eat fine flour, and honey, and oil; and thou wast exceeding beautiful, and thou didst prosper into a kingdom*". The great cultures of the past knew these foods had inherent qualities unlike anything else.

Bee Products

The magic of this category of food produced from the sacred bee hive appears to be the source in which they come from. Bees are cultivators and travel from some of the most mana-filled areas of nature. What this means is they are absorbing the intrinsic factors of nature and these energies are giving us that direct connection when we consume these foods raw. Each one of these foods has its own properties that make them complete nutrition sources. When combined, they become a power house of nutrition that could store in the body for future needs.

When Professor Nicolal Vasllievich Tsitsin from the U.S.S.R(Russia), a biologist and botanist, did a long term study on the longest living people in the Caucasus mountains of Russia, he was very intrigued with what reports have stated over 200 people living in the upwards of 125 years of age, some say even 150. The thing that was so surprising to Professor Tsitsin was all of the natives were still working well into what any common modern civilian would consider old age. This was a clear sign of remarkable health. The common theme he was looking for between the people was that they all owned bees and what they consumed regularly was the thick residual accumulation of honey they harvested fresh from the combs. Tsitsin was served a portion of what he would believe to be their longevity nectar, a sticky glob-like substance(honey) that had inside it noticeably large amounts of bee pollen. The product of the bee hive combined with the villagers' healthy lifestyle and clean air was what is to be believed to be the main ingredients to their impressive vitality.

Honey:

"The people of antiquity knew that both milk and honey are strongly connected with healthy human life force"

Rudolph Steiner

The sacred substance we call honey has had a long history as a revered food in different civilizations such as Egypt, the Middle East, Ancient China, mighty Rome, mythical Greece, and traditional Mesoamerica. Honey has had different uses than just food. In Egypt they used it for embalming the dead. It was used as an ointment for burns and skin rashes as well as helping to alleviate throat issues like chronic bronchitis and asthmatic conditions. Topical honey has been used in the place of topical antibiotics for diabetic ulcers. Honey is a verified antibacterial substance because of the natural hydrogen peroxide properties present in most honey. Honey has been used in Ayurvedic medicine and Chinese medicine through their thousands of years of history. I have heard that in China, as well as India, they would use honey to ball up certain herbs to make it palatable as the sweetness of honey makes for an effective delivery system.

The nutritional complex of raw honey is very impressive, far more than any other sweetener you can find. Honey is a far superior source of carbohydrates than heavier sources before and after workouts to influence muscle recuperation. The carbohydrates stored in the muscle (glycogen) help effective restoration. Most protein supplements contain a carbohydrate derived from corn called maltodextrin which is used to compliment protein intake. Studies have verified that using honey instead of maltodextrin has equal, if not better, effects for muscle repair.

Honey has a good response in moderation for those dealing with glycemic sensitivities due to the complex sugars it gradually releases into the blood stream, making it a sustainable source of energy. Honey is extremely enzymatic, making it much more digestible than most heavily concentrated sugar foods, specifically processed carbohydrates, which, in most cases, glob up our cells and can shorten our life spans if not balanced by other nutrients and minerals. The big problem with carbohydrates in conventional food practices is that they are void of complimenting nutrients which honey has in excess. High quality raw honey is full of B Vitamins such as Thiamin(B1), Niacin(B3), Riboflavin(B2), and Pyridoxine(B6). It has an impressive list of minerals which may vary depending on the source of the pollination. For instance, Manuka honey is said to have the highest concentration of minerals of any honey. The darker the honey, the more dense the nutrition is in most cases, assuming it is raw, organic, and unfiltered.

Bee Pollen:

One of the most extraordinary foods on earth is also one of the simplest and most accessible for human consumption. Bee pollen is one of the best sources of nutrition in nature. It can bridge the gap for almost anyone that is having nutrient deficiencies. The protein content is said to be around 40% free-form amino acids which means the protein is highly available and can act almost immediately in the blood stream. Bee pollen exceeds all animal products as a complete protein. Serious athletes and body builders are becoming more interested in its benefits. Muhammed Ali who is considered the greatest boxer of all time by many was known to start using bee pollen. This is possibly where he got the phrase "Float like a butter fly, sting like a bee".

"Honey bee pollen is the richest source of vitamins found in nature in a single food."
Institute of Apiculture, Taranov Russia

Many cultures around the world have been using Bee pollen for a long time to increase physical vigor, improve the immune system and increase endurance. Bee pollen is a complete nutrition sourcefor extending life span as bee products have been linked with some of the longest living people in the world. Bee pollen is one of the most concentrated sources of polysaccharides (essential sugars), helping our immune system and giving us long sustained energy. Bee pollen also contains a high amount of RNA(ribonucleic acid) and DNA(Deoxyribonucleic acid), nucleic acids that aid in the formation of healthy cells and can stimulate the growth of new skin tissue. Bee pollen is really an extraordinary food as it nourishes one at the cellular level. As a result of these unique nucleic acids, it can positively effect our genetic code. This food is so powerful that it is not to be abused; it must be respected like any of the foods we would deem "super foods", and therefore you would only require a decent amount to make a difference. You can mix half a tablespoon or possible even less with some honey or just eat it straight.

Royal Jelly:

When the time comes for the worker bees of a colony to breed a new queen they must select several small larvae to feed them generous amounts of royal jelly in order to initiate the transitional stages. Royal jelly is the secretion from a honey bee used as a high quality source of nutrition originally for the development of the queen. In asian cultures, royal jelly is celebrated as a longevity food, supporting fertility, immunity, and long life. Considering how this food in particular is reserved for the queen bee who lives exceedingly longer than regular worker bees, the queen also matures sexually whereas the worker bees do not. This presents an interesting idea, such as the doctrine of signatures, when looking at the potential of a food so unique and exclusive to the royalty of an entire species.

Royal jelly contains many of the same B-complex vitamins in honey and bee pollen along with sources of different amino acids, simple sugars(monosacharides), and a good source of fatty acids. The main constituent of royal jelly that causes a female larvae to develop into a fully matured queen bee is the individual protein *royalactin*. This protein seems to cause a phenotypical change in the bee, giving it a larger size and ovary development. Bee products have always been linked to increased sexual health and royal jelly seems to be no different. Royal jelly has also been shown to improve brain health by stimulating the growth of Glial cells (provide protection and support to brain neurons) and neural stem cells(self renewable cells). This can explain why the association with vitality has been so strongly linked to this substance.

If you decide to use royal jelly then do it sparingly since it is very potent. About the size of your pinky finger tip is enough to begin with. I have been known to throw a small spoonfull into my raw chocolate bars I make occasionally or just it eat straight.

Propolis:

Propolis is the resinous material that is collected by bees from a mixture of botanical sources. This waxy substance is used to provide protection from outside invaders as well as to seal up any holes or cracks in the hive. Propolis has been studied extensively for its unique anti-bacterial compounds that have been used all through human history as food and treatments. Bees are depicted on vases of the Egyptian because it is a well known fact that they used this product of the hive effectively for sores and ulcers. The Egyptians were also known to use strips of propolis on the bodies of the deceased in order to prevent decay from microbes and other bacterial infections. In the book **Health from the Hive,** *Carlson Wade* points out the recognition of propolis by the Roman scholar Pliny (A.D.23-79) as a medicinal tool to sooth pain, reduce swelling, and sores. *Wade* had this interesting observation, *"So we see that the beehive is a miniature city teeming with life. The temperature inside the hive is kept at approximately 95'F. With 90% humidity- a perfect breeding ground for all kinds of molds, mildews, and bacteria. Yet the hive remains the most sterile environment found in nature. Reason: Propolis has antibacterial and fungicidal agents and contains many different antibiotic substances.*

The nutritional composition of propolis varies from hive to hive, like most natural foods. Propolis is said to be approximately 55% resins and balms and 30% wax. These are considered to be the bacteria fighting compounds in this exotic substance. It is full of amino acids, minerals such as iron, zinc, manganese, copper along with most likely "undiscovered trace minerals" to note. Perhaps the most important aspect of propolis is its bioflavonoids, otherwise known in the medical community as "vitamin P". These flavonoids are a type of plant pigment found in certain fruits and vegetables as well as flowers found in nature. Our immune system gets attacked on a daily basis. Flavonoids add a tremendous antioxidant surge to our body, thus empowering our immune system to full strength. Oxidative stress on our internal system is a major issue in any city environment, especially considering the food choices most people are making. Terms some people may be familiar with are polyphenols (cellular restoration, blocks cancer cells from forming), quercetin (Anti-inflammatory, helps vitamin C work better), and epicatachin (supports heart health, circulatory health-also found in Cacao) which are different types of flavonoids that work to increase vigor and extend all forms of life!

The Karmic Perspective

Men are not punished for their sins, but by them.
Elbert Hubbard

Every action of our lives touches on some chord that will vibrate in eternity.
Edwin Hubbel Chapin

People pay for what they do, and still more, for what they have allowed themselves to become. And they pay for it simply: by the lives they lead.
Edith Wharton

There are no mishaps in nature. The flow of the universe is accurately delivering back to us the energies that we have sent out at one point or another. The hardest lessons are usually built up through constant resistance to the obvious. If we decide to live outside of natures balance we ourselves will always be off balance. Man-made laws hold little weight when stacked against natural law. Eventually we all must own our actions, regardless of how much we deny the unpredictable occasion for which karma will present itself into our path.

A simple principle to live by is "do not bring harm to the body by not doing harm to the body". Do not do anything that you are unsure will bring harm to the body, and certainly do not do anything you know will bring harm to the body. We must get clear on this if we are to progress in our personal journey of health. The energies we bring into our bodies eventually are shown to the world on outside the same way a house breaking down from the foundation eventually tarnishes the decadent coating.

No amount of cover up will cover up the truth, if you refuse to go within you will always go without.

The way in which we live our lives has much deeper implications than we like to admit or think about. The wheel of karma acts like a boomerang, finding itself right back where it started, emitting an enhanced version of the intention that sent it out. *Jim Rohn* once said "you do not reap what you sow, you reap double". Every seed planted has a gestation period where it must germinate before it can fully develop until one day it is in full bloom. It would be wise to look at our daily actions and thought patterns in such a way because something will always grow from our own creation. Whether you believe it or not, our thoughts are adapting its development according to the pattern of our life. If you center yourself around prosperity, youthful vigor, and service then frequencies of these virtues will be invited in. If you are centered around poverty, scarcity, and selfishness then you will force those energies in as well.

Our time on this earth is spent according to our value system which *Dr. John D. Martini.* Martini points out in his work that human beings conduct their lives based on what they value most. If a mother values her child most in her life then she will place the majority of her focus on her child's best interests. If one values finance the most then they will place most of their focus in that arena. This concept I find very important to analyze for our own lives because it gives us a tool in how to essentially build or rebuild the kind of life we want. You can design a personal pyramid that is broken up into your own priorities in life and direct your actions which most align to those. This is a very good way of getting on track and gaining clarity because it is easy to be confused in our society of high pressure and fast-food consciousness.

The way events play out in our lives can be related to the idea of having a personal karmic bank account. Actions, thoughts, and feelings are either building or decreasing the spiritual equity we have available as we go through our journey. The missing link in many perspectives on health is the most important one, which is the health of the spirit. If our spiritual life is full of abundance then our health will be considerable, even if we do not put much focus on it. In truth, the spirit is what we must feed first. The more things we do that are positive and heart-felt the more well intentions are deposited into your karmic account. I believe the old adage of patience being a virtue applies to this concept simply because it is easier to cheat than to fully develop yourself for excellence. Help someone in need if you have the opportunity to do it! If you have the opportunity to share a kind word of encouragement then do it! If you have the opportunity to help an animal then do it! Seize the moment to build your karmic account because it will act as a parachute when you least expect it.

Reverence for Life

If a man loses his reverence for any part of life,
he will lose his reverence for all of life.
Albert Schweitzr

If all the ancient traditions and teachings are in fact taken seriously then the key principle to practice is reverence for life in all its many forms. Human beings are custodians to the planet and have been given a powerful responsibility to share this land, not control it with an iron fist. We must remember as a whole that we are only as strong as the weakest link. We all feel it if any creature suffers. An idea came to me that when we feel upset or off balance for no reason it is because we are receiving the transmitted energy of another being in pain. The weather most likely shapes itself in response to the collective attitudes and emotions of the beings living below.

Life exists exclusively in each breath, and the deeper and fully focused the breath the deeper and centered the entire life becomes. The world is much bigger than we assume it is. The deeper we go inside, the bigger the outside becomes. When we become open to that world that exists beyond our current understanding we learn of all that life has to offer, and thus begin to respect it much more.

The subject of eating animals for sustaining human life is a deep and emotional one for many. I believe it goes much deeper than just pointing out the health and environmental challenges it poses. Truly it is a spiritual interference of the highest order. Many of the great religious and spiritual leaders, yogis, and transformative thinkers have suggested we move towards a vegetarian diet for the progression of the human race. Leo Tolstoy said *"A human can be healthy without killing animals for food. Therefore if he eats meat he participates in taking animal life merely for the sake of his appetite."* The desire for pleasure of filling our stomach has created a steady collapse in all human affairs and confused our understanding of where we belong in this world. To take part in the act of killing presents its own consequences, regardless if it is the offering or receiving. I have noticed that most people will give lip service, assuming their words harbor their power but without the understanding that it is in their conviction to a core belief and purpose that power is born. The reason people still consume meat, in my opinion, is a lack of belief. The powers that be have been overbearing and convincing that meat is synonymous with health. This lack in ones own power creates a cycle that is hard to break because the more product one consumes. the more one becomes addicted like a drug addict. This causes a tremendous strain on one's soul, causing illusions such as fear and doubt to flood the system.

The most important desire a human being has beyond food or water is the desire for love and happiness. The very fact that breatharians are living today, that Jesus and Moses did 40 day water fasts in the burning heat should begin to knock down the ivory tower society has created surrounding meat consumption needs. The great Greek thinker and mathematician Pythagoras said "*For as long as men massacre animals, they will kill each other. Indeed, he who sows the seed of murder and pain cannot reap joy and love."* When we inflict pain on another we feel that pain just the same. When we consume pain it becomes apart of the body and we turn on ourselves because a body that is out of harmony conflicts with the soul.

Truly we wish to be free of obscurities and negative influences of all kinds. We are ever expanding creatures of conscious evolution. In order to fulfill our gifts we must step out of the molds we have been placed in. In many ways we have been trained the same way a elephant is trained in the circus. The baby elephant's foot is tied to a pole to ensure it does not run away. As it gets older and realizes it is stuck to the pole the elephant releases its belief that it can be free. Even when the rope is taken off this magnificent animal has been programmed to stay where its at. Albert Einstein left us with this deep insight: "*Our task must be to free ourselves . . . by widening our circle of compassion to embrace all living creatures and the whole of nature and its beauty."*

The absolute truth of the matter is we become a mirror reflection of our individual integrity. The separation of spirit and expression comes from confused ideals. You may have a completely different perspective on this subject and I respect that. We are all where we are based on where we have been, and it is naive to ignore our past just because we have reached a new level of understanding. Exactly as Albert Einstein has said above: "*We must widen our circle of compassion to all living creatures from humans to animals to insects and all plant life.*" To live in such a way where we take time to consider all the living interactions of our day is where true beauty resides. It is such a pleasure to embrace life in all things, to bask in each breath of the concert of nature's orchestra beaming through the cosmos and resonating in every soul.

"The time will come when men such as I will look upon the murder of animals as they now look on the murder of men."
Leonardo Da Vinci

Ethical Nutrition

The idea of our food habits being in line with ethics and personal morality was never considered when I was first studying nutrition in school. The idea that we may be harming our health by taking the life of an animal was completely absent. The general thinking is that the body is its own domain, having little to do with beliefs and emotional stability. Luckily this cooked paradigm is being weeded out of the program because the overwhelming evidence to the contrary is flooding in. When we speak of developing an ideal nutritional program for someone, the ethical side must be taken in account if that is important to them. What is ethical for one may not be for another. We all have different belief systems that exist together and, instead of competing with one another, it would be intelligent to gather the body of data to find common ground where we can all stand on.

Since the beginning of recorded time the topic of food has been discussed in relation to spiritual health and clarity of mind. As mentioned in the chapter **Deconstructing the Die-it**, many cultures historically would work around the killing of animals for sustenance. The hindus did it with raw dairy products as they believed in a vegetarian lifestyle but also believed in the sacred offering that the milk of a cow could provide to their people. They worked in partnership with the cows, providing them with food and shelter where the cow would provide them with a nutrition source. This is an area that is not so black and white where many strict vegans ignore. If the cow was not cared for by people then it would be killed by wild animals. In the Chinese system of herbalism, health practice was not broken down in just animal and plant. The Chinese believed as the Hindus did that animals had an important role to play in the overall vitality of humans that are out of balance. Consider substances such as the deer's antler used as a tool for balancing Yang Jing, adrenal support, growth factors, as well as many other benefits that could save someones life in unique cases. The Chinese do not kill the deer to procure its antler. In fact, the antler of the deer will naturally fall off and grow back. From this observation, researchers found that the tip of the antler contains important anabolic pre-cursors that humans can substantially benefit from. The few services in which animals are involved, such as ethical bee keeping, can be of great service to the animals, not just for people.

I personally cannot bring myself to kill or consume the flesh of an animal for food. My belief is that flesh foods do carry a strong karmic energy and the bigger picture of my place in the world will not allow me to participate in that behavior. I know the upside of abstaining from meat and understand the downsides. The down side is that if you do choose to be a vegan or vegetarian then you must become your own nutritional expert. Since you are reading this book I commend you on educating yourself and working to further your own growth. Meat does contain "momentary" short cuts such as caloric density for those who may not be fully confident in making a vegetarian/vegan transition. The upside to abstaining from meat has been widely detailed in this book and many others. I would say one of the most obvious fact is that the higher up on the food chain we eat the more we become exposed to karmic repercussions and environmental poisons because all animals are affected in this way. I feel that the ethical and moral direction of diet in the future will not be bound entirely by being vegan or not; it is becoming a choice of either I live with killing or I don't.

The native american indians are an example I like to share with people in terms of reverence for life. These people were custodians of their environment and loved all life around them. They were guided by the stars and spent all of their day under the sun, soaking in the light the same way the plants do. In many ways they were much more conscious than most of us are in city environments and yet they consumed the flesh of animals. The difference with them is they only used what they required, never wasting a portion of the animal that was sacrificed for the survival of the tribe. They believed in contribution and living within their means, never going overboard as we cannot help but see in today's culture. A belief of many ancestral people was that the psycho-spiritual energy is imprinted into the flesh. This means that the consciousness of the animal cannot help but become one with the human who consumes it. The greatest disturbance in the circle of life was when the white man came to their land and wiped out the honored buffalo for sport and entertainment, leaving a field of death at their feet. This behavior ended up playing out into their interactions with the native indians themselves as they were eventually wiped out as well. I bring this example up as a way to expand our viewpoint of what may be ethically appropriate for one but not appropriate for another.

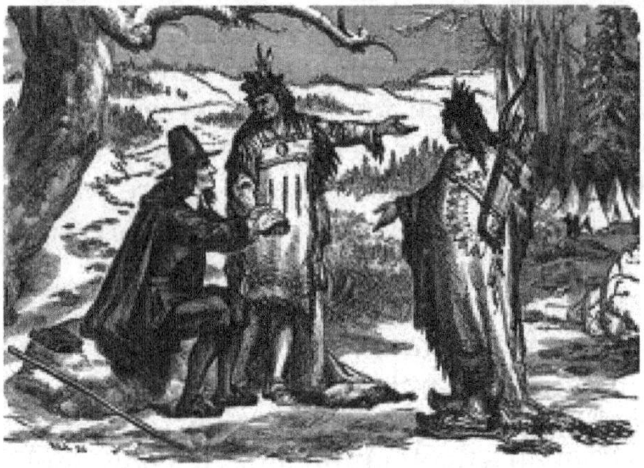

In the **Essene Gospel of Peace**, author and researcher *Edmond Bordeaux Szekely* speaks heavily of the implications of our food and spiritual path. This excerpt spoke to me and many others on a more naturalistic path: "And Jesus continued *"God commanded your forefathers: Thou shalt not kill". But in their heart was hardened and they killed. Then Moses desired that at least they should not kill men, and he suffered them to kill beasts. And then the heart of your forefathers was hardened yet more, and they killed men and beasts likewise. But I do say to you: kill neither men, nor beasts, nor yet the food which goes into your mouth. For if you eat living food, the same will quicken also. For life comes only from life, and from death comes always death. For everything which kills your food, kills your bodies also. And everything which kills your bodies kills your souls also. And your bodies become your what your foods are, even as your spirits, likewise, become what your thoughts are. Therefore, eat not anything which fire, or frost, or water has destroyed. For burned, frozen and rotted foods will burn, freeze, and rot your body also. Be not like the foolish*

husbandman who sowed in his ground cooked, and frozen, and rotted seeds. And the autumn came, and his fields bore nothing. And great was his distress. But be like that husbandman who sowed in his field living seed, and whose field bore living ears of wheat, paying a hundredfold for the seeds which he planted. For I tell you truly, live only by the fire of life, and prepare not your foods with the fire of death, which kills your foods, your bodies and your souls also"

Sacred Birth

The path of giving birth is a special one, a precious passage from one state of being to another. A new life that is born onto this planet is precious and should be viewed with the utmost consideration. The birth of all children are sacred, deserving a profound initiation from the mother and father. The choice to initiate entry of a new soul should be considered in all areas, and I am not referring to financial or time management. I am speaking of the cleansing process both parents would do well to involve themselves in before the act of love is made and conception takes place. The embryonic development of a child requires that it encodes its DNA with both the genetic make up of the man and woman. This stands to reason that whatever you put into your body has also been put into your future child. The foods and substances that influence our genetic code are determining the advantages that child has from the moment it takes it's first breath in the new world.

There are more and more babies being born with immediate deficiencies and illnesses before they take their first steps or say their first words. The same is true of babies that would have been born but the physical body of the mother could not sustain itself and miscarriages have taken place. The current living conditions most people are in is bad enough but then to compound it with junk food, toxic emotions, and negative associations is pushing it much too far. These are clear indications that the parents of the future that will inherit the earth must treat this experience as a ceremonial cleansing as the ancients did before.

The act of giving birth is such an important experience to endure and partake in that the right preparations should be made beforehand. When two people decide they want to have a baby I strongly suggest they immediately look into natural cleansing options (See Section: **Leaving Behind Excess**). The body is filled with toxins through the years and even if one has been on raw foods and involved with cleanses it is still a good idea considering the pollutants and pesticides we are exposed to regularly. A peer reviewed study was done from the University of Sherbrooke, Canada detecting an insecticidal toxin called "Cry1Ab" in the blood of pregnant woman and non-pregnant woman. This study covered 30 pregnant woman and 39 woman who came to receive a tubectomy. They were all eating a standard diet that was generally containing Genetically Modified foods(GMO) such as soy, corn, and potatoes. The umbilical toxin was detected in 93% of the blood samples from the pregnant woman and 69% of the non-pregnant woman. This is not just subject to the mothers but can be passed onto the child that is absorbing the fluids and nutrition that the mother intakes. The quality of a mans' semen is critical to the child's development and sparks the process. If the semen is full of vigor from highly mineralized foods and a healthy lifestyle, then baby will grow much stronger. For this reason alone it is recommended that men practice preferred times each year to abstain from sexual activity to reserve nutrition that is lost through excessive ejaculation and to keep the quality of the sperm which can become devalued if released too often. (See Chapter: **True Beauty: Abstinence**)

Each one of us has karmic energies we must face in order to move on with our lives and transform into the rightful ambassadors of this planet we were originally. I believe it is essential in our time to wipe away the karmic baggage before bringing a new life into this world. A child born of ones energy will carry that same energy whether that child is conscious of it or not. The emotional afflictions a mother deals with become hardwired into her child. The way the woman feels about herself will translate into the way the child sees the world before the child is able to see it. The best thing a man can do as a partner is to provide the highest emotional attitude possible. Despite all obstacles he must remain clearly focused on helping the mother remain calm and give her everything she needs, even when she doesn't know it. A man can rub her tummy with coconut oil or cacao butter to nourish the skin and the developing embryo. Talk to your future child with only expectations of love, joy, gratitude, and always express how proud you are for such a gift to occur. It is so important that we work to alter the cycle of karma in our world and the best way to do this is to begin with our own family.

For those who are at a place where they are able to make the decision to create a new gift of life, I highly recommend after you go through the physical and emotional cleansing you book a trip for the tropics. The best place to make love is where love is most concentrated: the negatively charged ionic field of the earth (negative electrical charge not to be mistaken for negative energies)! Setup an intimate and romantic area on the beach at the time the sun is dimming down. This is even better if you are able to do this with a full moon present. The moment that conception takes place the expansive field of cosmic energy becomes condensed and delivered directly to the mother to be expressed in physical form 9 months later. There are some truly amazing children walking this earth today who see, hear, smell, and touch the abundant nature of the universe in ways the most educated metaphysical philosophers still cannot. A child born from parents that take the time to prepare themselves in such a beautiful way will be nothing short of extraordinary!

Vision of Paradise

In each one of our lifetimes we must decide what our purpose is going to be all about. We have endless choices and directions we can take according to our beliefs, ethics, and personal desire to help curve the world in such a way that is compatible to all living beings. The deepest vision of paradise that we can hold in our heart is that which matches up with the types of energies we cultivate and express out into the world. If our hearts become more pure then our vision of the planet will match that just as the cynical-minded individuals perceive the world as a scary and uncomfortable mess. The idea of creating bliss on the outside radiates from a blissful nature; your heart must be tempered with the beauty of nature's genetic expression.

In nature all things just are. Animals do not take more than they require but if you domesticate an animal they will begin to take on the habits of the people they depend on. When a domesticated human steps out into the natural world they begin to feel ease and can eventually adapt to the energies of the environment. The reason why wars exist and why people are agitated and unhappy is because of our over-imposed concrete reality. This is exactly the same reason people take vacations; they have the deep need to "get away" and they never want to return once they do get away.

Real change will begin as soon as we begin to eat in a way that connects us to the earth and, in turn, the way we live will mirror this effect. The more we are connected to all things, and less attached to paradigms that no longer serve us, the more we will experience true happiness.

In order to create paradise we must understand what paradise is. The word paradise is referred to as a utopia where all life is positive and harmonious within the boundaries of all creation. All living things deserve reverence and respect, none being placed on a pedestal of hierarchy because nature's brilliance is equal to all life forms. The mother energy of this planet flourishes, nurturing all of its children without the suppression of chaotic theories and assumptions. The energetic panel of the earth's surface electrifies the minds of men to develop the most innovative ideas that are in line with the karmic understanding of life's natural cycles. There is no compromise in the true image of paradise. The tainted perspective of how life should be comes from a society that supplies substances that bring you high only to bring you back down. In all of natures wisdom there is only highs where the lows of the past only get higher, and we inevitably find ourselves laughing out loud for absolutely no reason. This is the vision of paradise I can see just across the horizon, an unprecedented time of uncontrollable prosperity elevating consciousness and imagination through the source field of the interconnectedness we call life.

The Triangle of Life

"Man is provided with all he needs in every corner of the earth, he only has to know where to look."
The Cancer Ward, - Aleksandr Solzhenitsyn

The biggest distinction between a fresh living plant-based lifestyle and the mass variety of try-it diets lies within the connection to the elements. The earth is a vast platform of electricity looking to resonate and support all living creatures ranging from humans to four legged mammals to the microscopic bacteria and fungi in the soil. The majority of the planet is a vast arena of consciously charged water that hosts life forms we still know nothing about. What we do know is that the most nourishing sources of nutrition come from the ocean. In fact, the great deal of minerals, proteins and brain oils we require like seaweeds of all kinds and algae's like marine phytoplankton are only procurable from clean waters. The sun sustains our life and ignites our soul when we learn how to absorb it properly. The moon is the sun's counter balance, calming us and tapping us into a deeper fascination for life and all of its intricacies.

The Earth:

This most magnificent planet we all place our feet on has a deep secret only a hand full of people are aware of at this point. Possibly the greatest discovery in health research comes from the last place most people would ever think to look: the ground we are stepping on. Thanks to the book **Earthing** put out by *Clint Ober, Stephen T. Sinatra, and Martin Zucker*, we have a tremendous body of research and information to let us know what our ancestors most likely knew in their time. The earth is the most powerful conductor of negatively-charged electrical energy available. Our bodies have been very depleted of negative ions that support every function of the body such as enzyme activity, nerve transmissions, muscular repair, inflammatory reduction, mental acuity, digestion, and improved sleep. Our bodies are operating primarily on electrical currents and this information has been suppressed in place of chemistry which has led to the pharmaceutical idea of healing. The outer atmosphere of the earth is positively charged (gravitational) and we have an over abundance of this suppressive force. In order to receive it's counter-balancing force, negative charges(levitational) that we require for optimum functionality, we are required to have a skin connection to the earth, especially in cities where we are completely cut off from the electrical currents/pulsations that the earth produces to shield us from the electromagnetic pollution of our high-tech devices like cell phones, computers, planes, wi-fi signals, hospital equipment, microwaves, etc.

The shoe is a major problem in this scenario because it acts as insulation from our feet to the ground. The bottoms of our feet contains the greatest receptor site for the entire endocrine system of our bodies. When we are disconnected from the earth's electric currents we are in a greater state of stress and our cells are being oxidized from all the toxicity of modern society and poor eating habits. This is where we start developing chronic conditions such as joint pain, old injuries that won't heal, muscle cramps, cloudy thoughts, indifference, and every single form of inflammation.

Disconnection from the earth actually translates into disconnection from the soul. Human beings have a deep affinity for mother nature as she has nurtured our bodies and spirits. if you add in the living foods into the equation, your connection to the planet gets even more deeply rooted because you are feeding the electric body fuel that contains highly charged negative electrons that promote the healing of every kind.

"All of nature begins to whisper its secrets to us through its sounds. Sounds that were previously incomprehensible to our soul now become the meaningful language of nature."
Rudolph Steiner

These recent discoveries have led us to new lifestyle changes, building upon the idea that we need to focus more attention on developing the soil of our earth. The true wealth in the world is not some material consumption outside of us like jewelry or precious metals; it is actually the high grade mineral matrix that we have inside of us. The greater your mineral quality the more efficiently the body and mind work. The mineral quality of our food is completely dependent on the soil quality. Unfortunately, most of the soil right now is highly demineralized and contaminated with pesticides, chemicals, and weak strands of recycled soil. We have to reintroduce ourselves to the earth as a vibrational partner of creative expansion. The best way to do this is to get barefoot on the grass or dirt, put your hands in the soil and start planting the seeds of future fruit.

The Water:

The essence of all life is blanketed throughout the world, crossing the barriers of thought, time, and space. The sacred flow of water is formless, able to adapt to any situation, breath life into a dying soul, flush out massive toxicity like a broken dam, absorb all energy surrounding it, and deliver it right back into whatever may consume its magic. The true nature of water has been grossly misunderstood by conventional standards. The average onlooker may see a glass of water as purely H2O(Hydrogen, Oxygen), thinking nothing of it other than something they should drink more of. The truth is just the subject of water alone is so vast and ever expanding that I do not believe it is possible to fully comprehend but definitely deserves our exploratory efforts.

The mystery of water is becoming less of a mystery as we dive deeper into it, pun intended. We are realizing that water has spiritual elements laced within its structural makeup. Water in its most natural form is pure consciousness. The breath of life I believe comes directly from the ground, from the water that has been harboring inside the earth, unaffected by light, heat, and oxidation of any kind. The trees dig their roots deep in the earth, absorbing the water which rises upwards, similar to how your blood rises through your veins and is dispersed throughout the rest of the body. The intangible consciousness of water infuses every cell in the human body with oxygen so it may perform at peak condition. The word hydrogen really means to generate hydration.

In the book **Your Body's Many Cries For Water**, author *Dr. Fereydoon Batmanghelidj, M.D* explains how the body tries to communicate to you that it is thirsty. Many times we misinterpret this by assuming we are hungry when the reality is we are greatly demineralized and dehydrated. Dr. Batmanghelidj explains the interaction water plays in our lives, especially the lack of water and how chronic dehydration contributes to all dis-ease. Many people try to substitute coffee, soda, tea, or even alcohol for water, claiming it has water in it and therefore it is just as good. This is a horrible assumption that is literally killing people in record numbers. One can of soda is so acidic that it takes 32 cups of clear water to offset the acid formation. What is even worse is that this figure that does not account for the chemicals the body is being exposed to when consuming soda. You are not just what you eat but very much what you drink.

Consider these words from Dr. Batmanghelidj in regards to dehydration: "*Since the water we drink provides for cell function and its volume requirements, the decrease in our daily water intake affects the efficiency of cell activity. As a result, chronic dehydration causes symptoms that equal disease when the variety of emergency signals of dehydration are not understood.*"

"Within these premises, the only thing one can be is an impeccable mediator. One is not the player in this cosmic match of chess, one is simply a pawn on the chessboard. What decides everything is a conscious impersonal energy that sorcerers call intent or the Spirit."

Carlos Castaneda

A prime example of the conscious aptitude of water is in the work of *Dr. Masaru Emoto* who wrote **The True Power of Water**, **The Hidden Messages in Water**, and **The Secret life of Water.** Dr. Emoto has been deeply fascinated with the interactive structuring nature of water and how our own intentions create personal imprints into it. He set up multiple experiments to test the response of water to our own intentions. One experiment was to have two jars of rice filled with water next to each other. One jar was labeled and applied with the intention of "Thank You" and the other "You Fool". After leaving the jars with soaked rice for a certain duration the one with the negative intention turned black and lifeless yet the other was still white. This is extremely interesting seeing as how 70% of the world is made of water, our brain is 70% water, up to 60% of the human body is water by weight, body fat contains around 10% water, and our bones are about 22% water. It stands to great reason then if our body is mostly water then the thoughts and feelings we generate have monumental effects on our health. We could literally be promoting alkalinity or acidity based on our most consistent emotional state. (See Chapter: **Alkalinity**)

Dr. Emoto in his experiments used a device called a *Magnetic Resonance Imaging* machine which could take pictures of the water molecules which are crystalline in nature. The way the water crystals would react to the vibration of the words and intentions people would place onto the water was astounding. The water that was positively focused was beautifully structured whereas the negatively focused water was yellowish and crude. This example shows exactly what is happening within our own bodies and mind as we interact with ourselves all day long.

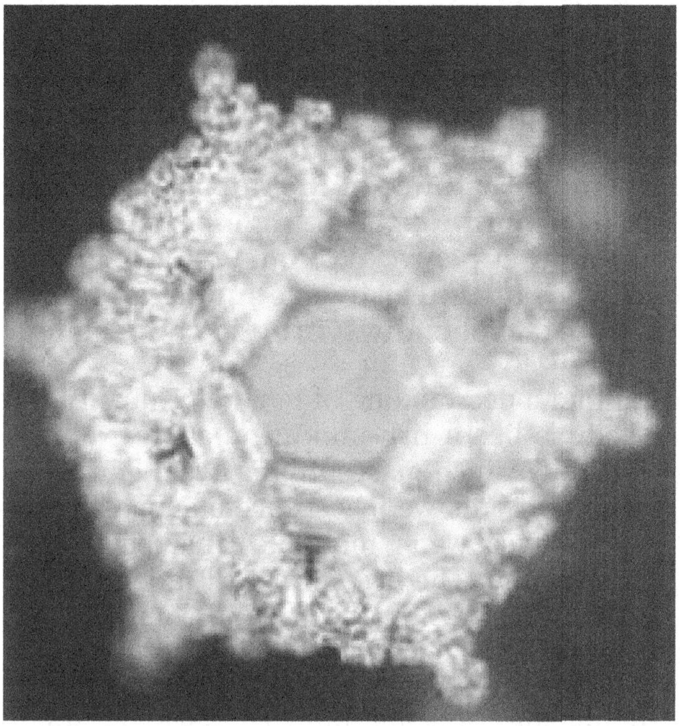

The crystalline structure of water molecules shaped from loving vibrations.
Water is not H2o; it is pure love!

These examples are phenomenal and I deeply appreciate Dr. Emotos work but I must point out that each experiment was done with distilled water, not pure spring water. I first heard about drinking spring water directly from the source from *David Wolfe* who has been promoting this idea for over a decade. This idea was originally brought out by *Victor Schauberger,* known as the water wizard, in the early 1900's. My own experience with drinking spring water directly from the source has completely changed me in ways that are so experiential. You will have to drink only spring water for at least 1-3 months to fully relate to this experience. One thing you begin to notice is you do not need to drink as much water as you did before to feel completely hydrated. I strongly suspect the idea that everyone needs to drink 8-10 glasses of clear water a day is based heavily on a cooked-food diet since water is being extracted out of the food, perpetuating dehydration. Also, I would suspect it is based on poor absorption by the body from lifeless water. The absorption of fresh spring water is immediate, causing you to receive hydration(hydrogen) at the cellular level instead of the water sinking to your stomach where it does not belong.

The best time to drink water is upon rising in the morning when your stomach is empty and your body is going through its detoxification process to move unwanted residue out of the body. Drinking a full liter (32 fluid ounces) to one and one half liters with sea salt will help flush out the system and sustain you well into the late morning.

When bottling water make sure you use glass, dark amber glass if possible. We know now that plastic is not bio-degradable; it is photo-degradable, meaning the plastic particles begin to leach off into the water upon contact by light. Plastic in the human body is one of the leading causes for hormone disruptions, endocrine problems and arthritic conditions. Plastics create what is known as xenoestrogens which deposit themselves into our fat cells. This leads to an extreme imbalance of the hormone estrogen. This has been shown to create an over feminensation in men where excess belly fat and even breast development appears. Women run a serious risk of increased chances of certain types of cancer by producing an imbalanced estrogen dominance, especially synthetic xenoestrogens.

The importance in the understanding of our water quality should be at the top of our priority list. Our body is like a fish tank in relation to nutrition. Water is being cycled and recycled constantly which makes up the overall environment of our internal ecosystem. The foods and nutrients we ingest take a supporting role to the crystalline structure of consciously charged water molecules that begin to replicate themselves within our own cellular structure. The big wave of filtration devices and alkaline water machines have created a major buzz in the healing community. These machines are great for transitioning out of the toxic municipal tap water paradigm but ultimately they exist primarily as technological attempts to replicate the recycling process in which spring water does naturally. Filtration and Ionizing machines are very much like a good cleanse; they are short term answers. Naturally occurring spring water that harbors within underground aquifers unexposed to the atmospheric influences is the long term solution.

Another interesting point about spring water is it is the most direct pathway we have to experiencing the true substance of nature. The water helps sustain the trees, the soil, all facets of the land, all the microbes, all the wild life including the plants, the animals, and creatures we never see. All of their individual experiences are directly absorbed into the microscopic fabric of the water that then travels from nature's canvas to our pallet. It will cause you to have much different thoughts than if you are from the concrete city environment drinking bottled water. I have led groups through hikes to the local spring and literally seen people go into euphoric-like states from tasting it for the first time. Spring water does something to you on a deep level, almost like being reconnected with the source of life for the very first time.

(Recommended Book: Living Water by Viktor Schauberger, Secrets of Natural Energy: by Olof Alexandersson)

The Sun:

"If I had to choose a religion, the sun as the universal giver of life would be my god."
Napoleon Bonaparte

Throughout history, perhaps nothing has been more revered and celebrated with great appreciation and curiosity than the sun. People have created shrines, monuments, pillars, and ceremonies all in favor of the immense life-giving powers of the sun. Nobody even knows exactly what the sun is. There are ideas and theories but its true identity is still unknown. We do however know a great deal of how the sun interacts with all life on earth and how it can uptake the activation of the human body simply by basking in its presence.

We have been told so many contradicting things about how the sun is a detrimental factor in our health and how it is a direct precursor to many different cancers. This is probably the most absurd assumption that has ever been told and the people behind these blanket statements seem to be making a decent profit from it. The entire dermatology and eye care industry has benefited tremendously with this idea that we need to shield ourselves from the ultraviolet rays of the sun. However, the facts have been coming out stating otherwise: 20-150,000 deaths in 2002 are believed to be the result of not getting enough sun exposure stated from an article in a journal on cancer. There are some validity to claims in overexposure being dangerous but when you look at the information. it becomes clear that it is not actually the sun thats the culprit, but the residual toxins accumulated from unhealthy lifestyles that are literally "cooking" under the sun.

The idea that the same source that gives life to creatures on earth could be working against life has always been suspect to me. The plants thrive tremendously under the sun all day long; nothing grows in the snow. Some of the most powerful plants in the world will only grow in warm tropical climates because they need the sun's energyto absorb carbon dioxide and turn it into oxygen for all surrounding life to breath. There is absolutely no mistakes in nature, only vitality as long as it remains as our creator intended.

The supposed dangers of sun exposure seem to come entirely from a denatured diet high in cooked and processed foods. When you are under the sun you are literally a beacon of light energy. If your body is filled with artificial substances like chemicals, refined sugars, inorganic salts, rancid oils, and undigested material that is being cooked inside of you then it becomes clear how problems can arise. When you rub sun lotion onto your skin it absorbs directly into your blood stream. Conventional cosmetic and skin care products are all full of foreign compounds the body will try to reject but if you are under the sun you are cooking chemicals into your pores which seems to be a common sense correlation to certain skin diseases.

The benefit of moving towards a dominantly sun food lifestyle is that you find yourself spending more time in the sun. I remember getting very sunburnt all the time when I used to be out at the beach or park for too long. Now I spend way more time in the sun and never get sunburnt. The reason I believe is that when you eat plant based foods that are full of chlorophyll(plant blood) which is almost identical to hemoglobin(human blood), your body is able to receive the rejuvenating force of the sun. The body should be as clear of obstruction as possible to reap these benefits. If there is too much acidity in the blood stream the cells that make up our body will react much like the molecules in food do when you cook them. That is why it is so important to eat water-rich foods high in minerals and chlorophyll like super foods, herbs, and green leafy vegetables.

If you are wiped out go lay in the sun for an hour. Your adrenal glands, mental faculties, and spirit will begin to recharge from the nourishment the sun provides.

The sun is the best natural way to get your vitamin D which, in many cases, cannot be effectively taken supplementarily because it is not always able to absorb into your body in artificial form. Vitamin D metabolizes calcium into your bones, promoting stronger bone health and it is now shown that vitamin D is essential for optimum health because it aids the immune system in protecting you from foreign invaders. (See Chapter: **The Sun Food Connection, Vitamin D**)

Sun gazing has become a popular topic and practice among raw foodist and many cultures alike. The native indians took part in sun dance rituals reserved for the men of the tribe who would paint themselves yellow representing the sun. This was a spiritual practice where the tribesmen would make an offering by cutting off parts of their skin and dance under the sun in order to receive visions from the spirits of the sky.

The ancient Egyptians have been involved in sun worship rituals since the beginning of their recorded history. They worshipped the sun god Ra for protection and acceptance into the after life. After looking at this topic closer some interesting information comes up. Perhaps the Egyptians were not simply worshiping a god but were gathering information from the sun. The king Akhenaten had ushered in a new time of peace and prosperity after Egypt stopped worshipping many different gods. Akhenaten was said to have brought in the light. There are many depictions of the Pharaohs making offerings to the sun or what could be perceived as communication. When we consume live plant foods we are absorbing the light of the sun which contains cellular education. Cooked food contains calories but living food contains information that literally connects us with the electromagnetic field of our planet.

We now know information literally travels at the speed of light and almost all cultures previous to the industrial age had formed practices relating to the acknowledgement of the sun. It is safe to assume since our human bodies are electrical in nature that we would need a main power grid to keep us powered up. It appears that the sun is just that. We are constantly being downloaded with ideas, thoughts, insights, and inspirations. The sun is our best friend and allows all life to flourish. Without it we lack enthusiasm and the energy to take action in our lives.

We have been told that the sun is damaging to our eyes so we must protect ourselves with darkened sun glasses. Although I do not recommend staring directly into the sun at first this is largely a myth or attempt to sell more merchandise. There are people largely from India and other parts of the world who are for the most part breatharians (See Chapter: **Deconstructing the Diet, Breatharianism**) who are baffling scientists. They claim to get all of their nourishment from the sun by looking deeply into the sun's rays. The problem with sun glasses is that they block out the full spectrum of light that is supposed to be absorbed by our iris or retina. 60% of this light is estimated to be blocked out by sunglasses. If you take off your glasses and try looking into the sun you will have trouble because your eyes are weakened and need to be reconditioned.

Sun gazing while grounded in the beginning of a sun rise and at the very end of a sunset can reset your circadian rhythms in order to regulate regular sleep cycles. Sun exposure also increases positive hormone production, digestive strength, elimination of toxic materials in the body, helps stimulate the capillaries, and allow more blood to flow to the skins surface. If you eat a lot of fruits spend more time in the sun as it helps metabolize the sugar more efficiently.

"The ancient people would call the sun the door way"
Nassim Haramein

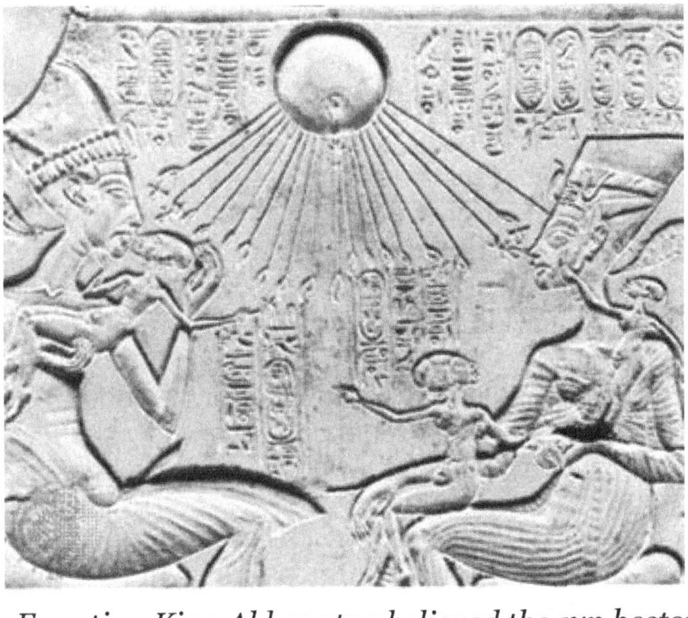

The legendary Egyptian King Akhenaton believed the sun bestowed messages

The Scientific Method

"A new scientific truth does not triumph by convincing its opponents and making them see the light, but rather because its opponents die, and a new generation grows up that is familiar with it."
Max Plank

"All truths are easy to understand once they are discovered; the point is to discover them."
Galileo Galilei

For most of us up to this point we have been taught strictly based other people's ideas, concepts, and theories that, in many cases, were passed on as strict fact. The perpetuation of theoretical statements that turn out to be mere assumptions has presented us the situations that we face right now.

Your unique perception shapes your own viewpoint of how the world is. Too many times we have locked ourselves into limited belief systems that may actually be contradictory to the way the world actually works and even our own best interests. The proposed ideas that are being over turned in each area of thinking is shining new light where there were once only outdated ideas.

In *Thomas Khun*'s ground breaking book **The Structure of Scientific Revolutions** he explains how the general scientific community adhere to the commonplace paradigms of what has been "proven" and eagerly sticks to these ideas in regards to opening the conversation to other possibilities. He implies that the job of normal science is to create solutions for designated problems while making as few changes to the given paradigm as possible. The problem with such a format is that it restricts all incoming information that could form solutions that the current way of thinking cannot provide; it is a limited and flimsy structure like that of a glass house. One of many descriptions of this are articulated in his book: "*Normal science can proceed without rules only so long as the relevant scientific community accepts without question the particular problems-solutions already achieved*".

We can see an identical conduct in every social community ranging from science, religion, martial arts, education, health care, politics, and definitely in the nutrition field. It would appear that even if an outdated theory is obviously not working anymore those that have created a career or personality surrounding it will fight tooth and nail to preserve its image. This attitude is a link to many of the nonsensical problems we face today. The solutions are sometimes so obvious that they stare us right in the eyes. I believe it is imperative to tear down, deconstruct, and completely break apart old ideas that seem to lead in the opposite direction to where we are trying to go in order to actually get there. The words of Frantz Fanon give us tremendous insight into the power of our core belief systems: *"Sometimes people hold a core belief that is very strong.*

When they are presented with evidence that works against that belief, the new evidence cannot be accepted. It would create a feeling that is extremely uncomfortable, called cognitive dissonance. And because it is so important to protect the core belief, they will rationalist, ignore and even deny anything that doesn't fit in with the core belief".

Lets explore some of these ideas that require a deeper probing.

Your Brain in the Dark

"You have more connections in your skull then there are stars in the universe"
Dr. Daniel Amen

The great facilitator of the human experience is the most powerful and complex organ not only in the body, but perhaps in the entire galaxy. The brain is designed to create an unfathomable amount of cellular connections each minute. The lenses in which we look out on life is largely due to the healthy interactions and communication of cells in our brains. There is an epidemic of neurological dis-ease and disruption in civilization at this point in time. In fact it is the very root of every breakdown in relationships, both personal and professional. According to a staggering volume of research in neuroscience that suggests every aspect of our lives such as relationships, behavioral tendencies, habits, thought patterns, and the regular choices we all make daily are effected by the health of our brain. There has been a long held doctrine in the field of brain science that once implied that all the required brain cells you will ever need or ever have already exist. This has been overturned by a study called "neurogenesis", which is when the brain creates new brain cells. The brain makes new connections in the hundreds of thousands every single day, assuming we are not losing more brain cells then we are creating due to poor diet, lack of exercise, negative attitude and relationships, and environmental factors. When we learn new and exciting things every day we promote neurogenesis to take place on a regular basis. This allows us to reach further into our potential as creative and innovative beings.

There is a revolutionary method of identifying the root of an individual's imbalances whether it is depression, chronic cravings, negative thinking, or a list of other detractors of health called SPECT, otherwise known as functional brain imaging device, which looks at the blood flow and functionality of the brain instead of just the image of it. Dr. Daniel Amen is the leading psychiatric doctor and researcher in the field of brain scan analysis. He runs the Amens clinic nationwide which houses the world largest database of brain scans. He believes the quality of the decisions we make every day are a direct reflection of the health of our brain. Dr. Amen in a lecture told a story of a couple that came to see him as they were going through marital counseling. Both of their brains were scanned for possible problems. The husband's brain, as Dr. Amen described, was identical to a long-term alcoholic or drug addict. When asked if he drank or did any kind of drugs the husband assuringly responded that he did not participate in these actions, as confirmed by his wife. As Dr. Amen was reviewing the possible reasons for the husband's brain to have degraded he asked, "what do you do for a living?". The husband told Dr. Amen that he currently works in a furniture factory and his role is to finish furniture all day long. As the connection for his brain health reduction was becoming clear, Dr. Amen asked the wife when did problems in your marriage began. While the wife was recalling their history, she made a startling realization. She responded that her husband's drastic change in behavior began about five years ago when he started working in the furniture factory. People that work in buildings or professions that are giving off toxic materials, such as inhaling airborne solvents, are extremely susceptible to brain deterioration. Professions such as painters, conventional farmers, construction workers, exterminators, and those who work in hair salons are only a few among the population that are being exposed daily.

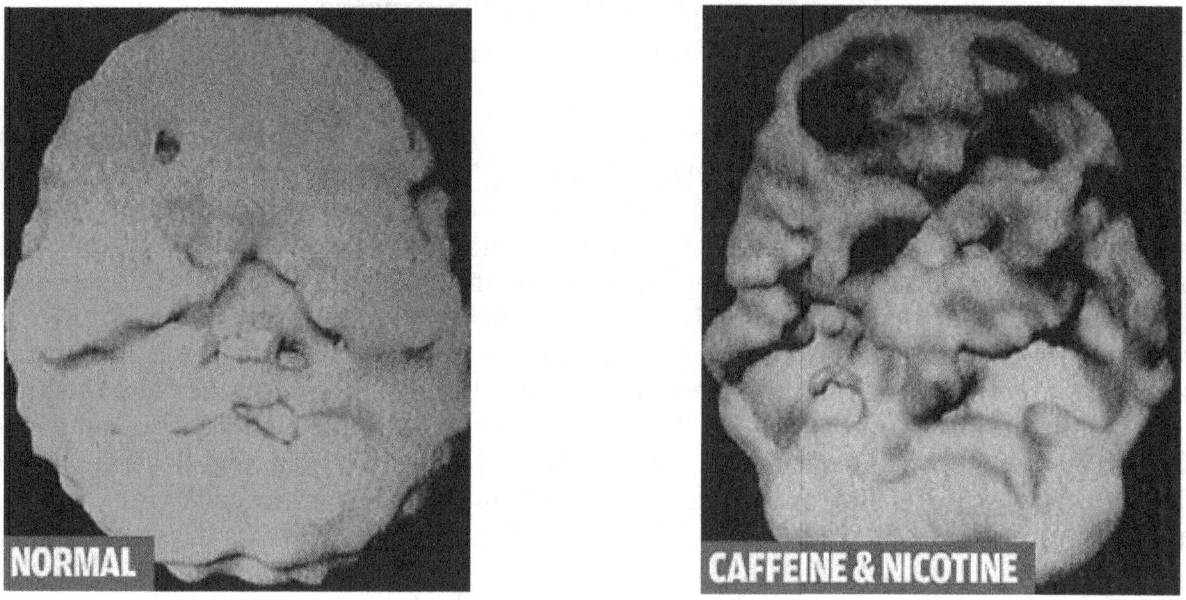

The comparison of a healthy brain scan and a severely unhealthy brain scan

Fat stores toxic material in the body and increases inflammation. When our body is induced in an inflammatory state cells begin to die, including the cells in our brains. Generally people do not notice the significant accumulation of toxins that develop the health crisises that are claimed to be "age-related" dis-eases. This is why people are shocked when they are somehow sidelined with a report stating they have diabetes or cancer, for example. Our thought patterns are being influenced by the inner environment we set up for ourselves, allowing someone to simply assume there is no immediate problem until that fateful day presents itself. It has been estimated that Alzheimer's begins in the body 20-30 years before symptoms physically arise. Every ailment starts from a seed planted in the fertile soil of our body. In order to evade such conditions we must avoid the action steps that lead to these problems.

There is now new research that shows a powerful correlation between obesity and brain damage. As unnecessary weight gain increases the physical size and function of our brain decreases. It is shown that over 300 million people worldwide are considered obese (BMI>30) and a million more are simply considered overweight (BMI>20-25).

The effects of memory loss as aging occurs have been shown to be directly linked to excessive caloric intake. A study was conducted in Olmsted County, Minnesota involving 1,233 people between the ages of 70-89 completely free of dementia. Of this group, 163 people had "MCI" which is the stage of cognition between "normal memory loss" and that of accelerated aging from a dis-eases such as Alzheimer's. The participants of this study logged what they ate and drank in a food questionnaire. They then where divided into three separate and equal groups based on their regular caloric intake. One group consumed between 600-1,526 calories per day, another group consumed between 1,526-2,143 per day, and the final group consumed between 2,143-6,000 calories per day. According to the study, the chances of developing MCI more then doubled for those individuals consuming the highest calorie percentages in comparison to those consuming the lowest calories. Please review the section on calories in the chapter **The Sunfood Connection** to find more information on the benefits of lower caloric intake and higher nutrition intake.

Although the brain is only 2% of your body's weight, it uses 20-30% of the calories you consume. The quality of the food we take in soon becomes the quality of everything we experience thereafter. This fact successfully bridges the gap between the two most powerful laws we know of which are "You are what you think about" and "You are what you eat"!

Leading researcher and UCLA professor Paul Thompson and Cyrus A. Raji authored a journal titled "Human Brain Mapping" which compared the brain tissue reduction of obese and overweight individuals with those who are considered normal weight. In a neuro-imaging study they found those people that were simply "overweight" had a 4% reduction in brain tissue then the normal-weight group. The people who were considered obese had an upwards of 8% loss in brain tissue than those who were normal weight. The significance of this study could go misunderstood unless one considers that, according to the researchers, 8% loss in brain tissue translates into 8 billion neurons lost. The human brain is being reported as containing about 100 billion neurons. In order to drive this idea further, the researchers selected brain scans from a previous study conducted on 94 elderly people in their 70's who were all clear of any cognitive impairments. This was done five years prior to the scans being taken. The researchers then converted the brain scans into detailed three-dimensional images that are designed to offer high resolution mapping of the anatomical differences in the brain. The discovery that these researchers uncovered was that those obese individuals lost 8% tissue in the brain primarily in the frontal and temporal lobes. These specific regions are responsible for planning and memory. Also the regions dealing with long term memory, movement, and attentive functions were affected as well.

(Recommended Book: Change Your Brain Change Your Life by Dr. Daniel Amen)

As I have drove deeper into the scientific theories, as well as the immediate effects nutrition has on our lives, I was exposed to the work of *Tony Wright*. Wright wrote the book **Left in the Dark** and actually holds the world record for the staying awake longer than any human, which is currently 12 days. He is also a long term live foodist. In Tony's book, he focuses on the nature of the left and right hemispheres of our brain. He beautifully shares the patterns of human behavior based on the function of our brain and how humans have, as he believes, actually devolved based on the tampering of our food supply. Despite conventional wisdom that says the human brain has increased in size relatively recently and that we are at the pinnacle of evolution, Wright says human beings were much more evolved biologically 10,000 years ago when eating a much more natural diet that was believed to be primarily of fruits.

I believe the problems that have arisen in our world over the last few hundred years originate heavily from the misunderstanding of how our brains work. The right and left hemispheres of the brain perform completely different functions yet they rely on each other for optimum balance. The left side of the brain is primarily focused on details and calculations, making specific coordinates to get from one point to another. The right side is associated with creativity, expanded imagination, artistry, and deeper layers of connectivity with life. This is important to understand because our brain uses food to not only sustain itself but to function in unique ways, with the possibility of unlocking areas of consciousness not yet explored on a modern diet.

Wright discovered that when humans consume a dominantly altered (processed) and cooked-food diet it disturbs the psychology in a way that makes someone become left-brain dominant. This is an idea I have intuitively understood ever since becoming a sun food practitioner. When you clean up your food intake, your thoughts, feelings, actions, and emotions dramatically change from lack to abundance, from pain to comedy, and from sorrow to inspiration. The majority of society seems to be running a left-brain program, one of a short term viewpoint fueled by immediate results. The right hemisphere is more mysterious, allowing access to a much broader picture of life. Not everything has to be validated by general consensus or a majority-rules style of making judgements.

In the book, **Left In The Dark**, another confirming discovery that live foods is the obvious fuel of choice for human progression was that of Tony Wrights' experiments into sleep deprivation. It has been hinted in many raw food circles that the higher quality living foods you eat, the lower your requirement is for sleep. I have talked about this earlier in this book in the section (See Chapter: **The Sun Food Reality**). What has been found out is that the left side of the brain requires a tremendous amount of rest in order to recuperate. It expends an enormous supply of energy calculating and formulating. This is exactly why most Americans come home right after work dead tired and retire in front of the television- they need to shut their brain off. The exact opposite is true of the right brain. It requires little sleep in order to function at maximum capacity. The right brain can create the most inspiring and exciting experiences all day long and you never get tired. Ask yourself how many times you have come home exhausted and got a phone call or had the idea of doing something you were passionate about and all of a sudden you got a surge of energy. How is it that the most successful people in the world can stay up all day and night doing what they love while completely forget about eating? This is an interesting question to ask yourself the next time you feel sluggish.

This single discovery ties in with the idea that our conventional theories and scientific methods may in fact not be perfect after all. The "general" idea of how the diet does not make a difference, you can eat whatever you like, and if you get sick the doctor will make it all better is false. Getting sick at all, for any reason, is a false assumption only acceptable based on a highly-structured cooked-food theory. All unfounded assumptions of the past are being overturned every single day due to a reintroduction to living-food understanding and common sense consciousness.

The Calcium Theory

In recent years there have been numerous discoveries in all fields of health overturning previously upheld theories, and none, in my opinion, more immediately needing our attention than that of the calcium supplement theory. We have been told for many years that we need to consume more calcium simply because our bones are made of calcium. This idea is not only suspect at first glance, it shows this idea is missing key elements. It becomes apparent that this idea is flawed when we understand that the mineral composition of our bones require magnesium, silica, zinc, phosphorus, boron, manganese, selenium among others, including, of course, calcium.

This idea appears to come from **Lavoisier's (Antoine Lavoisier) Law** which states nothing is lost, nothing is gained, everything is transformed, in this context it is saying an element may change it's shape or form, yet it's original mass remains the same. This idea has been overturned many times. The plausible theory on biological transmutation where one element/mineral can transmute into another was presented by Dr. Louis Kervran. In the book, **Silica The Forgotten Nutrient**, author *Klaus Kaufman* explains one of the most interesting examples of Kervran's belief of biological transmutation going back to Kervran's childhood recollection:

"His parents kept chickens that never received any limestone, nor was their diet in any way supplemented with limestone. Yet every day during the egg-laying season those chickens laid eggs with calcareous shells. Young Kervran observed that the chickens were incessantly scratching for fragments of mica that were strewn around the yard. The boy knew that mica, with feldspar and quartz, contains silica. Why did those chickens search for mica? He watched his mother open the gizzards of slaughtered chickens, finding small grains of sand, but never any mica. What had happened to the mica? How did the calcium get into the eggshell in an area lacking calcium?"

I find it especially interesting that the famous philosopher, activist, and agriculturalist Rudolph Steiner felt most forms of calcium were accelerators of gravitational forces. Gravity has toxic effects on the body when unbalanced by the earth's inherent levitational properties. These properties, sometimes referred to as "Ormus Elements", are heavily concentrated in organic vegetable juice, super foods, medicinal mushrooms, wild grasses, organic raw bee products, and living spring water. It is possible that the counterproductive effects of "gravitational forces" on the body are nothing more than what is now called *calcification*.

Calcification is the excess of bad calcium in the body brought on by what is called calcium-forming organisms or nano-bacteria that was brought to light by over 30 years of research that has been compiled in the book **The Calcium Bomb.** It was one of the first works to really explain the dangers of calcium in isolated supplemental form which, is in most cases, derived from rock sediments mined from the ground or, in many cases, coming from oyster shells or coral, causing coral-stone formations in the bones and joints leading to major arthritic conditions, hardening of the arteries by chalky build up in the arterial walls or otherwise known as arterial plaque. Calcification is being linked to nervous system disorders such as strokes, Alzheimer's disease, and brain tumors. Things such as gallstones, kidney stones, bone spurs are stoney build ups coming from nano-bacteria that, over time, has taken residence in the body, literally furnishing it with terrain modifications that make it more comfortable for the invasive calcium grouping bacteria(parasite) but make it deadly for the host.

As the progress of over calcification continues throughout the body, these bacterial organisms will attract heavy metals such as lead, mercury, cadmium, steal, inorganic iron among other known toxins, such as pesticides and plastics, as a base to fortify themselves in a particular area which eventually leads to skin problems, stiffness of the joints, brain problems, cataracts, heart, and circulatory disorders and even reproductive disorders. These opportunistic organisms seem to gravitate most often to areas in our body where we have scar tissue built up from past injuries making it near impossible to rejuvenate our torn tissues unless we implement strategic tools to break down these calcified walls and escort the nano-bacteria out of the body.

The assumption that we need more calcium in order to produce stronger and longer lasting bone health continues to lead us astray. Bone density is only part of the equation. Bone flexibility is the most important factor in structural health. This is an obvious observation if you look at the nature of a bamboo tree, for example. It is one of the strongest trees in the world not because of its hardness but mainly because it can adapt to the changes in nature where a mighty oak tree might be torn down by a vicious storm. If your bones are over silted up with concrete or calcium-forming organisms then it will restrict your ability to adapt to the changing weather climates and to immediate changes in physical movement. It will also reduce your cells' ability to carry information from one point to another in the process of healing, and the years in your life and the life in your years. Green vegetable juicing is a vital piece to increasing ligament and muscle flexibility. Practicing yoga for increased pliability is highly suggested as improvements in the flexibility of your joints will help release circulatory stagnation and help keep the unwanted guests moving.

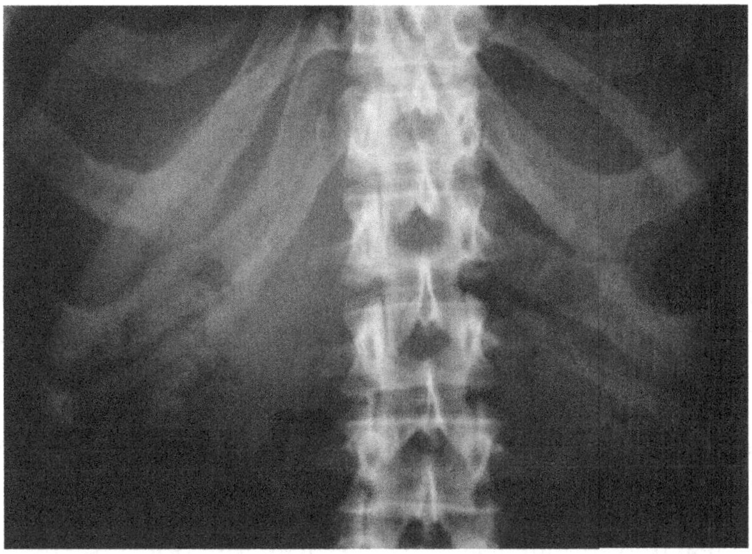

The white spots indicate calcium deposits in the costal cartilage of the sternum Associated with Thyroid disorders

Dr. Robert Thomas, author of the book **The Calcium Lie** admits to prescribe his patients with calcium supplementation for years through his own misinformed education in the medical background. Through his study of tissue mineral analysis, he discovered that excessive calcium in the body was in fact causing the many disorders stated above. Osteoporosis which is a loss of minerals in the bones is not a loss of just calcium. He states that 90-95% of the American population is mineral deficient while having an excess of calcium. If this is not compelling enough then you may find Dr. Thomas' book along with **The Calcium Bomb** available on the internet.

Calcium carbonate is a very commonly found compound in calcium. When heated for the use of the chemical industry it forms marble, chalks, and limestone. If you ever see calcium or carbonate in any ingredients be aware of this. Calcium, when formed with phosphate, creates a form of whats called hydroxlyapatite. This is a mineral portion found in bones and teeth and also has been found in corals. It is found that up to 50% of bones are comprising of inorganic forms of modified hydroxlyapatite which is also a main ingredient in dental enamel and dentin. This inorganic substance is very toxic, especially in high dosages. Mercury fillings from the teeth leach off into the mouth making a bedding ground for nano-bacteria(calcium forming organisms) which disables brain activity. This partial mineral substance hydroxylapatite has been found to leave small calcification crystals in the the pineal gland, contributing to mental disorders such as corpora arenacea otherwise known as "brain sand". It is literally causing sand in the gears of our bodies!

Now it is important to clarify that calcium is extremely important in the human body but the correct source and form of calcium that is completely organic and absorbable. The dairy industry has claimed for years that milk is a great source of calcium. This is simply not true and it is becoming known that the animals being raised today are over calcified as well. Plants have the best and most recognizable forms of calcium which, on an organic living foods diet, is extremely hard not to get more than you need- it is in all green leafy vegetables. I would highly suggest anyone interested in this topic invest into David Wolfe's **Longevity Now Program** that has based years of intensive study on the subject of calcification and how to drive it out of the body.

The Pineal Gland

This tiny gland in between the two hemispheres of our brain is responsible for serotonin release in the brain as well as initiating melatonin, which is believed to be the hormonal response that modulates waking and sleeping cycles. For a long time this small endocrine gland seemed to not be very intriguing, getting overlooked by more "interesting" areas of the body. We have now learned that the function of the pineal gland far surpasses the original speculations and may be the most important area of focus moving into the new conscious transition in our world.

We are now learning about the physiological functions of the pineal gland and coming to a better understanding of how it affects us. Interestingly enough, there has been much discussion and debate regarding this single topic perhaps dating back to biblical times. The pineal gland has been referred to as the "third eye". In the early 1600's, the French philosopher Rene Descartes believed it to be "The Seat of the Soul", feeling that it was the exact point of connection between the intellectual mind and the body. Descartes had an interesting perspective, believing that the pineal gland is positioned in between the two opposite sides of the brain to bridge the gap since we can only have one thought at a time. It makes sense that this gland would be that mediator.

The physical structure of the pineal gland would appear to be the shape of a tiny pine cone with nothing but a watery substance inside. Inside the structure is what is called pinealocytes, the main cell divisions that secrete melatonin production in the brain. These cells have been linked to the photoreceptor cells which are neurons found in the retina of the eye allowing the process of phototransduction to occur. This is the process in which light is converted into electromagnetic signals in the retina of the eye connecting back to the visual cortex of the brain. The pineal gland is stimulated by light. Complete darkness promotes melatonin release which the reason why we have trouble sleeping when we have computer screens or artificial lighting.

David Wilcock, author of **The Source Field Investigations**, has done extensive research on the pineal gland and its relationship with our higher mind or intuitive abilities. He claims that *"the Pineal gland physiologically is the center point in the brain that connects the physical body and the astral body"*. This idea connects much of the historic speculation on the purpose of this gland and how we can actually utilize this information to our benefit in life. The emergence of this subject in such detail is also in my opinion the biggest area of concern when we look into human behavior symptoms. Due to the toxic lifestyles we have become accustomed to, our ability to use our pineal gland productively has been greatly reduced. It has even become completely shut down in many people as they age.

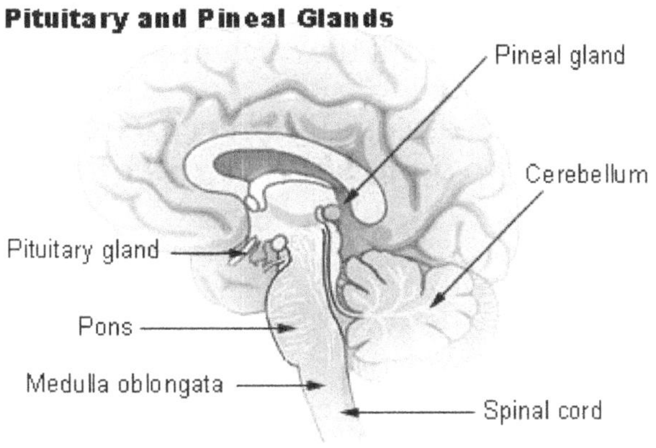

What is actually happening to our pineal as we age is calcification, causing the pinealocytes and other crystals in the water of the cone-like gland to crust over and become deactivated. This is the exact reason why people get age-related mental illnesses: a tumor is created from the microscopic coral shells pushing against the brain. Calcification is not restricted by the blood-brain barrier (the brain's filtration mechanism) and therefore the dangers of a conventional diet will without a doubt contribute to the reduction of one's ability to gain clarity over their life. Your ability to draw ideas and intuitive nudges will become drastically decreased, lowering your spiritual powers. This information directly ties in with Tony Wright's findings about the influence diet has on the brain's focal positioning in terms of intuition or rationalization.

The biggest offenders to the health of our pineal gland are refined foods of all kinds, especially white flour and sugar. All artificially processed foods and fried foods containing trans-fatty acids corrode our cells. I strongly suspect that most cooked foods will have negative effects on brain chemistry (specifically the pineal) based on Paul Kouchakoff's findings (See Chapter: **The Raw Naked Truth,** Section: **Cooked Food**). When our body is in too much of an acidic state (See Section: **Alkalinity)** calcium begins to get pulled from our bones to offset of the overbearing effects of acidosis. This is just my own idea but I would presume that much of the calcification we see may be linked to calcium particles that were once naturally occurring in our bone structure but have become denatured by an acidic reaction, creating an inorganic mineral in the body that re-attaches itself to other regions in the body. Food for thought!

The water from municipal pipes are harshly contaminated with all kinds of chemicals, pharmaceutical residues, chlorine, and fluoride (neurotoxin). The structure of the water is being affected by straight pipes. Conscious water responds to spirals and upward motions as observed by *Victor Schauberger* (See Chapter: The Triangle of Life). The best water to consume is spring water that is coming from the source of the earth. If you are unable to tap into that resource then distilled water that you personally remineralize with natural sea salt and MSM may be your best option.

Eating as much "organic" raw foods, super foods, and immune-boosting-herbs as well as engaging in detoxification protocols are definitely the best way to break up bad calcium deposits in all areas. The modus operandi of this strategy is to give your body the nutrients it needs while crowding out the calcium-producing agents it dreads.

The light of the body is the eye: if therefore thine eye be single, thy whole body shall be full of light.
Matthew 6:22

The Genetic Expression

The study of genetics is the biological focus that deals with heredity and the variability of hereditary traits passed on by very similiar or related organisms. In order to further understand the deeper intricacies of life on this planet, science has used this study to explain the genetic expression of all living things. This is a universal approach to exploring the biological fabric of viruses, bacteria, plants, animals, and most especially human beings since every organism has its own genetics. The idea that a baby inherited certain traits from their parents was very familiar, dating back to ancient times. It was used in attempts to improve crops for agriculture and the selective breeding of domesticated animals. Although this basic understanding has been prevalent throughout time, the modern scientific theories on this subject began in the mid-1800's with the work of Gregor Mendel, an Augustinian priest and scientist.

Mendel is widely known by genetisists as the father of modern genetics. His unique process of discovering what we now know as genetics has been labled as the Mendelian Laws of Inheritance. Eventhough Mendel was unaware of the term "genes" during his time, he was able to determine the genetic inheritence that was passed on from a parenting organism to its offspring. Mendel performed an experiment out of curiosity where he cross-bred pee plants in order to determine how inherent traits are found from one generation to the next. It took about 8 years and 30,000 plants for Mendel to conclude his experiment. Mendel took the tiny reproductive organ(the flower pollen) of the male pea and attached it to the female plant. The mass assumption in those days was that the blending of a male and female resulted in the offspring inheriting equal halfs of each parent. This idea was disproven in many examples. One such example was a black sheep appearing in a consistent offpsring of pure white sheep. A recent experiment was conducted to mimick Gregor's original study by combining wrinkled peas and smooth peas while expecting to get a blend of both. The study conductor was surprised to find the result was almost entirely smooth peas. The following offpsring produced about one third wrinkled peas and two thirds smooth peas. This showed that the previous "dogma" of the day was not accurate, and was merely the constructed belief for which no other answers existed at the time.

"Genes are not destiny!"
Bruce Lipton, Ph.D.

The accepted explanation for all activities within the human body is that our genetic disposition controls who we are. In many circles of the scientific community, the idea that our genes determine every aspect of our personality is even being accepted as a fact. The only alternative theory for our "fixed" genes would be in the rare case of a random genetic mutation. There is a worldwide epidemic that has been pervasive throughout recorded history. This epidemic is perhaps the most destructive of all known dehibillitating occurences: the complete and utter acceptance of bad information. The vast exploration into the field of genetics and biology has provided us with one of the most inspiring ideas of our time: despite physiological setbacks, every human being has not only the power to alter their attitude but to also create a new genetic expression which we call our phenotype. When we are born we inherit certain traits given from our parents gene pool. These traits can vary depending on multiple factors (environment, diet, lifestyle). The human phenotype is simply the physical expression in which certain genes are activated and can be visably seen. For example, your eye color, hair color, complexion, and physical build are all phenotypical expressions. Based on what is easily observable, this is the common method in which modern medicine is operating at. Behind our physical traits there is our genotype, which is simply the genetic make up of an organism, cell, or individual. The health and intelligence of our genes will determine the apptitude in which our physical characteristics can express themselves. It is true that some individuals are gifted with certain genetic advantages like athleticism, smooth skin, thick hair, clear eyes, and strong bones while some individuals may be born less fortuanate. However, the deep hidden truth is that how you entered this world does not have to be the way you leave it.

One of the most basic assumptions pertaining to genetic dispositions is the idea that we undoubtably take on the conditions of our parents or our parents' parents. There is a vast body of research that indicates the above assumptions are accurate. The problem in this scenerio is the relunctance to investigate this situation further.

The manner in which our genetic material is able to fulfill it's potential is most influenced by the environment in which we are consistently exposed to. Throughout evolution, spanning eons of time, certain species have developed physiological traits that allow them to more readily adapt to their surroundings with upgrades such as horns, claws, and fangs. In this same way, all organisms are easily suseptible to devolution as well, which is the regression of optimal traits such as strength and speed. In the human condtion, traits such as emotional integration, brain activity, and ultimately the healing process are also subject to devolution. If we look at this topic objectively, the root of the problem becomes undeniable obvious. If the phrase "you are what you eat" is actually taken seriously, then we may discover one of the greatest truths that exists in each of our lifetimes.

The most obvious factor in relation to adopting the genetic fate of our senior relatives is less about heridity, and almost entirely on whether we adopt the lifestyle habits that created the poorly functioning genes we blame for our setbacks.

In order to take a step further into the great mystery of human potential as it pertains to the increasing of our genetic intelligence, we must first explore our DNA. DNA(deoxyribonucleic acid) structuring in the human body was first discovered in 1953 by geneticists James Dewey Watson and Francis Crick. This was a powerful discovery and has led to the expanded understanding of who we truly are at the microscopic level.

Every one of our genes carries with it information that is stored in unfathomably long strands of DNA. The human DNA is structured like a long spiral ladder called the double helix. Each step of the double helix ladder is made of four key chemical bases which are Adenine, Cytosine, Guanine, and Thymine. The combination of these four sugar/phosphate molecules determines our genetic output(phenotype). The entire DNA sequence that takes place along this double helix ladder is what we now call our genome. According to the most recent analysis, the human genome is constructed from 3,200,000,000 base pairs. The reality of this has been noted as saying for someone to type out the length of our DNA, it would require a typing speed of 10 words per minute for 8 hours a day over 50 years. If you unwrapped the the composition of your DNA from only one single cell it would span 6 feet long. If you unwrapped your entire DNA structure of every single cell in your body it would reach the moon 6,000 times! This fact may not mean a lot to the average person, but when we consider how extremely expansive the human genome truly is, it may create a surfacing curiosity as to how and why the prevelence of mediocrity in the human culture has reigned over us like a dark shadow. As curiosity grows, the proposed paradigms that pose greater questions than they are capable of answering begin to break apart. One of those pervasive paradigms is the idea of "Junk DNA".

The term "junk DNA" is a loose non-scientific term that is basically attempting to classify a multitude of our DNA that is believed to hold no biological function, otherwise known as "non-coding DNA". The best example to describe this idea is to open up a mainstream magazine where the bulk of the pages contain content that is relevant to the magazine like articles and stories. This what would be considered the coding DNA. Non-coding DNA or "junk DNA" would be the non-relevant advertisements that have no connection to the content of the magazine; essentially it is empty matter. The basis for this theory can be more vividly explained by some of the biggest proponants of its validity. Biologist John Avise of the University of California had this to say: *"Non-coding repetitive sequences-'junk DNA'-comprise the vask bulk of the human genome"*. The world-recognized biologist Richard Dawkins is quoted saying "*It is a remarkable fact that the greater part of the genome might as well not be there, for all the difference it makes"*.

The concept sustaining the theory of junk DNA seems to rest on the premise that human beings could not possible have been constructed out of an intelligent design based on the fact that 95% of our genome contains 'non-protein-coding DNA (junk DNA). Many view this as prime evidence that Darwinian evolution was accurate because if we were created from an intelligent designer then how could the bulk of our genomic material be useless? I do not presume to have the answers to seal this controversial debate within the biology community. I am not a biologist yet I have observed the varying opinions, attitudes, and speculations that dominate this field. The very idea that a biologically active human being could delete a vast portion of their DNA structure and be no worse off for it is, in my opinion, at the extremes of unconsciousness. It once took a tremendous amount of time for new research and differing points of view to be widely accepted in place of long held beliefs.

In the last ten or so years a new perspective on the entire field of genetics has taken shape known as Epigenetics. The original idea of each human having fixed genes is now being overturned due to a revolutionary new method in which science can identify the markers for not only a bigger picture of what our genetic potential may be, but also how we can willingly alter our genetic expression through lifestyle modifications. Epigenetics is the study of the change in gene activity that are caused outside of the DNA sequence or gene code but still pass on to the successive generation. Epigenetics explores a vaster picture of the human genome through the discovery that certain genes can be turned on and turned off like a light switch. The natural patterns of our genetic expression has been indicated to be the result of the cellular material that rests directly on top of each gene. The information that is carried through each one of these cells creates the markers that inform our genes whether to turn on or turn off. Biologists in the field may compare epigentics to a computer. The computer hardware(genome) remains the same but the software(epigenome), which programs the computer, can differ greatly, altering the characteristics of the computer based on the programming. The idea that we can program and reprogram our most delicate cellular material to produce a variety of results is not only a powerful discovery; it should be blatantly obvious to anyone who has gained or lost a considerable amount of weight. There is strong evidence that all lifestyle factors have deep implications on which genes are signaled for activation and which ones are silenced. Behaviors such as smoking, over consumption of alchohol and food, along with heavy amounts of stress, all influence our genetic expression. The epigenetic markers can literally trigger genes that are programmed for obesity if they are expressed too strongly which, in contrast, depresses the genes that are meant to trigger longevity.

A key factor that has been brought to light is the subject of telomeres which are repeating DNA sequences residing at the end of each of our chromosomes. Their function is to help protect the chromosomes from cellular deteriation and to stop our chromosomes from fusing to each other. It has been shown that as our telomeres shorten, the aging process accelerates. Telomeres shorten when there are "cell divisions" occuring. The replication of our cells is what allows our molecular clock to keep on ticking. When our telomeres become too short the chromosomes reach their peak and are then unable to replicate. This translates into the death of a cell due to a process known as apoptosis which is a "pre-programmed" death of that cell. New research is consistently coming to light that these telomeres are the missing key to our genetic advancement. This is being dubbed by some scientists as the "immortal cell theory".

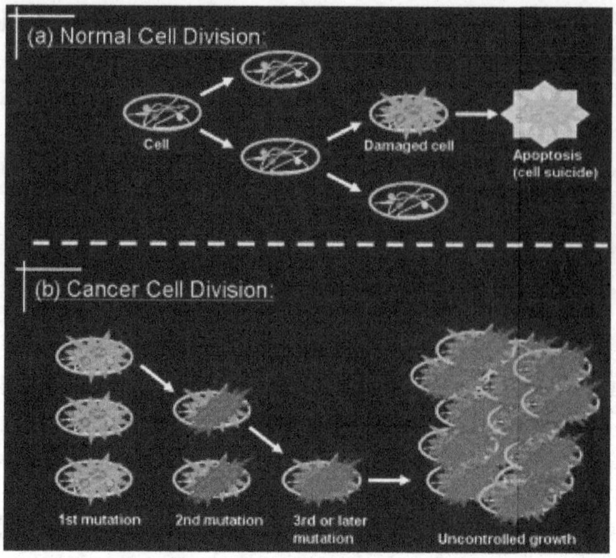

Compare the difference in cell division growth between normal cells and cancer cells. Once a cell becomes influenced by a cancer it begins to replicate out of control eventually taking over it's host. The information delivered to a healthy cell is replaced by an invasive organism preprogramming it's host for sickness.

The power that this information provides lies in whether or not we can reverse the aging process or, better yet, reverse the process of telomere shortening. The lifespan of the telomere is dependant on an enzyme known as telomerase, which is inactive in most people. This enzyme can become triggered by the reduction of what caused it to deactivate it and the inclusion of what encourages its expression. Before the discovery of the Hayflick Limit in 1961, the point in which normal cell division production ends due to the shortened telomeres, there was a belief that vertebrate cells carried an unlimited ability to recreate themselves. If anyone looks onto the general public for evidence it may become very obvious that this theory is not true unless the premise this theory was built on was excluding the most critical factor in the validation of this idea. The long held consensus on genetic potential for human beings has never really been explored. The true markers for genomic variability are environment, diet, lifestyle behaviors, and psychological stressers. The very idea that was announced not long ago that cancer or even diabetes could be strictly based on genetics calls into question the entire structure of which this paradigm was constructed. The word cancer implies a variety of dis-eases that have become worldwide epidemics in only recent historical times. Cancer in the way we identify it did not exist over one hundred years ago and certainly not in the prevalent manner taht it does today. The word cancer implies a replication of "misinformed cells" that perpetuate a cycle of growth, continuing to spread throughout its host. Every epidemic form of dis-ease is literally a cancer, therefore basing it on heredity alone makes little sense considering the exceedingly different forms of dis-ease that have only recently spread through the western world.

Consider this paragraph from *A. True Ott, Ph.D* from his book, **Wellness Secrets for Life:**

"Always keep in mind and understand what causes cells to mutate. To prevent cancer from forming you need proper virus controls, proper pH levels, low pollution levels, and proper nutrition. It is a fact that most people in the West have been 'inoculated' with 'live cultures' of certain bacteria and viral infections (i.e. polio, measles, rubella, etc.). It is also a fact that these 'live cultures' very often 'hide' in one or more of your major organs and/or spinal fluid and are totally impervious to your immune system. Some organ 'problems' often appear years later and such problems are caused by these 'hiding hosts' introduced by well-meaning health practitioners.

A great wave for change in our current and ever-evolving understanding of biology was created over four decades ago by the former stem cell biologist, Bruce Lipton. He performed an experiment where he isolated a single stem cell culture and placed it into an empty petri dish. Lipton observed that the stem cell would reproduce itself every ten hours and, after a number of days, there were thousands of cells in the dish. The real discover came when Dr. Lipton removed a number of cells from the original petri dish and placed them in three different dishes that all had different "growth mediums". In other words, the cells were placed in different environments. These cells all contained identical DNA structures and, according to the original theory, these cells should develop in identical fashion despite the environment they grow in. The result of this experiment took Dr. Lipton by surprise. Cell Subject A formed muscle cells, Cell Subject B formed bone cells, and Cell Subject C formed fat cells. This showed that the popular idea that the nucleus in the cell performed an identical to the brain in a human was inaccurate. The nucleus actually functions more like our reproductive system, producing new proteins (building blocks) and new cells. It turns out that the mitochondria of our cellular structure is more appropriatedly considered as the brain of the cell, and this is the cells skin coating which is the most receptive signaling agent translating messages from our outer environment into our inner environment. Human beings are basically skin covered petri dishes as Dr. Lipton explains. The skin is the largest organ in the body and is "inheriting" all of the influences it comes into contact with.

The greatest "culture medium" within the human body is our blood. If our blood is too thick and acidic we will experience degenrative effects in the body. This is why chlorophyll and oxygen therapies are tremendously effective- they help build back our blood. In order to reprogram the genetic code that is playing on repeat within each of our cells we must wipe the floppy disk clean. We must flush out the system by examining the foods, liquids, and environment we expose ourselves to. Drinking the best quality water you possible can is essential to cleansing and rebirthing our body- nature's solution to pollution is always dilution. Water is the greatest transportation vehicle for carrying information into our body through the blood. In fact, as you saturate yourself with water (or whatever liquid you drink) it becomes your blood. If you drink water that is carrying the toxic residue of municipal waterpipes and recycled city reminants, your internal environment will be constructed out of these materials. Since 2009 it has been stated by the Environmental Working Group(EWG) that there is over 300 known pollutants in tap water.

One very well known contaminant in tap water is chlorine, which is an antibiotic in it's 'chemical' nature as its purpose is to eliminate bacteria and microorganisms in the water supply. Chlorine initiates free-radical production in the human body, compromising the immune system, and thus accelerating the aging process. It has been estimated that taking in chlorine from showering is the equilvelant to drinking eight glasses of unfiltered tap water. Hot water vapourizes chlorine, creating a toxic steam similiar to poison gas in a gas chamber. The skin opens up due to heat and absorbs toxins directly into our intracellular structure, creating a genetic disposition that not only the person themselves must contend with, but will be expressed in future generations as the cycle persists.

Probiotics are extremely valuable tools to help assist the beneficial bacteria inside our bodies. It is estimated that the bacteria that lives in our body out numbers our cells by a factor of 10:1. Chlorine, anti-bacterial soap, and pharmacutical anti-biotics deplete our digestive tract of these much needed bacteria. According to Dr. Joseph Mercola, 80% of our immune function is based on the health of our digestive system.

Historically, the use of pesticides, herbacides, and all kinds of chemical fertilizers was non-existent in traditional farming. People consumed these foods along with wild foods that grow in nature with no assistance from human hands. It was not until the widespread popularity of clearing out large stretches of land for mono-cropping that people stopped growing food in a normal and integral way, a method which has been lost through time due to supermarket-focused agricultural practices. The very first step everyone must move towards is completely organic foods. The weaker and sicker the plant the weaker and sicker the person who eats that plant. Pesticides have been widely known to severely impair our nervous system (neurological), reproductive system, endocrine system, thyroid, and literally shut down our entire immune function, resulting in many common auto-immune conditions. Farmers and gardners who work closely to chemically treated crops have been known to be far more likely to develop neuro-degenerative disorders such as Parkinson's Disease. Chemicals of all kinds disrupt our DNA strands by intruding into our cells, turning certain genes on (cancer cells for example) and switching others off (immunological cells), causing the deformation of our phenotype(gene expression) into what we know as a dis-ease.

What is possibly the most obvious deterent to our health and genetic potential is the introduction of genetically modified foods(GMO). Genetically engineered foods are created in a laboratory where the genes from one organism are taken and artificially implanted into the genes of an unrelated organism. Genetics from insects, animals, viruses, bacteria, and humans are mixed and matched to create artificial trans-genetic deemed as food. The implications on our own DNA by consuming genetically and artificially altered foods should be half-way evident by now. According to the Institute For Responsible Technology(IFRT) the current highest commercialized GM crops in the U.S. are soy(94%), cotton(90%), canola (90%), sugar beets (95%), corn(88%), Hawaiian papaya (more than 50%), and zucchini and yellow squash (over 24,000 acres). The IFRT has documented an enormous supply of information regarding the health aversions related to GM foods and products in studies done on rats such as:

- GM soy drastically reduces digestive enzymes in mice. If it also impairs your digestion, you may become sensitive and allergic to a variety of foods.
- Rats fed GM potatoes had smaller, partially atrophied livers.
- More than half the babies of mother rats fed GM soy died within three weeks.
- The DNA of mouse embryos functioned differently when their parents ate GM soy
- By the third generation, most hamsters fed GM soy were unable to reproduce.
- Babies of female rats fed GM soy were considerably smaller, and more than half died within three weeks (compared to 10% of the non-GM soy controls).
- The longer mice were fed GM corn, the less offspring they had, and the smaller their offspring were.

The fact that our DNA is and has been changing due to the introduction of toxins, mediocre diets, GM/processed foods, radiation, and electromagnetic fields is being brought to the forefront by scientists in the field of epigenetics. The very future of the human race depends on healthy people reproducing into healthier and more intelligent people. Health must be an evolution and not a devolution as we move into the future. The greatest example of adverse genetic changes show up in the acceleration of chronic illnesses across all ages, regardless of culture. Infant mortality rates appear to be at the very peak of the list in terms of major markers for downward changes in the United States, a country that was once number 1 in health has now dropped to number 50. The average sperm count has dropped 50% in only a few short decades, and the human immune system has dropped even further below that. This means that much fewer people are capable of reproducing children and the ones that do will produce genetically inferior models.

According to the once held belief of evolution by Charles Darwin, "survival of the fittest", those who are the strongest and best adapted will have the greatest chance to survive and thrive. If this is even remotely true then it would indicate that future generations would gradually improve as they progressed along the evolutionary track. In our case, we are going through dramatic devolution, where the proceeding generations are getting weaker, less adaptable, and unable to reproduce for the future.

While the influence of outside factors has been shown here to heavily impact the potential of healthy genes, what is affecting us on the inside may be even more urgent. One of the reasons I have chosen to leave meat out of my lifestyle indefinitely is due to the high concentration of parisitical organisms that reside in all meat products. Meat/fish coming from supermarkets is left out in an open air environment susceptible to a variety of pathogeons (bacterial organisms). The utensils used for cutting and preparing meat, such as knives and wooden cutting boards, can retain microscopic parasites that get into our food from constant use. Parasites manipulate a person's DNA by influencing the internal environment to suit its own needs. It uses a host primarly as a housing station to sustain its own life with no regard for its host. Human beings, when healthy, operate on a negative electrical charge. Parasites operate at a positive electrical charge, meaning that in order for this organism to sustain itself, it must create an environment(acidity, heavy metals, plastics, sugar, rancid oils, stress) that is counter conducive to the health of its human host. Parasites thrive in pollution where bacteria, yeast, and fungus are prevelant. The amount of people harboring these creatures in their bodies is staggering. If someone gets a colonic and is heavily loaded with parasitical organisms, then that person may be able to see these organisms pass through the extraction tube as they are released from the body. One of the key reasons why children inherit the same viruses or de-habilitation as their parent is believed by many to be because of "genetic parasites" passed onto the child through the umbilical cord. The function of a parasite, whether we are speaking of a bacteria, viruses, or lengthy parasites such as tapeworms, is to inhabit a viable host and replicate itself for breeding. If our immune system is already compromised by a detrimental lifestyle and diet, parasites can slip past the guardianship of white blood cells and creep into our organ/glandular system. In the hallmark book on the subject, **ParasiteRex**, author *Carl Zimmer* states *"They use their hosts-their fellow genes-to get themselves replicated. Like more conventional parasites, genetic parasites can harm their host. As they insert themselves at random places in the genome, they can cause disease. Because genetic parasites can replicate at a faster rate then their fellow genes, they have swamped the genome of many hosts, including humans".*

Parasite cleanses are a critical area to look at for the rejuvination of our bodies and minds. When we clean up the inner ecosystem of our bodies we naturally clear out the food supply that these organisms thrive on and they will no longer have a hold on our health or behaviors.

The information that has been presented through this specific topic leads us to the very core idea that as we identify the triggers for gene mutations and cellular atrophy, we may begin to see how we can change our general outline of this story. When we explore the different ideas that surround the concept of "free will" we may discover things we once did not consider, such as the idea that going against the grain of mainstream promotions we can actually become something far different than we once thought was possible. The idea of "genetic determinism", where genes determine your phenotype, has long held a pigeonhole in the minds of people for the entirety of modern scientific inquiry. This idea provides comfort for the "victim attitude" to sustain itself. Victimism is convenient because it supports complacency and irresponsibility which also supports the need to be rescued. This creates a wide open door for corporate entities such as the supplement and pharmaceutical industry to flourish. There is no longer any question that the frequency/vibration of our thoughts and emotions do alter our genetic make up through time, programming us to display certain characteristics of attitude which allow us to broaden our view of life. Napolian Hill once said, *"What the mind of man can conceive and believe, it can achieve".* If you can begin to believe the possibility of altering your phenotype is real you will instill the sense of self-reliance into your physical make up, through consistency and patience results will begin to prove this point.

Human beings are the only life form on the planet that is known to be fully aware of our own mortality. The victim mindset is deeply rooted into the consciousness of almost every person through generational imprinting. The fear of a life that is fleeting can cause one to allow complacent actions to increase, believing there is no way out of our destined outcome, or it can begin to shift someone in the direction of action steps leading them to higher and higher possibilities for their extended life. The raw food/vegetarian path is philosphically based within the "culture of life" whereas the dead-food diet is based within the ever prevalant "culture of death". The corellation between our biological aging(physical state of aging), psychological aging(mental state of aging), and chronological aging(age measured by time) is important to examine. The psychological stressers can create biological markers such as wrinkled skin, dark puffy eyes, hair loss, and lack of sufficient movement over the duration of our lifespan. The most accepted theory of aging is based in chronology, which attempts to predict the general markers for aging based on number of years one has lived up. From 1912-1940 a Nobel Prize laureate Dr. Alexis Carrel performed an experiment where he kept cells from a chicken heart alive and reproducing for 28 years (the average life span of a normal chicken is eight years). He was able to do this by keeping the cells in a clean environment with the proper nutrient/mineral balance, pH, appropriate temperature, and replacing the solution daily to remove any toxic wastes. The cells actually did not die on its own after this 28-year experiment, they simply stopped the project. This is one more indication that we are not inherently programmed for age-related dysfunctions or possibly even death as we may have believed.

The cell is immortal. It is merely the fluid in which it floats that degenerates. Renew this fluid at regular intervals, give the cell what it requires for nutrition, and as far as we know, the pulsation of life can go on forever."

Dr. Alexis Carroll, Nobel Prize Winner

The general paradigm that is now taught in the western culture is based on the Newtonian understanding of our world at its core which is entirely mechanical in its philosophy. While Newton was a great mathematician, his ideas on physics where very much at an entry level understanding compared to the progress we have made since then. The approach to standardized medicine is formed around the idea that our bodies are a machine. If you want to fix the machine then you have to go into the machine, take out the malfunctioning parts and replace them with new parts. The discovery of quantum physics shows that there is a magnetic field that links all living organisms together. Without this field, the individual parts loses their ability to function correctly. Albert Einstein brilliantly drove this point home when he stated "*The field is the sole governing agency of the particle*". This single idea then opens the door where we may find a new realm of possibilities to exist, not only for the rehabilitation of any health aversion but, perhaps, for exceeding the genetic limitations we have been imposed to believe that we have up to this point.

If you look back on the section, **Cooked Food**, there may be no examples more clear as to how the quantum reality can be more practically implemented. The introduction of kirlian photography as an art form broke the visual barrier towards the intuitive nature of our food beliefs and showed that raw and living plant foods do indeed hold the most electrically charged field in which ionic particles can exist. Kirlian photography, as a science, has explored situations where two individuals displaying anger towards each other and situations where two individuals expressing love for one another. The difference in energy emitted in these examples are as profound as the differences Dr. Masuro Emoto's experiments on projecting opposing emotions into water. The actual structure of water molocules change their shape while greatly enhancing the DNA of the water by the influence of energetic imprintations of a human being's emotions (See Chapter: **The Triangle of Life, Water**). As I have mentioned in the previous chapter, our body is mostly concentrated water. When healthy, each cell of our body may in fact be a structured water bag. This example serves to drive the critical importance of saturating your body with raw plant foods, especially water rich fruits and vegetables that are grown with love, reverence, and free of all chemical add-ons.

Overview of methods to prevent cellular damage and healing protocols for healing genetic weaknesses:

Habits to Avoid:

- Cooked/oxidized oils (canola, vegetable oils, cooked olive oil, etc.)
- Genetically Modified Foods (corn, potatoes, soy products, sugar beets, papayas, seedless fruit)
- Raw Meat & Farm Fish (heavily concentrated with parasitic organisms)
- Conventional Produce (make sure the label begins with a 9 to indicate organic)
- Contaminated Water (tap water, plastic bottles, etc.)
- Processed foods and Artificial Ingredients (High Fructose Corn Syrup, aspartame, fast food, soda, sports drinks, artificial flavoring, etc.)
- Conventional Dairy Products

Habits to Increase:

- Super Foods (algaes, green powders, medicinal mushrooms, goji berries, marine phytoplankton, aloe vera, noni fruit, camu camu, coconut products, hemp seeds, chia seeds)
- Green Vegetable Juices (no less than one green juice a day)
- Super Herbs (pau d'arco, he shou wu, mucuna, cat's claw, ashwaganda, ginseng, astragulus, tribulus, deer antler, etc.)
- High Grade Water (natural spring water, distilled water)
- Sea Salt (salt water flushes are incredible for mineralizing the body and helping to abstain from heavy foods)
- Pro-biotics & Fermented Foods (improves the gut flora which houses the majority of our biological functions)
- Meditation (focus on your healing process)
- Support (surround yourself with only positive and supporting people!)

Peak Performance

"The most important skill of the future is being able to learn and master information immediately"
David Wolfe

I believe within every person, regardless of circumstances or setbacks, there is a specific set of skills that are intrinsic to that person. Each one of us is special, we all have an inner light that carries subconsciously recorded knowledge of the ancient world. Awareness of this fact is awaiting permission by the beholder, similar to that of the samurai's yielding the impeccable craftsmanship of the katana that can only be wielded by the one who knows how to draw upon its brilliance.

We are accomplishment-driven creatures, only truly satisfied when our energy is being poured into the focus of our desires. The unease some feel in life can be attributed to the direction they have chosen to focus their lives. If what you do from day to day does not cause impulsive moments of creative inspiration then it is possible you are on the wrong track. Everyday should bring circumstances, people, events, and new ideas that stimulate higher levels of performance in the chosen venue of your life. The limits of human potential have yet to be tapped. Many people think they know what the limits are but fail to realize that any limits imposed are coming from a limited frame of reference. Be rest assured, you have no limits at your best. You can re-map your life in a way where you can have all the time, energy, resources, and assistance to write all the books, read all the literature, travel through all the countries, meet the most amazing people, and excel in any field you pour your life-force into.

The world opens up its doors that were once unavailable when you do what you love. The structured nature of how we view time completely stops, and we begin to live outside of rules, regulations, and restrictive patterns. The level of performance you are able to achieve is in direct proportion to how much passion you have for something. How much of yourself you are willing to give is only half of what you will receive; you will actually double your investment by developing your strengths instead of focusing on your weaknesses. You already have the power inside, it will be up to you to recognize and then actualize.

Physical Efficiency

The human body is truly an amazing work of art from all angles. Every area of the body from our nails, fingers, eyes, arms, and hair follicles are, at the microscopic level, formed from tiny atoms. These atoms form together to create our cells which are essentially the blueprint of our entire body. The efficiency of your cellular health will dramatically improve every single aspect of your lifestyle. The way we interact with the world around us physically, visually, vocally, and collectively is greatly influenced by how well the cells in this body are communicating.

In 1859, Charles Darwin, famous for the Darwinian Theory of Evolution, believed that the traits and character behavior of an individual were determined by genetic disposition. Modern science is deeply rooted in this theory and through the study of cellular biology we are finding that your genetics can be altered naturally if you understand the ways in which the body operates, especially in terms of how your cells influence your digestive system, reproductive system, excretory system, circulatory system, muscular system, endocrine system, respiratory system, and all additional functions of the body.

One may have thought of a cell as a seemingly insignificant particle in the body when considering how there are trillions of them circulating depending on who you ask. In truth, these cells are extremely intelligent, constantly moving and absorbing new information in order to build new cell factions that are geared in that particular direction of development. The interesting thing about cellular functioning in the body is they seem to form micro-communities that split off into new regions of the body to perform specific actions much like a community of people all serving different functions in society or a tribe. Cellular Biologist *Bruce Lipton* in his book, **The Biology of Belief**, likens cells to humans in their identical nature. Cells, like humans, are directly influenced by their surroundings. If the environment in which the cell is in is toxic then cell becomes toxic, and therefore its ability to carry out tasks for the body becomes weakened. Cells are like humans in the way they learn information and use it in order to produce similar results, much the same way a parent will pass on their experience to a child whether it is accurate or inaccurate information.

We are the result of what we repeatedly do. If this statement is true, which I believe it is, then our physical make up is the result of what we habitually think, say, do, and eat. Whenever you think a certain thought it creates a wave of information that is sent through the nervous system. With time, more thoughts and words of that nature will have physical effects because the body always follows the mind. The food or substances you put into your body over time will prove their worth. Physical deterioration is absolutely inescapable when you are constantly picking up the bread crumbs that lead to its doors. If you have built up these habits over time, you now have the choice to begin reprogramming your genetic make up to work for you instead of against you.

I strongly believe that the key to spiritual activation is through the body first. In fact, it is infused with the spirit- there is no separation when one's nutrition is aligned with the physical body and the light body. I have seen many people in the 'spiritual' community who believe the highest form of being is leaving out the physical and only focusing on the etheric realms. This is an interesting point of view, but as a life long martial artist and athlete, I have to beg to differ. We are on this planet in these bodies for a reason. I say instead of neglecting them we should find out as much as we can and use them as best we can by challenging them with multiple forms of exercise and experimenting with the highest quality food the world has to offer.

The body is able to adapt to almost any circumstance and environment if given the appropriate time and conditions to do so. If you are just starting to change your dietary patterns you should do it at the pace you are most comfortable with. Of course there will be changes that your body must process so be patient with it because you will soon notice incredible results take over. If you are coming from the standard diet then the chances are your cells have been dealing with a level of toxicity that has been overwhelming. There has been an inner war going on because when your cells detect foreign invaders they immediately dispatch defense squads (white blood cells) to resolve the issue. Imagine if this is happening every day- that is a lot of stress on your digestive track followed by your entire body.

Keys to maximize physical efficiency:

- **Eat only what you require:**

Generally speaking, people are consuming calories several folds over that which their bodies are even close to needing per day. If you begin to drink clean or preferable spring water(add sea salt) when you feel a little hungry, that will give you a good signal if your are just thirsty or actually hungry. Space out your meals by 3 to 4 hour or longer on a given day in order to maximize the digestive power. If you compound too much food on top of left overs it will block up and interfere with absorption, causing decreases in energy, inflammation, and reduced brain function over time. I find myself having more energy when I eat less. I feel more on point and can stay up longer even without adequate rest as long as I am consuming nutrient-rich plant foods and super foods.

- **Drink Most of your Meals:**

It has become my own personal experience that if you can turn 60-75% of your meals into liquid such as smoothies, teas, and vegetable juice then the feeling that comes over your digestion is nothing short of incredible. You will have regular bowel movements signaling that the food is moving right through as it should. Also, if you do splurge once in awhile you will not feel the effects as much because the intestines are clear of corrosive residue blocking the pathways.

The food we eat must be broken down into a liquid form for optimal digestion and absorption. We need to pre-signaturize everything we put into our bodies since our cells are so intelligent that they will either accept it or attempt to reject it. Human saliva contains electrolytes, mucus, antibacterial compoundds, and enzymes. It is recommended to chew your food until it is completely liquified. Chewing can be even as high as 50 times per bite! By doing this you are coating your food with extra bacterial disinfectants as well as enzymatic aid for breaking down food. By focusing on chewing up your food you indirectly increase serotonin production in the gut.

When you turn your meals into liquids you are increasing your water intake and therefore do not have to measure how many cups of water you drink each day.

- ◦ **Barefoot on the Earth:**

As mentioned in the section **The Triangle of Life** it is crucial for us to get connected barefoot on the bare earth for maximum health potential. Our bodies require the electrical currents from the earth to offset the abusive force that gravity places on us. Gravity is the force in the world which keeps our bodies stuck to the ground and levitation is the force that uplifts the body(at the cellular level) which brings life to all of the internal functioning. If you always have shoes on your feet there is an extreme gravitational force suppressing your body's ability to heal itself which actually causes more physical problems. Rubber-soled shoes are insulators to your connection to the earth's ability to balance the atmospheres of negative(levitation) and positive(gravity) currents. Levitation is uplifting, affecting the fluidity of your body and joints, influences blood thinning(smooth blood), and brings stability to the right and left hemispheres of the brain. When you are barefoot in nature you are deeply connected to all the animals, flowers, plants, trees, and all creations of life like a web of consciousness that heals and builds at the same time.

The most obvious observation when looking at the biological constitution of our body is that we are actually a mobile column of water which is vibrating at a frequency that is being influenced by our environment and, in this case, the earth's magnetic pulse. Most neurological conditions come from a few different areas such as refined and artificial food preservatives, excessive simple sugars, heavy metals, lack of brain oils (EPA, DHA), mineral deficiencies, and lack of negative electrical charge from the earth for the assimilation of nutrients needed by our brains and body. When we connect barefoot on the earth the charge is lifting through our bodies, the very last place it goes is to the head. In order to maximize the potential of your health it would be a wise idea to lay down on the earth or grass with your head touching directly in order to get the full benefits. If you have a headache then do this to feel the difference it can make!

"When you run on the earth and run with the earth, you can run forever"
Born to Run, Christopher McDougal

- **Effective Exercise:**

Exercise is critical to the human body for strengthening, increasing bone density from weight-bearing movements, and actually becoming more intelligent. Aristotle once said "you must be fit in order to think". Aristotle had his philosophy students train with the olympic athletes because he knew that real thinking requires full engagement of the body, not just the mind as some would assume. Bruce Lee, one of the greatest thinkers of the last century was as finely tuned physically as anyone could be. He wrote many great books, developed a unique system of martial arts and philosophical ideas that revolutionized the martial arts and fitness approach.

Now before you run out the door to the gym it is paramount to understand what types of exercise are productive for your body and which ones are destructive over the short and long term. It seems many people are focused on cardiovascular exercises like long distance running, the treadmill, the stationary bike, triathlons, etc. I see most people doing long intervals of cardiovascular exercises which are really burning calories. An overly excessive regimen of aerobic exercise can break down muscle fibers, joint health, and can accelerate the aging process as I will explain below. The constant wear and tear of long distance single-motion activities can leave one with an extremely thin look if not coupled with anaerobic exercise like weight training or short explosive types of exercises.

The problem with most exercise regimens is that they are only working on slow muscle fibers whereas the optimal health benefits lie within our "super fast muscle fibers". The types of exercises I would have people incorporate would be short-burst sprinting, box jumping, squats, hill running, high-intensity short-period intervals on the stationary bike or incline treadmill(raised up), fast-paced swimming routines, and other routines that can be done in a minimal time frame and exert the maximum amount of energy. If you are not out of breath by the end of your routine then you are not putting forth enough energy. Higher intensity plus minimum output of extended time has been shown to produce Human Growth Hormone(HGH) in the body. This increases testosterone levels which is anabolic, meaning it increases muscle growth, strength, bone density, and increased maturation of the sexual organs.

As someone who has been deeply involved and dedicated as a high-performance athlete in multiple arenas of sport I can say that my own experiences confirm this information. I have successfully healed two knee surgeries through corrective exercise, grounding my "electrical system" to the currents of the earth, and becoming a passionate sun food and super foodist. Now as I age, I seem to be getting faster, stronger, smarter, more efficient, adapting almost immediately to all situations. This is all done directly through fine tuning the physical vehicle so our higher awareness, enabling us to execute our intention as directly as possible.

(Recommended Books: Biology of Belief: Bruce Lipton, Born to Run: Christopher Mcdougal, Earthing: Clint Ober, Steven Sinatra)

Athletic Performance

The emergence of the meatless and raw food dietary approach to athletic performance has become ever more popular in recent years. Athletes of all ages, ranging from young teenagers to olympic gold medalists, are discovering the value of a primarily plant-based lifestyle. This is not an entirely new concept in the sports arena. In terms of publicity, the raw and plant-derived approach has received little to no attention. The overwhelming acidification brought on by the conventional diet takes an increased toll on the body of dedicated athletes, mainly for the reason that as we demand more from our bodies, our bodies demand more from us in terms of nutritional-fuel. Young athletes can get away with the indiscretions of a poor diet with seemingly unnoticeable symptoms, especially if they are naturally gifted. As the physical demands increase and we move up in age the body begins to show signals that we must adjust our nutrition practices, most noticeable in the forms of lactic-acid accumulation, muscular fatigue, delays in recovery, irritability/frustrations, chronic and nagging injuries, brain-fog, and stagnant/creaky joints(calcified-joints).

The accepted projections for the general lifespan of a professional athlete is between the ages of 25-35 in most cases. I believe this is a terribly inaccurate determination of human potential based on the poor standards that society is currently operating under. Generally 25 is the age a dedicated athlete begins to fully integrate the mental acuity of their sport with the physical application and evolve into a well-rounded athlete. I know from my own experience as a life-long driven athlete I only came into the wider spectrum of athletic capabilities at the age of 24. The body is designed to regenerate itself in response to wear and tear. In fact, there is emerging research indicating that when we do vigorous exercise our muscles require a consistent routine of equal or greater exercise to simply maintain itself as we move up in age. There is a large number of professional athletes re-instilling their careers in their late thirties and even late forties by changing their dietary practices. Many of the proposed theories and ideas on nutrition that have saturated the sports field have greatly limited the full potential of dedicated athletes. The corporate sponsors that help fund athletic endeavors from middle school sports all the way to the olympics are synonymous with the root cause of the cancer, obesity, and diabetes epidemic. Professional and Olympic athletes are not allowed to criticize their sports sponsors, and the individuals who compromise their integrity in endorsing soda, fast food, and sports drinks are rarely making those products a part of their daily routine.

The first key for the success of an athlete is optimal hydration before, during, and after their activities. Our bodies have a built-in cooling system that attempts to regulate body temperature as to avoid overheating. When we sweat the body is sending signals to cool down. If our sweat begins to evaporate during exercise this means we are most likely well hydrated. If our sweat is dripping profusely from our head we are most likely overheated and must hydrate in order to create balance. The popular sports recovery drinks that are generally marketed as "electrolyte enhanced" are actually overburdened with false sugars that stimulate false energy production. What we actually want are full spectrum salts that help our body hold onto water when we exert our bodies.. When we become dehydrated it can be because we either have too little quality salts or have an excess of refined false salts(table salt). When I finish a long cardiovascular workout I enjoy a celery-based vegetable juice, mainly in part because celery contains good amounts of sodium which helps to rebalance optimal hydration and recovery. If you consume a wide variety of water-rich fruits and vegetables you will naturally become more hydrated. However, make no mistake as this does not replace good quality drinking water. We need to consume both to maximize our results.

The foods consumed through the day should be in accordance with an athlete's specific exercise agenda (weight training, running, endurance, explosive, etc.). The main goal is to consume foods that are rich in antioxidants, amino acids, essential fatty acids, and are all around anti-inflammatory. The culprit that gets most athletes in trouble is inflammatory foods which promote the breakdown of the body, especially in addition to rigorous exercise and dehydration. Due to the biological individuality among the human species, the foods that most serve someone will be dependent on their ideal macronutrient ratio: the unique balance of carbohydrates to fats to proteins. Effective energy production and long term sustainability is going to be found by identifying what will work best for each person (See Section: **The Sunfood Connection, Calories**).

When an athlete chooses to approach a raw food lifestyle, it becomes even more important to understand their dietary ratio largely because they are removing heavily concentrated caloric sources from their diets. When we exercise our bodies go through a catabolic process of breaking down larger food molecules into smaller molecules as an energy source. The body performs efficiently by absorbing easily digestible food and shipping the biologically broken down nutrients to the muscle groups that are exerting energy. In order to activate our anabolic state, which is the growth of muscle tissue, bone density, metabolic regulation of macronutrients, and healthy hormone levels, athletes must consume nutrient-dense foods. The general idea in sports nutrition is that athletes(or anyone) can induce a prolonged catabolic state similar to starvation if they deprive themselves of necessary calories for a long period of time. The body begins to use its own healthy fat reserves along with muscle tissue to survive, leading to extreme weight loss and fatigue. If one replaces the simple calorie concept with nutrient-dense calories, then they will automatically reap entirely new results in their ability to sustain longer intervals of energy and initiate recovery much faster. The most biologically available nutrient-dense foods are plant-based foods. Plant-based foods are the most identifiable to the human body and require the least amount of digestive effort in comparison to animal foods (excluding bee products).

When presenting the idea of raw plant-focused foods as a superior model for enhanced athletic performance, it is not to be attempted as merely a general concept. It must be carefully thought out and executed as strategically as a skilled tactician of chess would methodically choose his moves with direct intent. The standard model of diet (conventional meat, dairy, cooked, processed, junk food) provides a young athlete with the illusionary sense of invincibility in the form of empty calories, believing that they can eat anything they want and maintain performance. There have been extraordinary athletes who have had great careers with little alterations to their diet but as soon as a serious injury occurs, usually from a lingering fracture or ongoing inflammation, serious nutrition must be implemented in order to offset the cause and eventually rejuvenate the body.

The multi-branched compounds known as glycogen is used by the body during exercise as the primary fuel (glucose) storage in the liver and muscles for fast-release energy. It is used for long-term sustainable energy second to fat deposits stored in the body. Glycogen that is present in muscle cells act as an immediate reservation for glucose to enter muscle cells. The liver breaks down glycogen into glucose, sending it through the blood stream to enter the brain and muscles. The factor that allows a malnourished athlete to sustain their activities is dependent on the glycogen that is available in the body. When glycogen depletes from the body without glucose and protein synthesis takes place, we may experience what is known as "hitting the wall". This is when the body becomes far too fatigued to continue the normal pace of exercise. When we use food as a tool we can replenish muscle and liver glycogen, resulting in decreased inflammatory response given off by the catabolic state (breaking down) and in turn increase our anabolic state (building up). The increased energy demands requires an increase of energy-replenishing nutrients. If we can decrease glycogen depletion in the muscles we will increase endurance capacity.

The effective absorption rate for greater athletic performance is based on nutrient timing, a planned out strategy on food intake from three phases of the day: Energy Phase(pre-workout), Anabolic Phase(post workout, 45 minutes), Growth Phase(remainder of the day). If we follow out this idea regarding increases in athletic performance then we can see how we could begin to implement the most powerful raw foods and super foods as our main source of fuel. When applying the first phase of a workout it is important to note that we do not want to ever work out on a completely empty stomach. Instead of using glycogen as the primary fuel for energy the body will end up using its own muscle tissues as fuel to compensate for the absence of glucose. The immune system can become suppressed if this is repeated for too long. It is recommended that you consume a carbohydrate such as fruit or honey at least 30 minutes before your pre-workout warm up. During the workout, while your body is in it's most catabolic state, it is important to replenish the muscles and keep your blood sugar levels high to resist fatigue. Honey mixed with a small amount of bee pollen is a great choice to help carry valuable amino acids to the cells and keep energy levels high. Continuing to stay hydrated throughout the entire work out is paramount to the body's ability to produce results. When the workout is finished there is a "window of opportunity" which lasts 30-45 minutes where the cells are very sensitive to insulin (insulin transports glucose into the cell). An athlete wants to take full advantage of this window by consuming a high-glycemic drink that is dependent on your ideal ratio. For example, higher in carbohydrates to protein. A smoothie containing a higher ratio of berries (carbohydrate) to chia seeds (protein) as the caloric base works great for me. When formulating a post-workout drink you want to limit the amount of fat as fats take the longest of the three macronutrient groups to digest. The goal here is to drive the necessary nutrients into the cells with the lowest lag time possible. The growth phase is the rest of the day after the workout, we want to consume foods rich in full-spectrum nutrition such as amino acids(protein), antioxidants(anti-inflammatory), essential fatty acids (hemp seeds, algae oils), and micronutrients (minerals, vitamins, enzymes). A big salad that is layered with fresh organic green vegetables, walnuts/almonds/brazil nuts, hemp seeds/pumpkin seeds, and your favorite cold-pressed oil will work great.

The information that has been provided above could easily become seen as merely a theory unless it has been put into consistent practice. Carl Lewis, 9-time Olympic gold medalist, is one of the most well known vegan athletes. He attributes his best athletic performance from the age of 30 to his dietary change from meat and conventional food options to beans, lentils, salads, fruits, and vegetable juices. Robert Cheeke is a famous bodybuilding competitor and author who, in 1995, asked himself a simple question: "can I build muscle without eating animal products?". He found out the answer for himself as well as hundreds of other bodybuilders following his example. The accumulation of vegan/vegetarian professional athletes are growing as the trend expands. The short list of recent and long term athletes include Serena and Venus Williams, Brendan Brazier, Alexander Dargatz, Nick Diaz, Matt Frazier, Mike Mahler, Mac Danzig, Kenneth G. Williams, John Salley, Marcus Patrick, Bill Walton, Robert Parish, Joe Namath, Tony La Russa, Salim Stoudamire, and so many more.

Activating Genius

"What to the physical mind seems to be the ceiling, to the higher mind is just the floor"
Bashar

Looking back throughout history, there have been both men and woman who have transcended all expectations that came before them. Somehow these bright individuals unlocked their treasure chest of unexamined abilities that they put into use and created legacies that have endured the test of time. The most exciting thing I believe looking back on these characters of the past is that they were all normal people with fears, insecurities, and faults like the rest of us. The only difference is that at some point in their lives something clicked and the padlocks of restraint were broken. If you can look at yourself as a locked treasure chest that just needs the right combination, the right insight or tool, that can turn on the triggers, then you will be able to become a true genius.

What is it to be a genius anyways? I believe a genius is someone who has become fully aware of their inherent gifts and have accepted their personal legacy. The idea of achieving genius is nothing more than coming to terms with who you are, with what your life mission is all about, and how you are able to communicate this to the world. There are multiple ways to bring yourself into this state but I would say there is no more direct avenue than what you put into your mouth. Our state of consciousness can be greatly enhanced by the food we put into our bodies. It can also be greatly reduced by the same accord. I find nothing more influential in the human experience than the subtle energies of our food which in all cases becomes our thoughts, feelings, and actions.

The idea of "activating genius" has a lot to do with "activating genes". Our genetic expression can exceed itself from the influence of plant medicines found specifically in the true super foods and super herbs.

Once someone has activated a level of genius inside of themselves everything begins to slow down. The clock may seem to speed up on occasion but that is because you are fastened tight into the flow of imagination. The energy that comes from being on purpose is infectious and, because of this, you begin attracting all the resources needed to keep the flow in motion. The goal here is to see things happening as they come or even before. The deep implications of each decision you make becomes clear in order to keep you on track. The disconnection of our abilities comes from rushing and ranting in a disenchanted world.

Keys to Activate your Genius:

- **Active Meditation:**

Meditation is simply the act of focusing all of ones attention on any given task, to be fully emerged in the process of creation. Whenever you are focused on something you are actively creating, whether it be sitting down in the silence of each breath or putting one foot in front of the other along the coast while soaking up the surrounding noises. A true master or genius has learned to be aware of their surroundings at all times. Beyond that, they are fully aware of themselves. It is easy to let our thoughts get away from us. This is why it is important to develop a tunnel vision focus so all of our thoughts and emotions are singularly aligned for the purpose of whatever we are putting into the world. We now know that when our mind is at ease and relaxed our brain waves are in an even flow, undisrupted by the unbalancing of negative or tense thought forms.

The ultimate goal would be to allow ourselves to be fully present in all activities like folding laundry, doing the dishes, reading a book, having a good conversation, preparing a fresh salad, and anything else that may come along. When you begin to pay more attention to the details of your life you will begin to activate subtle differences in those details. As Wayne Dyer once said, “when you change the way you look at things, the things you look at change”. Many times people overlook important pieces of their own life puzzle because they are simply not paying attention. They are putting their moment to moment attention on things that aren’t even happening, either from the past or in a uncertain future.

- **Tap into the Universal Intelligence:**

One of the greatest insights I have gained in my life is the idea that I myself am not as smart as my ego would like to believe. I have discovered that I do not know all the answers in life. The more I acknowledge this fact the more life confirms it for me. I used to believe that I alone was responsible for not only my actions but figuring out the best way to direct the sails of my ship. I have found out that the universe has an intelligent design I am unable to predict, and the more I try the more I get in my own way.

It is a true blessing to allow the world to take shape around me without my constant interference. We are taught that we must take action on every decision, that if there is a problem then we must jump up and enforce our will until the problem is solved. I have found that this is not always the case. Almost always the events that come our way are in our best interest and we just need to be accepting of this if we are to gain the spiritual rewards. In tapping into the universal intelligence that is seeking to move through us, it is important to listen to your heart when making tough decisions. Your gut feeling will never lead you astray; it is the chatter of the mind that gets us in trouble. A lifestyle centered around raw plant foods and super foods will help channel the heart connection while a diet high in cooked and processed foods will keep one at bay from their center and remain in their mind.

- **Interaction:**

The most repeated interactions of our lives will eventually shape our viewpoint in which our life is shown to us. In most cases I believe people are interacting with the world in self defeating ways which will hold them off from the possibilities they desire. The people we interact with will determine our personality traits, our confidence, our use of language, and our social awareness. The environment we interact with will determine our most frequent energetic disposition, our natural awareness, our connection with the planet, and general reverence towards life. The interaction we have with food will determine our perceptions, our chronic thoughts, our overall health, and our eventual legacy.

The Creative Flow (Zero Point)

There is a space in between our physical atom-based reality and the empty freely moving dream-like state which I consider to be the creative flow. In almost all cases we are spending our time in either one or the other state, rarely fusing them together to pull the forces of creation into their most appropriate destination. We are taught to respond and react to what we can see happening in front of us. We are not shown how to actively pursue the circumstances we can see as clearly when we close our eyes and open our hearts. Some spend most of their time inside their mind playing with ideas, dreams and wishes which I highly encourage all of us do. However, when inspired action is lacking then the dreams go unfulfilled. The creative flow is all about finding ourselves in synchronization with both fields of space. The ability to use what we can feel, see, and touch as building blocks to construct our dreams is where the heights of joy, abundance, and creative expression exists.

Keys to Maximizing the Creative Flow:

- **The Infinite Exchange Cycle:**

The unbreakable bond that each one of us shares with each living creature whether person, animal, plant, or tree is a continual feedback of energy from distributor to receiver. Everything is energetically connected, constantly attaching itself to similar frequencies that match, never attempting to hold space with a vibration that is out of harmony. What we put out into the world we do indeed get back at alarming speed. Our world is in a hyper flux of conscious awakening and, because of this, we are all being affected by the energies we allow into our reality. When we give a smile we are feeling the smile. When we give a hug we are feeling the hug. When we give our love we are living our love. The infinite exchange cycle is the flow of energy that is being put out into the world and coming back to you in which you give it out; it is the ultimate boomerang effect. No matter what you put out into the world it can be turned into a higher state of vibration. It can be elevated at all times and the results you wish to seek in your life can be heightened as long as you put out the most harmonic intentions that lines up with your hearts true desires. When you feed the world with your positive direction it will feed you right back like a powerful fire ignited by the passion of of the soul.

- **Transformation:**

All of the problems in our world stem from our own reluctance to do the inner work that is a prerequisite for true transformation. The issues of humanity are simply the collective mirror for all of us so that we can see the truth of our lives and make the changes in order to literally change, not only in our results but the greater display of the world. Each and every one of us has our own personal journey that is encoded in our DNA. Only we can find out what this is by taking one step at a time towards its realization. As we take these steps into uncertainty we find out about ourselves. True transformation is uncovering the shadows that keep us blind and rediscovering the light that is lit in our hearts.

When you take the focus off of changing other people and direct it towards your own development, those around you begin to catch on. The people that were not meant to share your space will be removed naturally and the ones who are deserving will learn to build themselves up simply by watching you do it first. The great tendency is to point out the faults of others, implying there is something wrong with them. If you look back on your own life I figure you could detect the moment you decided to make changes and I bet it wasn't done simply by a "Eureka" moment. Most likely someone or something aided you along the way. You must do that too by setting an example as most people need to see someone doing it first before they believe they can do it too. Almost everyone deep within their souls want more out of their life but the insecurities that are imposed upon us in society hold us hostage to mediocrity. Be the light you wish others to shine in the world; be the change you wish to see first and foremost. True transformation will occur only when we all take a focused and responsible role in our own personal lives.

Accelerated Learning

The way in which we all learn is completely specific to our personal needs, preferences, interests, and associations. We have been taught to learn through the methods given to us in traditional education structures such as text books, employed teachers, and a very basic slow-paced forms of processing information. In all honesty these techniques of learning are inferior to the way in which a human being was designed to break down, absorb, and assimilate information, exactly the way we do with food. We must pre-signaturize information by investigating it through our own experiential filters. Only then do we break it down by absorbing what is specifically useful for us and removing what is not. At the end of this process the information is only valuable once it becomes part and parcel to our personality at which point we are able to call upon it like second nature. We have been more or less dumbed down by lazy tactics that slow our brain waves, causing us to think slower, feel less, and do nothing. This is changing now and all of us can take action to activate our true potential.

In the book, **Outliers**, *Malcolm Gladwell* says that it takes approximately 10,000 hours of dedicated time to master any one specific practice. I believe this to be very true as I also believe by implementing certain techniques coupled with superior nutritional practices this process can be dramatically shortened.

As the gap between informational resources and accessibility become smaller, it becomes very clear that the confusion in our world cannot overlap common sense for much longer. We do not suffer exclusively from nutritional deficiencies. In most cases, we suffer primarily from informational deficiencies. The beginning cause of all disease is a closed mind.

Keys the Accelerated Learning:

- **Speed Reading:**

The ability to obtain information is vital in such a time where all information is widely accessible. I myself could never understand the vast groups of people who decided to remain sedentary while a small percentage of interested people took hold of the wheel that eventually steered them in the direction of their dreams. If you are one of the rare individuals who seeks knowledge then you can become massively talented at whatever you choose in a relatively short period of time by learning how to saturate yourself with proper information; saturate your mind with the ideas that the great minds that came before left us.

Learning how to speed read is an excellent tool to gain an advantage. Given the impossible task of absorbing all the ideas, insights, experiences, and literature in the world. we can at the very least stack the chips in our favor every day by getting a little bit better. There are different methods used for speed reading. I personally like to engage in multiple books at a time. I will sometimes pull out a book that is more like a story, another based on nutrition, and another on a different subject, going in between them as I see fit. By doing this, I noticed that I can absorb different information as my mind becomes stimulated by different ideas. Actually what this does is it trains my mind to plant new neural pathways in the same way introducing new exercises to your routine will train your muscles to be stimulated differently. Remember the brain, although technically an organ, acts like a muscle as it becomes stronger with exercise. It is always advantageous to your learning process to bombard it with multiple ways of integrating information.

If you can get into the habit of reading multiple books on different subjects you will be surprised how many books you can finish in the time it would have taken to read just one. There is nothing wrong with just focusing on one book at a time. I do this specifically if the book catches me in a certain mood or it is important I only focus on that particular book. You can use your left finger to scan through the lines of the book to enhance the speed, the eye traces the information much faster without losing track of what your reading.

- **Slow Reading**

The flip side to speed reading is attentive meditative reading. Speed reading is great as a technique for filtering information but slow reading is especially important for retaining and examining information. The grand mysteries in life make themselves known to us when we exercise patience and a genuine curiosity for the journey. When you find a book that strikes your curiosity I suggest you examine it sentence for sentence, picking up the subtle cues that may not be obvious at first. I have found myself discovering hidden meanings in literature that I have read multiple times but was unaware of it the first time around. For example, lets say you read only 12 books a year- that would mean you averaged one book per month. This may seem like an under accomplishment to some, but consider that if each book carried only one key piece of information that could shift the way you produced results then consider how valuable would that be.

As a martial arts student I was taught to value down time and use my time wisely as to further my understanding of the art. We would spend considerable stretches of time sitting in one position in deep meditation, freeing the mind of frivolous thoughts in order to allow deep insights to take shape. It is this attitude to learning that will produce a heightened awareness which, in turn, will allow you to pick up on the gems of wisdom most people overlook frequently. I remember one of my instructors told me he would read only one passage from his book per day and would spend the rest of the time contemplating the meaning within the words. Attention to detail is everything!

- **Auditory & Visual Learning:**

There are many different ways to learning information which can benefit all of our personal learning styles. Some people are more prone to grasping information through auditory learning such as lectures, audio tapes, and speaking words out loud. Some people are visual learners primarily. They can learn easier from watching information programs like documentaries, movies, or attending lectures. I personally believe if people would practice all of these different methods of learning they would far exceed all of their peers who only do one form of learning. Human beings are multi-dimensional in all ways and, in terms of integrating new information, this is no exception. I personally read, write, listen to audios every chance I get. I also watch a lot of movies and documentaries on subjects that captivate my interests to gain a wide array of perspectives that cannot attained from just one point of view.

Double your Failure Rate

"I've missed more than 9000 shots in my career. I've lost almost 300 games. 26 times, I've been trusted to take the game winning shot and missed. I've failed over and over and over again in my life. And that is why I succeed."

Michael Jordan

I remember being at a personal development seminar many years ago, hearing from the guest speaker, Darren Hardy, who is the head publisher for Success Magazine. He touched on something that has stuck with me to this day: "If you want to be successful in life you must double your failure rate". I immediately got excited hearing this advice because it clicked with me that you will eventually reach goals if you just keep moving forward in the pursuit of your objective. Everyone who ever did anything significant in life did not always know how to do it. However, they kept trying even when failure was repeatedly knocking on their door.

Thomas Edison, who created the first powered light bulb, is the perfect example of failing your way to the top. He failed over 10,000 times in creating his idea. Never once did he believe he was a failure though. Every time a mistake was made he calculated it and reworked his plan until the final failure turned into a massive success. I have had this experience in my athletic career, losing many basketball games and many Tae Kwon Do tournaments for extended periods of time until I was able to develop myself into a winner. That is when the winning streaks began. Those who are merely spectators might say it is a lucky streak but little do they know the blood and sweat equity that goes into becoming a success. You can take this approach in your entire life, your health, your nutrition, your lifestyle choice, and your passionate pursuits. The more you are willing to make mistakes the better equipped you will become for the fateful day you learn how to succeed!

Highs and Lows

In life we all experience a wide assortment of high points and low points. When we feel the highs, it can be like putting the gears into ignition, breaking through old barriers that once held us back. When we feel the lows, it can be the exact opposite, like an anchor rooting us deeper to the ground, making us feel unable to spread our wings. I believe a big part of peak performance is learning how to not only navigate through these stages but also how to use them to your advantage. I have learned through personal experience that live foods makes this so much easier to experience, cutting through the buffers that insulate us from our higher potential. Denatured, damaged, and de-mineralized foods absolutely contribute to the lack of creativity and enthusiasm, increasing the experience of passivity and boredom. Life requires movement and, to do this, you must have high energy that is circulating through the body and encouraging the flow to continue. This is exactly how you get higher, by moving your body through physical activities, your mind through different stimulating methods, and your spirit by engagement in life however that looks for to you.

When you get onto live foods and super foods your entire experience can be greatly enhanced for a number of reasons. The effect of this can sometimes be abused or become addictive because many of us in western society have been raised in what is called the alcoholic consciousness. This is the idea that when you experience highs in life you will be brought down to earth with a harsh crash or a massive headache as the case may be. What is the reason people are smoking marijuana, doing chemical-laden drugs or abusing alcohol? It's because human beings want to naturally feel high- it is definitely a normal state to be stimulated and feel like everything is good, like the world is not crashing around us and we actually do live in a blissful state of paradise. There is a saying that ties in with the idea of highs getting higher and lows getting higher: "We are not human beings having a spiritual experience rather we are spirits having a human experience". It is our inherent birth right to feel as high as possible, not in the artificial sense, but in the way that brings us closer and closer with our true emphatic state of being.

Keys to create harmony in your life:

- **Flexibility:**

Harmony in life is about bringing all factors of living together collectively, not just the ones that are most attractive and leaving out everything else. As I have mentioned earlier in the book, one of the most important tools one can use to their advantage is adaptability. Regardless of what life throws your way, your ability to remain flexible to the changing tides will allow you to get to where you are going. Flexibility is very important in all areas of life and. in terms of health, it is good to look at how it improves by implementing more foods rich in chlorophyll like green vegetables, juicy hydrating fruits, and important lubricating fat sources like avocados, olives, and coconuts. After becoming raw for a considerable amount of time, I noticed how limber I was without having to continuously stretch or warm up before workouts. This was a profound discovery as I have been into martial arts most of my life. I have had two serious knee surgeries and a lot of lactic acid built up regularly when I was on the standard cooked diet. I had no idea that another possibility existed. Although I do advocate working at your own level and practicing good body mechanics such as static and dynamic stretching exercises, one thing you will notice over a short period of time is that your need to stretch every day falls away.

The mind becomes much more flexible in its approach to processing information and handling everyday situations. Most people are stressed out, tightened up from head to toe, and stuck in mind games they play with themselves. I know the feeling all too well. The seeds of inadequacy stem from the energies we allow into our space. The outside influences like people, television, talk radio, etc. promote stress by lowering our naturally enthusiastic frequency. It can take years to reverse this condition and change the dial if you are attempting to do it by shear will power alone. The food helps ease the pressure of hypertension-related conditions and actually promotes more heart-felt living. When your heart, mind, and body are aligned in unison instead of separation, not only does true healing begin but a flexible approach to life is easily taken and there is little will power involved.

A skill I would seriously suggest every reader develop is flexibility in dealing with all types of varying personalities. We live in the most multi-faceted society in all of history where ideas, paradigms, and cultures collide. Peak performance is not just focused on the body, but a great deal must be directed towards our interactions with other people we share this planet with. I have found in my own experience that being adaptable to the different perspectives of others has proven beneficial in many ways. I have a goal to share this powerful information on nutrition and an upgraded lifestyle with as many people as possible. I have noticed the less judgements I have about the behavior of others, the easier I am able to slip my message into random conversations with those that may have not given it a second thought previous to our interaction. Another way we can become the benefactor in such situations is by adopting the idea that each human being has something of value to share, even if it is merely to show us the contrast of our personal beliefs. When we are only willing to converse with those that agree with us, we run the risk of overlooking gems of wisdom that can loosely fall out of someone's mouth. By paying attention we can gleam tiny nuggets of insight to apply in our widened view of the world around us.

- **The Miracle in the Struggle:**

The gifts in our lives are given to us in many different forms, one of the most profound is the miracle of adversity. Adversity is our greatest teacher. It allows us to face ourselves in a way that is so real and direct that we can see the truth in a situation where if everything was the way we ideally conceived it there would be no space for growth and, in turn, our journey on this planet would be less meaningful. What I find especially exciting about accomplishing goals is the effort towards them. If you knew no matter what lies in front of you and your goal that you will get there, come hell or high water, wouldn't you go full force towards it?

The struggle I see most often in people is in their health challenges, whether it be weight loss, reversing dis-ease, or poor self image issues. Even if you have the cleanest eating habits and take all the outside precautions to keep a healthy temple, that is only half of the equation. The biggest hurdle to overcome is our inner self and the emotional tendencies that come along with it. Sometimes people can become somewhat neurotic about their health journey as a replacement for the emotional voids they feel. We all go through adversity but it is how you deal with it that defines the outcome. Actually, it is how you are able to embrace it into your experience and use it as a tool to prosper instead of continue to struggle that defines character. It is rarely those who have the highest intellectual intelligence alone that succeed- it is usually those with the greatest emotional intelligence that make it to the top of the mountain. The rational mind always seems to get in the way of great achievements for some reason.

Along our health path I believe a part of it is to take on the role of the wounded healer. We are always healing ourselves of one thing or another. The scars of our past show up in interesting ways, sometimes physical, sometimes emotional, and sometimes mental. It is our job to find the remedy that works for us and apply it at every given opportunity. The more you can use tough times to your advantage the more you will attract situations that no longer call for you to learn those lessons.

Adversity is the state in which man mostly easily becomes acquainted with himself.
John Wooden

Raw Philosophy

"Learn to see everything accurately, learn to see what is not obvious"
Miyomoto Musashi

"Success is a refined study of the obvious"
Jim Rohn

The times we live in are by far the greatest and most exciting time to be alive in all of history. The ability to research any subject is fully available and the choices that make themselves to our door step could never have been fathomed by our ancestors. The technological innovations that are being sent our way are outstanding to say the least, the ability to outlive prior expectations with an even greater quality of life is here. There is no need to look left or right; it is staring you in the eyes and always has been.

We are finding ourselves delving into deeper advances everyday and it is not always by complication. In most cases, it is by getting back to basics and being able to build upon what has been done in a way that is intelligent, simple, and most importantly fun. The raw food lifestyle looks very different than it did 20 years ago. It definitely is different than it was in the 1960's when Ann Wigmore pioneered the health movement by introducing living foods and vegetable juice to the public. The beauty of our current times is that we have learned so much and come so far that more and more people are becoming living food advocates almost over night. The unexplainable power of raw organic produce, super foods, conscious water, and herbalism is so profound, so deep that it is completely experiential.

In the older days it was almost a last resort for those who were in need of immediate healing because, compared to the conventional menu of society, it wasn't that appealing. Many people had to be in a dire situation to be converted into living food supporters. Now it is becoming almost effortless for many because of the vast and growing options we all can pick from. The introduction of super foods has created some of the most amazing options for healing, sustenance, flavor, and superhero-like activation no one could have guessed was available. Before people knew about raw chocolate the possibilities were only so high but now anyone can have their favorite dessert with pleasure, love, and joy, putting away thoughts of guilt or fear. The introduction of ancient herbal infusions has elevated a level of personal healing that the options of the past could not penetrate alone. As we move forward into the realm of zero limitations, all ailments can be healed and improved on indefinitely for all time.

The choice to become a completely devoted living food practitioner is an intimate one and is entirely dependent on your own inclination. There are many in the community that frown upon some for not going completely raw. This is very disappointing behavior considering how not everyone is metabolically designed for this or even wants to be 100% raw. It is so crucial to remember that all lifestyles are a personal choice and all dietary patterns have holes; no approach is foolproof. However, I do believe that a raw living lifestyle can be the closest to perfect if done appropriately for ones own preference, non-dogmatically, and that will be an individual experience. The important thing is that we move closer towards a lifestyle that is in accordance with the laws of spirit, the planet we live on, and the intricate web of life that keeps us all connected.

The great discoveries in the field of health and nutrition is that it is becoming easier and easier for those who do want to be raw to do it effectively without feeling like they are missing something in their diet. I have seen a lot of people in this community who try so hard to be completely raw while sacrificing their health in the process. This is based on a simple principle of life that the more you push against a brick wall the more you push yourself out of alignment with spirit. It must be a decision that comes from within for it to be real. It cannot be based on some pseudoscience or just on someone else's experience. Any transitionary move that does not take place in the heart first will always backfire in the body eventually. It might take going back and forth between some cooked food before you find yourself in that place of absolute grace, where you smoothly move into a complete sun food lifestyle. If this becomes your reality then it will be for all the right reasons and you will no longer have the attraction to the old foods you once had partaken in. This is the disconnect with all diet programs; they focus entirely on physical appearance and disregard the spiritual aligning of the human condition. It is always based on getting results the fastest, and that approach can never get you where you truly desire to go.

I believe the drastic times we are living in has sparked a massive surge in the way we look at our lives from all areas, none being more important and sacred than what we put into our mouths. Speaking from my own experience, the greater part of society has spent most of their time eating for all the wrong reasons: "being hungry", "needing protein", "boredom", and for social gatherings, but very rarely is it focused intentionally on the needs of the individual. The food we put into our temple is meant to be a sacred offering. The food should be coded with its own consciousness that aids us in reshaping our entire food reality. In fact, everything we considered food in the past escapes our reality altogether.

The enchanted beauty that a lifestyle in which is built from the juiciest, most flavorful, living and electrifying foods in all of the world is something you cannot get from any other dietary approach, guaranteed. I have seen people's lives healed instantly upon sipping fresh spring water from the source, grounded by the earths energy. I have seen spiritual afflictions vanish from the introduction of fresh vegetable juice or a super food smoothie. The effects of adding in all the good stuff is that it begins to allow you to get onto the correct program by literally deprogramming you from the old paradigms of the past. It wipes the slate clean, the physical issues, the emotional baggage, the mental chatter, the spiritual burdens all leave you and it happens without struggle; it happens naturally the way nature was intended to operate.

Many people feel like they do not want to be in this world because it is so full of greed, sickness, and war. Once you begin this journey you quickly find out that the greater part of the world is at war because they are ingesting substances that promote the problems. They are at war with themselves and this causes outward manifestations of how they feel inside. Living foods not only cleanses the body, it replenishes the soul. In fact, it can light a fire so bright in someone's being that it sparks an illumination of the soul. Instead of someone wanting to get through life and go to heaven (somewhere else), they slow down and begin to do their real work here on earth, wanting to make this heaven as it was intended to be all along.

There is no telling where this journey may lead, but as you take steps forward, it will certainly help you get off the fence of confusion and desperate actions that lead nowhere. In *Paulo Coelho's* beautiful book, **The Alchemist**, there is a passage stating "*You'll spend the rest of your days knowing that you didn't pursue your Personal Legend, and that now it's too late*". In life it is true that you usually only get one or maybe two chances to pursue your personal legend which is ultimately your gifts in life. I have found from personal experience and watching others that living foods can give you another chance at life if you have felt like time has run out. It is never too late to be the radiant beacon of loving light you were born to be, not only for yourself but for the world.

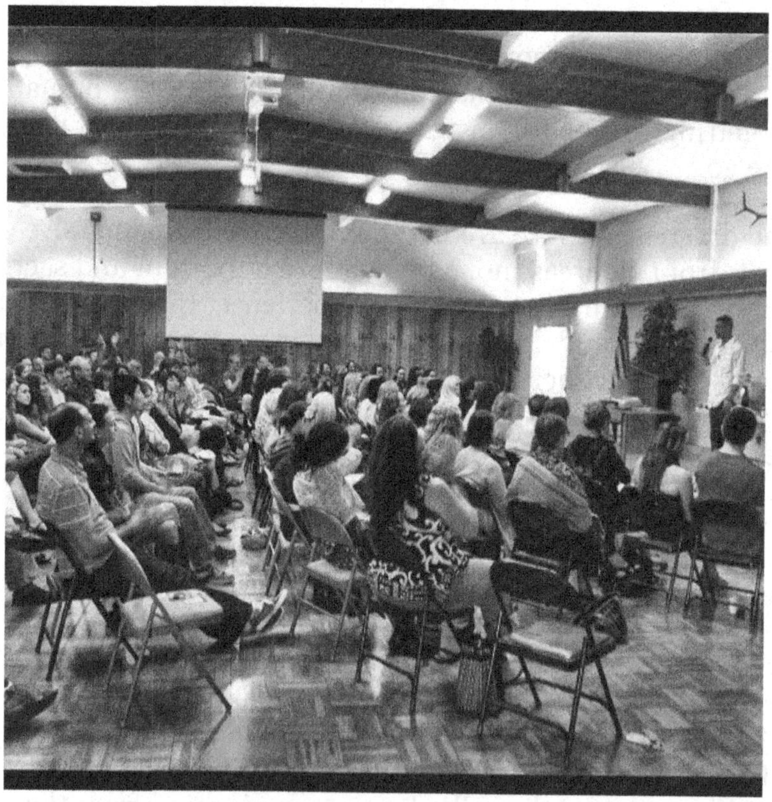

I have had to become someone completely different in order to become a voice for this message

Becoming Raw

The journey I have taken into raw foods has been one of inspiration, self revival, self reflection, and creating a new story for my life. Finding out that this lifestyle would be the centerpiece for everything I do in life was not only powerful but it was also unexpected. I have gone through many experiences that have given me deeper and broader insights for anyone who is becoming raw. This way of life is full of beauty on all fronts along with many challenges along the way that should be discussed as the path leads out.

When one follows out some of the proposed philosophies and ideas circulating in the raw food community, one thing becomes clear: most of the focus is on food. Anyone can look at this book and believe it is all about food but, in reality, it is not about food at all. Food serves as a tool or connection point for delivering results we wish to experience. Food, like any other piece to the puzzle, should serve as an integration for whole body enlightenment, not merely as an isolated factor.

Initially, the biggest obstacle is yourself and any kind of preconceptions you may be working through. I suggest in the beginning someone adds in any kind of raw foods they are most attracted to, with a completely zero-resistance attitude. It is a good idea to determine what your lifestyle requirements are ahead of time because the deeper you get into raw food living your day to day structure may experience some adjustments. You will find yourself visiting health food stores and markets more than before, sometimes several different stores in one day. I began to map out my day according to my shopping needs. It was not uncommon to find myself hopping from three to four markets in one day to find what I wanted. This can seem fanatical to many and in some ways it is. Raw foods is so much fun to jump into because it gives you a new perspective of what food is and drives the desire to explore the endless possibilities. My only disclaimer here is that you enjoy every bit of the process, savor every juicy fruit, and keep an open mind. The one thing that turns off people from becoming more raw is the unnecessary fanaticism that is associated with the health culture. When the mind becomes rigid then so does the body. Flexibility in all things is the great spark to accessing dormant layers of genius.

One of the most important and less talked about themes in the health/diet world is the distinction between short-term diets and long-term diets. A large number of people discover the magic of live foods through enduring some type of physical dis-ease and, if given a specific program to follow, can generate outstanding results they would not have experienced within their accustomed lifestyle. This, in most cases, can be considered a short-term healing diet, usually not designed for the sustainability of an individual's long-term lifestyle. A true long-term lifestyle approach must be developed long term as someone goes through life, fitting to their changing needs. This brings up the conversation regarding how much raw one should be for optimal health in the short and long term. There is a wide disparity of results from long-term raw food enthusiasts on all kinds of approaches, making it near impossible to give a definitive answer, although many people like to claim absolutism. I definitely do not agree with the traditional Natural Hygiene approach, a restrictively focused excluding all supplements, medical innovations, all animal products, and anything viewed as toxic. I believe many people get wrapped up in the all-or-nothing attitude towards raw foods and become confused as time goes on. In the short term (1-2) years an all raw food diet can be ideal for anyone (in my opinion). However, in the long term, many people may find themselves developing challenges that lead them to question the efficacy of this lifestyle and have them turning back to cooked foods.

The road blocks I see people get stuck with are actually very simple as long as one is willing to step outside the box, so to speak, and expose themselves to additional tools to keep them on track. The winter time seems to be one of the hardest times for many raw foodists to endure. Many people have a strong proclivity towards warming foods in cold climates. This can be worked around somewhat easily with the introduction of herbal wisdom by adding in warm teas. I like to make super food tonic teas that can be like meals in the winter time. If you let the water slowly heat just beneath boiling to avoid damaging the water molecules you can create a great warming drink. Another great option is using a dehydrator to warm your food instead of cooking food in a microwave or oven. Dehydrators are great because they warm the food up to the point that the enzymatic integrity is fully intact. Even slightly steaming vegetables can be a big help for many. Make sure you do not disregard the water because so much of the nutrition from the vegetable extracts into it.

Lifestyle needs must be addressed due to the versatility of physiological and social conditions. As an athlete I had challenging moments where the eating habits that gave me great results began to not meet up to my new requirements, forcing me to adjust. I said it before and will repeat it once again: as we change our lifestyle must change. If we are not growing we may be dying, or merely just dieting. When I was still in professional basketball training I began to notice after a while I was getting skinnier and skinnier, even as I put myself through a rigorous weight lifting program. I have heard this same complaint among many vegan and raw food athletes. This came as a result of both cleansing and a poor understanding of my core caloric needs. I was feeling small bursts of energy being followed by muscle fatigue, weakness, and light headedness on occasion. I went through the multitude of thoughts such as not enough protein, B-12, too much fruit, not enough fruit, and anything else that may have popped up. I actually found for myself, at that particular time, that adding in a few raw unrefrigerated eggs from a local farmer into a smoothie now and again had helped me get back into balance. This was an experience that allowed me to relieve my lingering notion that all animal products were detrimental to health as many of the raw food and vegan advocates tend to proliferate to the masses. The deep study into super foods, followed by herbalism, came to me which opened up another door. After adding things such as soaked chia seeds, hemp seeds, maca, spirulina, bio-fermented raw rice protein, goji berries, quality salt, and vegetable juices, my physical needs have been fully covered where I do not feel a strong urge for frequent animal products. A quick note: since I do not carry an ethical barrier with raw goat's dairy or unfertilized eggs I leave that screen door open for when it is useful.

Lifestyle has shifted dramatically while writing this book in this period of my life. I am not in constant training, working out 2-3 times a day, so my caloric needs are not as intense as someone who is under a heavy athletic regimen. As mentioned in greater detail in the chapter: **The Sun Food Connection, Section "Calories"**, your key to maintaining a lifestyle that you want is identifying your caloric ratio needs and then exploring a wide range of foods that fall into those categories. The more you can space out your food sources the more availability of different nutrients you will find, allowing you to cover bases you may have been unaware of. A popular tendency for raw foodists is to derive heavy caloric resources from bulks of fruit as a source of energy and sustenance. The problems with this approach long term and many times short term are detailed in the chapters **Deconstructing the Diet (Fruitarianism), Health Begins in the Mouth (Teeth Health),** and **The Sun Food Connection (Carbohydrates).** It is more important for someone to define for themselves what the line in their dietary lifestyle is going to be, high raw some cooked, all raw no cooked, all raw some animal products, all raw no animal products, etc. and then find out how that plays out in your own life. Do not use this as a straight-jacket, merely experiment with these "titles" and see how effective it is for you, both in the short term and the long term.

The phase you are at in your life is a factor I have considered for much of my own nutritional studies, yet it is not talked about in many health circles. As I have been exposed to many spiritual practices and eastern cultures from my involvement as a martial artist and an instructor, I have seen people of all stages develop in different fashions. I do not broadly advise everyone become a raw foodist overnight. I ask everyone to consider their personal needs and evaluate the platform in which they are living from. This means looking at all factors such as transitioning into a new lifestyle which will always create discomfort. You must be mentally aware of this and prepared to process through it. Factors such as the relationship status of someone is valuable to consider, the spiritual state they may be in, their career path is part and parcel to the direction they wish to go.

If someone is a seasonal athlete, for example, I would suggest they ease into it if they are in a heavy training routine. After the regular season would be a more appropriate to go fully in and experience the detoxification effects rather than attempt to balance this out through the stressful demands of performance. Super foods are the best aid in balancing the effects of detox while keeping the body and mind aligned. Without that added buffer of nutritional support one can lose focus of their immediate goals. Raw foods can be difficult to maintain until you find the right ratio of food groups that fit your individual needs. Do not burden yourself with guilt or negativity if you seesaw between cooked food and raw food for awhile. It is completely normal and eventually you will find the perfect place you fit in if you stick with it!

Avoiding Extremist Behavior

I have discovered many invaluable insights in my health journey as to what the seeds of sickness really are. The deeply ingrained behavioral tendencies each of us have must be identified and addressed in order to fulfill true health in the long run. A word of caution for those who are new to the health food culture, and especially the raw food culture: I have pointed out in different areas of this book that there is a heavy religious attitude that lends itself to the dietary field. There are divisions of certain camps that act as proponents for a specific dietary approach and, in many instances. veraciously attack those who subscribe to a different protocol. This single behavior is the downfall of many raw food, vegan, and paleolithic practitioners who, in many cases, are jumping from one band wagon to another. I have spent years trying to make sense of this irrational behavior as it has little to do with health and more to do with marketing and self-superiority. The conclusion I have come to is that when one is displaying these frequent tendencies it can only be identified as extremist behavior. Regardless of any health approach one chooses they want to avoid falling into extremes, jumping from one diet to the next, much like the way some people jump from one business opportunity to the next. The most appropriate way to follow dietary change is to piece it together one piece at a time. There is no golden prize at the end of this journey. Be easy with yourself. If you are not in a healing crisis then take your time to find what feels right for you. If you are in an immediate healing crisis then you will need to take more drastic measures but all bear in mind that you do not have to become rigid. Flexibility of then body and mind is recommended for overall physical and emotional health.

My Personal Diet

It would be near impossible to give a completely accurate break down of my normal dietary patterns simply because they are anything but normal. I have chosen to use myself as a human nutrition experiment, playing with many different approaches to find what works best for me. I have determined that there is no set system out there that I fit perfectly in. I have found that I produce energy on a macronutrient ratio that favors high protein, high to moderate fat, and moderate to low carbohydrates as a normal caloric spread. This is the very basic idea but does not even provide a clue as to what foods I am actually eating. Below I have put together a more in depth idea of my dietary lifestyle depending on the unique phase in my life I may be experiencing. I believe in eating for purpose and that changes with the seasons and periods of intention in my life.

Eating for Athletic Training

When I am in heavy training for sports I usually do a wide arrangement of activities to improve my body in many different ways. For example, just for basketball training I may be doing swimming/pool work training, weight lifting/explosion/body mechanic training, running/cycling/sprinting/endurance training all on top of my demanding basketball workouts and games. A lifestyle like this requires a well thought out ratio of foods to not only recover but to produce the right kind of energy for me to maximize myself.

A regular day may look like this:

- At least 1/2- 1 liter of clear water with MSM, lemon, and celtic sea salt.

- I may snack on a piece or two of fruit such as apricot, apple, peach, plum, or a small bag of cucumbers.

- A recovery smoothie, example (Coconut water with coconut meat, cacao powder, maca powder, mesquite powder, spirulina, high-grade protein such as hemp, brown rice, pea, a handfull of soaked goji berries, 2 tablespoons wild blueberries, 2-3 spoonful of soaked chia seeds)

- The next 3-5 hours may be snacking on any kind of nuts, seeds, berries, grapes, celery with almond butter, vegetable juices, or simply drink water.

- If I have another workout I will make another drink that is geared towards either cardiovascular/endurance exercise such as basketball where I will make a heavy green smoothie (kale, cilantro, avocado, cucumbers, etc.). If it is more weight-bearing exercise then I will concentrate on a much more wide assortment of protein-dominant foods like I have put together above.

- If I have a late night meal then it will generally be a big salad of green leafy vegetables, sun dried raisins, raw walnuts, 1-2 avocados and/or some avocado or olive oil.

Eating for Cleansing & Clarity

When I feel the need to bring more clarity and focus into my life I do so through nutrition as a first step. The foods that we eat can have a weighing down effect as well as a lifting up effect depending on which side of the spectrum we spend more energy on. When I choose to connect more deeply through meditation and creative insights I will minimize the density of my food and incorporate wide variety of power plants/vegetables/juices.

A Regular Day may look like this:

- 1-2 liters of clear water with MSM, lemon, clay, and sea salt.

- Anywhere from 40-80 ounces of vegetable juice (celery, cucumber, dandelion, parsley, apple, lemon, ginger, fennel, sprouts, etc.)

- I may snack on some fresh water-rich fruit through the day. I will abstain from heavier foods such as nuts, seeds, and thick smoothies to give my digestion a break. I suggest studying the chapters **Leaving Behind Excess** and **True Beauty: Abstinence** for a clear understanding of why this is beneficial for mental and spiritual clarity.

- To cap off the night I may fix a warm tea with herbs such as yerba mate, nettles, pau d'arco, horsetail, goji, he shou wu, etc. or 1/2-1 liter of clear water.

Eating on a Budget

I have found myself many times having to adjust my lifestyle due to financial downturns, especially through the greater duration of writing this book. Its a true blessing to have all the exotic raw foods, super foods, unique herbs, and supplements available through the most powerful medium called the internet but when we cannot take full advantage of these things then simple living is in need. These are the times I allow myself to venture into all kinds of markets I may have passed up before. The truth is, I found that many of these markets had better food than the higher end health food stores. Making great use of any farmers markets in your general area is a must, and developing relationships with those that grow your food becomes a very good idea!

A regular day may look like this:

- I will drink a little more water when I need to conserve food which can be a good thing! 1- 1 1/2 liters of clear water with MSM, clay, celtic sea salt, and lemon.
- I may have a tall glass of vegetable juice or a pint jar full of soaked goji berries and water. (Dried goji berries expand in water and increase life force, "Water Content")
- I may make a small meal out of raw almond butter with any kind of cut vegetables I enjoy such as celery, cucumbers, carrots, bell peppers, etc.
- At some point I will more than likely make a smoothie depending on what I have to use. I usually always make it a point to have soaked chia seeds and blueberries around as my base. I almost always have cacao in different forms (powder, butter, paste, beans) on hand at all times. This can be a good opportunity to use the things you may have had pushed to the side for awhile.
- The last meal of the night may be a big salad of mixed vegetables, sprouts, sun-dried raisins, sunflower seeds, coconut oil or avocado/olive oil.

Eating for Brain Boosting & Creativity

A huge focus in my life is now increasing the efficiency of my mental ability by gearing my nutrition towards brain health. I believe one key sign of health is in one's mental acuity, focus, and retention of information. Everything I do is actually moving me into this space but there are times when I become hyper-focused on building this factor in my life. I may take an entire week to create a day to day plan for stimulating the neurotransmitter production and other factors that go into brain building. I suggest you look over this section in particular and apply it to the information in the chapter **Peak Performance** for alternative tools aside from just nutrition alone. Keep in mind that most days under such a focused routine I will sometimes depend almost entirely on liquid nutrition because the oxygen is supplied more thoroughly to the brain the less we eat and more liquids we take in.

A regular day may look like this:

- I will drink 1 –1 1/2 liters of water with MSM, lemon, sea salt, and clay. I will not consume anything else usually until I have a full bowel movement.

- I will put together a late morning/afternoon super food smoothie (cacao, maca, blue green algae, sea salt, coconut water or spring water, honey, blueberries, marine phytoplankton, chia seeds, algae oil, noni extract, hemp seeds or hemp/flax oil, etc.)
- If I am snacking on through the afternoon it may be walnuts, jungle peanuts, goji berries, cacao beans, hemp seeds, bee pollen, or pumpkin seeds. These are all strong brain foods!
- I will most often make a strong green vegetable juice. Chlorophyll is one of the most powerful brain supporting substances/antioxidants/blood cleansers known in human nutrition. A typical juice may look like 3-4 stocks celery, 4-6 apples, ginger, burdock root, cilantro, collard greens, kale, etc.
- I find for myself that I do some of my most creative work/writing in the evening so I like to make high-grade raw chocolate with all my favorite ingredients to carry me through my furthest imagination. This may look like maca, goji berries, spirulina/blue green algae, honey/palm sugar/yacon root syrup, lucuma/vanilla bean powder, hemp protein, or bee pollen. I also use a wide variety of herbs in my chocolate such as mucuna, he shou wu, astragulus, ashwaganda, reishi, gingko, bacopa, etc. (See Chapter: **The Sun Food Connection: Adaptogenic Herbs**)

The Symptoms of Society

"Everything man needs to sustain health can be found in nature. It is the job of science to find them."
Paracelsus

Hypoglycemia

Hypoglycemia is the clinical term for low blood sugar (glucose) levels in the body. Glucose is one of the main sources of fuel. When the body does not receive adequate amounts the brain sends out signals to inform us that there is a problem. These signals may vary depending on the individual but always resulting in the increased desire to feed our cravings due to extreme malnourishment. The use of 'essential sugars' in the body is very important such as glucose (monosaccharide) and the long chain sugar molecules known as polysaccharides. (See chapter: **The Sun Food Connection, Carbohydrates**) The body is designed to create store houses of sugar in the liver known as glycogen. In an emergency situation, the body can pull from these reserves to convert it into useable fuel sources. When glucose enters the blood stream it requires the hormone insulin to act as a delivery agent, assisting fuel into our cells. Insulin is released from the pancreas when the blood stream is overloaded with sugar while unused sugar molecules are stored in the liver and muscle tissue for later use (glycogen). When the body senses blood sugar is too low another hormone is initiated by the pancreas known as glucagon which breaks down the stored sugar in the liver helping to release glucose back into the blood stream to regulate blood sugar levels. This can occur when hypoglycemic or diabetics go long enough stretches without food to supplement this condition.

The best form of sugar as I have pointed out before is natural sugar coming from plant sources. Plants contain information that can educate our biology in ways that exceed our understanding of how nutrients interact with the body.

Hypoglycemia, which is a precursors as well as a condition of diabetes, has become one of the biggest health epidemics today. The root cause of this condition is lifestyle choices either created by the individual or passed on from the parents. The entire lifestyle picture is of considerable importance as our stress levels greatly effect the bodies ability to absorb nutrients and relax as needed for repair and maintenance. The most obvious factor is the types of food choices the average individual takes into their life. The cooked, refined, and artificial carbohydrates such as bread, pasta, grains, baked foods, excessive sweets, and dehydrated foods that contain high calories with little to no minerals are major factors. As mentioned in the **Sun Food Connection: Calories**, the current nutritional theory on caloric intake is completely suspect and in my opinion has created a society of diabetic patients. The reason why many people experience hypoglycemia is largely due to lack of nutrients(minerals, amino acids, nutrient co-factors) and intake of empty calories along with debilitating substances such a rancid oils, conventional dairy products, refined sugar and salt, and improper medications that may have an effect on our kidney, adrenals, and/or pancreas.

The absence of quality nutrition in most conventional food choices leads to extreme binging when one in this condition has gone a short time without any kind of food consumption. Food addictions keep many people prisoners to their own easily reversible ailments causing a revolving door of sick care type of lifestyle opposed to a dietary ease and flow. The best advice I can give someone right away with a hypoglycemic condition is begin switching out the stuff you know is contributing to the problem. If you are craving something such as bread, potato chips, carbonated soda, or candy go with its most appropriate upgrade. Instead of binging out on a bag of chips get out a big bowl of blueberries or cherries and eat as much of that as you like. Discover whatever fresh vegetable or fruit you gravitate towards most, maybe its a cucumber, celery, a tomato, an avocado, coconut, or a hydrating watermelon. The suggestion of experiencing a wide assortment of natures palate in the beginning of this journey will take you along way if your struggling to make better food choices.

After awhile of doing this you may notice you do not experience intense hunger cravings as you did before due to the high nutrition your body is being fed. When the body is given what it requires to operate at optimal function it does not continue to request more than it needs.

Diabetes

Diabetes affects 25.8 million people of all ages
8.3 percent of the U.S. population

DIAGNOSED
18.8 million people

UNDIAGNOSED
7.0 million people

NDIC-National Diabetes Information Clearinghouse

The dis-ease known as diabetes has become exceedingly harder to deal with in our world, especially because the lifestyle choices many are making often times perpetuates the problem. The medications people feel locked into such as high blood pressure pills and insulin shots are merely band aids to a wound ready to heal itself if given the chance. The ways in which such conditions as hypoglycemia and diabetes have entered our lives are placed evenly on our own shoulders, its through giving our responsibility to corporate spokespersons that would appear to know more about whats right for us than we do, right? The biggest underlining message of this book is taking back our power by reclaiming our self confidence and strength through assuming full responsibility. This is done through making conscious choices for ourselves. If you or a loved one is enduring this ailment right now know there are many doors open to you to not only keep it at bay but to alleviate yourself completely and walk along a path of self healing that was never sold to you in a shiny capsule.

Diabetes is a metabolic disorder stemming from an individuals inability to produce either enough insulin or the cells cannot respond accordingly to the insulin that is produced in the blood stream. Diabetes type 1 was once termed 'juvenile diabetes' because it was most prevalent in children although can be found in all ages alike. This occurs when the pancreas is no longer able to produce whats called beta cells which are in charge of making and releasing the hormone insulin. The glucose molecules in the blood stream, over time, become overbearing on the system without insulin to escort it into the cell so energy conversion may take place, this is how "high blood pressure" happens. Diabetes type 2 is when the body does not produce enough insulin or the minimal amount of insulin being produced is ineffective, this is known as 'insulin resistance'. Immediately after we eat, our normal blood glucose levels rise, and with that so does our insulin levels. Insulin acts as a key to open up the cell in order for glucose to make its way in. When there is a resistance to the insulin that our pancreas is trying to produce, the receptor site on the cell may be able to use some insulin, but not nearly enough, therefore trapping these glucose sugars in our blood stream.

When our blood sugar reaches extraordinarily high levels, far exceeding our bodies ability to handle the excess glucose a process known as glycation occurs. Glycation is when sugar molecules non-enzymatically-bond with protein molecules in the blood stream, creating a combination of enzymatic and cellular confusion within the body. Due to the poor functionality of our enzymes to deal with the linkage of glucose and proteins in the blood, our body begins to create non-functioning proteins which over time can leak into other areas of our body haphazardly, such as the kidneys. As this condition of glycation is allowed to carry itself out our red blood cells become excessively "globbed up", creating "sticky-blood", making it impossible for these red blood cells to travel through tiny entrances into areas such as the big toe, the kidneys, and the capillaries of our eyes. At this point a process known as AGES(Accelerated Glycation End Products) has begun. This is simply an accelerated aging process that begins to produce markers on our skin, white spots, or "liver spots", or signs of damaged skin resulting from a type of retardation of our "epithelial cells", as toxicity fills our inner terrain we experience a loss of "cellular-intelligence". The epithelial cells contribute in the formation of our connective tissue and skin, along with a host of other functions such as the secretion of hormones, sweat, mucus, and enzymes. Large dosages of concentrated vitamin C plant powders are advised to help restructure damaged skin and reeducate tissue cells as well as provide important antioxidant support.

The long term effects diabetes can have on ones health are numerous including kidney failure, severe nerve damage making it hard to recognize if there is any kind of injury until its too late in many cases. Diabetes is currently one of the leading causes of feet amputations and damage to the retina of the eye. This is also a leading cause of heart problems such as heart palpitations, atherosclerosis, heart attacks, high blood pressure, and hyper tension. These effects are generally the result of an over growth of sugar (glucose) floating in the blood stream attaching themselves to areas in the body they do not belong such as the heart and the tiny blood vessels in the eyes leading to possible loss of vision.

The realization from the diet community that the western world has completely blown themselves out on carbohydrates had led to the stream of low carb diet approaches for weight loss and "dis-ease control". This makes sense from the vantage point we are exploring noticing that an over abundance of sugar in the blood stream causes metabolic disruptions leading to the health issues stated above. The factor that is almost completely missing from all health perspectives is that every person giving professional advice is doing so through their own perspective filter. A good example is the explosion of the controversial "Dr. Atkins Miracle Diet" which stood on the premise that carbohydrates were creating too much insulin in people leading to a condition called hyperinsulinism from too much glucose and we need to dramatically limit our carb intake. He argued that we must consume much more protein rich foods and saturated fats. This idea makes perfect sense when you look at it from the surface, if your blood sugar levels are high you don't want to compound more sugar so consuming more protein and fat makes sense. The problem with this idea is that through his perspective filter that means low carb donuts, more bacon, ham, and steak. From my perspective filter that would mean lowering the heavy consumption of all animal products, refined sugars, refined flour, most fruits and fruit juices and increasing the high protein containing carbohydrates such as green vegetables, sprouts, and vegetable juices. A "low carb" diet is not the key to alleviating a diabetic condition, the most up to date research is finding it is most likely the complete opposite.

Dr. Neal Barnard author of **Dr. Neal Barnards Program for Reversing Diabetes** has pointed out that in countries such as Japan, China, Cambodia, and Thai Land the populations have the lowest rate of diabetes as well as consume a tremendous amount of carbohydrates, these countries also consume a very low amount of fat in their diet, traditionally speaking. The people who have adopted a western diet of refined carbohydrates and processed foods of all kinds begin to reflect the conditions we find common place. Dr. Barnards research has found that the reason the insulin receptor gets blocked up is not because too many carbs but too much fat in the diet, specifically coming from animal products and rancid oils. This is not to say quality fats are bad at all but in the case of a diabetic condition the consumption of saturated animal fats, oxidized(cooked or spoiled) oils and fried trans fats reached its limit and now must be cleared out in order to start brand new. In a study published in august 2006 in an issue of *Diabetes Care,* it was found that patients following Dr. Barnards program were at least three times more effective than the American Diabetes Associations dietary guidelines at controlling blood sugar, he advocates a completely vegan diet. The American Diabetes Association has been quoted as saying *"Diabetes is a chronic disease that has no cure"*. With this kind of unconscious approach its no wonder why it takes the dedicated work of individuals to step outside the mainstream problems and find the most obvious solutions.

"Society is always taken surprise by any new example of common sense"

Ralph Waldo Emerson

The diabetic condition is not inherently a blood sugar problem, that is the obvious symptom. Diabetes is the most appropriate designation of a lifestyle that has gone far out of balance with nature and is beckoning for a wake up call. Those in high places that claim diabetes is incurable are easily swayed by the funding of certain companies that are at the very root of the problem. If our goal is to completely remove the problem we must address the roots in which the problem has risen from, the longer we treat symptoms the stronger the roots dig into the ground and eventually refuse to move out.

Dr. Gabrielle Cousens author of **There is a Cure for Diabetes** and operates the **Tree of Life Rejuvenation Center** in Patagonia Arizona is perhaps the most well known and successful physician working with diabetes patients. His approach is entirely based on live vegan foods and helping others understand what diabetes truly is by creating a lifestyle that removes the dependency on insulin. Dr. Cousens describes diabetes(specifically type 2) as one part hormonal imbalance between leptin(helps inhibit appetite, the absence of it can lead to uncontrollable food intake) and insulin, another part metabolic dis-regulation, accelerated aging due to inflammation, and involves a genetic disruption. The discoveries being made by Dr. Cousens and many others in the healing field are absolutely relevant to every human being living in society. The absence of quality nutrition is the issue, with this understanding we now know the number one cause of all health related deaths are the medications being prescribed both long term and short term. According to recent statistics 1 out of 3 children will be diagnosed with a diabetic condition, this is completely preventable with the right tools and knowledge to apply them.

Diabetes has many commonalities all of which have been shown to drastically improve on a live food lifestyle for a number of reasons. Those suffering from any disease are highly acidic causing chronic inflammation which impairs our bodies ability to effectively heal itself through the use of enzymes(See Chapter: **The Sun Food Connection, Enzymes**). It appears that because of the backed up amount of glucose(sugar) in the system, the sugar molecules actually begin to unnaturally bind with certain proteins unwinding enzymes, disassembling the insulin receptor cells and leading its way into the malfunctioning of our own DNA. This is what the acceleration of the aging process looks like on the inside of our body. When toxicity becomes so harsh it sets up a catalyst for these type of problems to occur. What may be at the root of this enzymatic problem is the severe lack of minerals in the body, diabetes like most health issues can be traced back to mineral deficiencies. When our body is well mineralized it helps enzyme activation in the body, when enzymes and minerals are decreased the body becomes less intelligent therefore performing at a subpar level. The best foods to add for remineralization are green leafy vegetables, green juices, sea weeds, sprouts, and super foods(in moderation) such as Spirulina, Blue Green Algae, Marine Phytoplankton, Cacao, Goji Berries, Bee Pollen, Aloe Vera, and Noni Fruit.

The omega 3 to omega 6 ratio(See Chapter: **The Sun Food Connection, Omega Fatty Acids**) becomes very important as the research indicates that omega 3's reduce insulin resistance and improve overall brain and nerve function. Walnuts are a good preventative and healthy fat source as they contain a good amount of omega 3 fatty acids. Raw Walnut and Almonds both contain an amino acid known as arginine which has been shown to decrease inflammation substantially, raw almonds have been shown in some cases to decrease insulin resistance by 23%!

Some of the most common factors that have been shown to increase insulin resistance are the best place to start working on yourself or a loved one. A diet that is low in fiber (cooked meat & dairy) can weaken the digestive system and cause blood sugar increases. Excessive caffeine can cause huge increases in insulin resistance up to 30% in some people. Smoking of all kinds easily impairs our insulin receptors, smoking has a thickening effect on our blood stream causing clotting not to mention over 4,000 known chemicals that are concealed in an average cigarette. Chemicals, Pesticides, herbicides and heavy metals all increase insulin resistance so shopping organic has never been more important. The fluoride in normal tap water has also been shown to increase our resistance to insulin. These facts and figures are in large based on *Dr. Gabrielle Cousens* extensive research and clinical experience over his career on the subject of diabetic conditions. Anyone who is dealing with a diabetic condition or knows someone should immediately go online and look into the eye opening documentary Simply Raw: Reversing Diabetes in 30 Days and find information on Dr. Cousins Tree of Life Resort in Arizona.

Diabetes Type 1 with Children

Diabetes type 1 which is found most prevalent in young children or teenagers although also found in adults as well has some very common triggers to be aware of. Children are being diagnosed as a diabetic younger than ever before because of the habits taken on by a nurturing mother and what is being given to the child at the moment of birth. The popularity of soy based baby formulas in place of a mothers natural breast milk has risen to outlandish levels. Almost all soy based products in the US are genetically modified and greatly increases the estrogen levels in both men and woman, this results in severe hormonal imbalances. It has been determined that 1 bottle of soy formula or "soy milk" is the equivalent to five birth control pills. According to Dr. Joseph Mercola (mercola.com) babies fed soy formula have up to 20 thousand times the amount of estrogen circulating in their blood stream than infants that are fed mothers breast milk. This is thought by many to be the reason so many girls are reaching puberty much earlier than ever before. Soy also contains whats known as a trypsin inhibitor that blocks the absorption of essential proteins. Soy is definitely not the health food we were led to believe for many years, the form of soy that many Japanese consume is completely fermented and at much less quantities than in the western culture.

One of the biggest triggers for diabetes is directly related to food allergies coming from contaminated dairy products. Conventional dairy products are contaminated with all kinds of environmental toxins, injected growth hormones, and loads of bacteria that is treated with antibiotics. This is an overwhelmingly dangerous combination for any full grown human to contend with let alone the fragile body of a new born baby. When a baby is born it has not had the opportunity to develop a defense shield known as the immune system. Just as a baby calf requires the inherent in-between breast milk colostrum when it's born we require the same substance from our own mother. The immune system must be preprogrammed like an empty floppy disc, a mothers milk has the correct genetic information for a babies body to uptake and develop into a shield. When we attempt to replace this act with synthetic soy formulas or the milk of another animal we interrupt the program by introducing a foreign compound and ultimately producing an inferior result.

When scientists were developing theories for why children were getting diabetes type 1 conditions they originally believed it was from dairy consumption. The problem they came across was that they found children in Japan were developing diabetes and never consumed any dairy products so they initially threw that theory out. The interesting fact they came across was the mothers who birthed the babies had all spent time in the US eating a western diet and consuming milk. The scientists analyzed the mothers milk and found a certain protein found specifically in cows milk called "Casein". Long time Vegan advocate and health educator *Dr. John McDougal* explains in many lectures that when certain viruses and bacteria enter the blood stream the body knows to eliminate them as they are considered unknown and harmful. After enough exposure to viruses, toxins, pharmaceuticals such as antibiotics the cell lining that normally protects us begins to weaken, especially if a baby that has not created a strong immune system is exposed early on. When certain proteins coming from meat or beta casein coming from milk enter the blood stream antibodies are created to ward off these foreign proteins. The problem is even though these proteins are being identified as unknown, the 'antibodies' can begin to identify our own amino acid(protein) profile that rests on the surface of the beta cells of the pancreas which are the cells in charge of making insulin. This sets up the babies immune system for failure in the early stages of life and can begin to initiate what is known as an auto immune disease.

(Recommended Books: There is a cure for Diabetes: Gabrielle Cousens, Dr. Neal Bernards Program for Reversing Diabetes: Dr. Neal Bernard)

Overview of Diabetes Prevention and Healing Protocols:

Habits to Avoid:

- Remove all processed foods from the diet (artificial carbohydrates, soda, sports drinks, candy, etc.)
- Remove all dairy and meat products from the diet.
- Remove as much high sugar foods as possible, even high sugar fruits.
- Remove all Soy-Based foods from the diet
- Remove activities that promote the increase of caffeine, nicotine, alcohol, and any other form of artificial stimulation.
- Remove negative associations from your core circle of influence(negative people will only keep you stuck)
- Remove the television from the area in your house you spend the most time in, the bedroom is for making love and sleeping!

Habits to Increase:

- Increase the consumption of raw plant based foods
- Increase green leafy vegetable juices
- Increase the consumption of fresh organic berries in place of sugar cravings.
- Increase the consumption of fermented vegetables.
- Increase protein rich super foods (spirulina, chlorella, hemp seeds, chia seeds, walnuts, brazil nuts)
- Increase the amount of positive uplifting people you surround yourself with.
- Increase the pleasurable activities in your life(meditation, walks in nature, exercise, reading)
- Increase the time you spend focused on your goals and legacy you wish to leave the world.

Drug Addictions

"It is no measure of health to be well adjusted to a profoundly sick society."
J. Krishnamurti

The subject of addiction is a very elaborate one and spans across many different platforms. Addiction is never as cut and dry as many would prefer to believe, it must be approached from all angles. The way in which our society defines a "drug" must be examined and understood before any real head way can be made. There may be no greater confusion among popular culture than what actually constitutes as a legitimate drug or addictive substance. The term drug has been described as "A chemical substance used in the treatment, cure, prevention or diagnosis of disease or used to otherwise enhance physical or mental well being". The popularization of chemical laced substances in the form of "medicine" have created a distortion of reality over the last century. Everyone should engage in critical thinking when it comes to the proliferation of synthetic drugs masquerading as remedies or outlets for any kind of healing relief. Observationally speaking, the biggest scam the western world was sold is the idea that drugs are to be outlawed when in reality we are being sold drugs at every corner we turn. As the content of this particular subject evolves the underlining idea behind serious addictions are resulting from essential nutrient deficiencies, imbalance of brain chemicals, misleading information, excessive stress, and a lack of purpose or not following ones mission in life.

At the cellular level there are biochemical reactions that are orchestrating situations to fulfill an addicts need. We know now from cell biology and the discoveries coming from our more recent understanding of physics that the information that is feeding our cells actually begins to influence how we perceive the world around us and this creates our reality. If someone is consuming an addictive substance they will be fed information that feeds their "bias" and eventually situations will be presented to them that confirm this, situations that offer what that individual is reaching for from a thought form perspective. The most direct and surest tool for reaching the heart of any addiction must be the introduction of higher quality nutrition, most specifically in the form of raw foods. Highly charged mineral rich and enzyme active plants hold the trophy for alleviation of all disturbing behavior. I have never in my life seen someone go from raw foods to street drugs but I have seen people go from destructive street drugs to raw foods and never go back to "drugs" ever again!

This is a quote I pulled from *Dr. Hyla Cass's* fantastic book **Natural Highs**;

In an average week, Americans drink, smoke or consume;
◦ 1 billion cups of coffee;
◦ 3.4 million cups of tea;
◦ 4.5 billion sugared or caffeinated soft drinks;
◦ 2.3 billion alcoholic drinks;
◦ 8.25 billion cigarettes;
◦ 400,000 tons of sugar;
◦ 20 million pounds of chocolate

"On top of this we take 20 million antidepressants, puff our way through 25 million joints and pop 1 million tabs of Ecstasy. Whether it's to relax, get a boost or just plain feel good, it is clear that we are dependent on chemical stimulants."

I do not personally believe in the conventional attitudes towards drug addiction such as strict confinement whether it be a jail cell or a conventional rehab center. I do think that when someone has pushed the hot button too many times extreme measures may need to be taken initially but the long term success is not going to be achieved with a straight jacket. The cause for most addictions in my opinion starts with what we put into our mouths. I have not seen any other approach that can have such an immediate effect as raw plant foods. The predictable result of habitually using denatured and chemically altered foods, excessive sugar, rancid fatty oils, animal products, coffee, alcohol, and extreme stagnation(especially in front of a television) will be kidney, liver, and adrenal failure(See Chapter **Leaving Behind Excess: The Adrenals)**. The serious depletion of minerals in the standard lifestyle has lead to addictions of "all" kinds, especially attachments to calorically dense cooked foods. The average American, based on the conventional food supply, is at best getting 4 minerals they require for proper balance, the body is shown to thrive on up to 90 known minerals in order to operate functionally on all cylinders. Magnesium is perhaps the most critical of all(in compliance to the others) fulfilling a wide range of physical, emotional, and psychological imbalances. The foods that contain the highest concentration of bio-active minerals are the absolute first resort in creating a solution to addiction through nutrition.

(Recommended Book: The Magnesium Miracle, Carolyn Dean)

The fat sources in ones diet are one of the most crucial element to investigate. The electrolytical activity within the brain is being facilitated by fatty insulation, this helps maintain nerve impulses and increase the neural protective integrity within our brain and nervous system. Those on the standard american diet are not the only ones who must pay attention, many vegetarians and vegans can run into these issues without ever knowing it. The popular vegan dietary protocol is usually the "low fat vegan" diet which is great for short term and detoxification but in the long term we know that fat soluble nutrients such as Vitamin A, E, & K2 play an important role in health. I have seen time and time again many raw foodists attempt to adopt the low fat or no fat propaganda only to develop food addictions to hybridized fruits, processed "raw" bars, excessive juicing, or heavy cuisine raw dishes to compensate for caloric replacement. Although I do not advocate meat, fish, or fish oil it is neural protective which is why if someone becomes a vegan the long term calorie sources should be examined.(See Chapter: **The Sun Food Connection: Calories**) The fine nerve fibers in the body require protective layers, otherwise they can de-sheath and become unbound creating disturbances in behavior and personality. Nerve damage leads to nervous system disorders, this can create cravings for heavier meals to feed or dull the pain. The addition of Long Chain Fatty Acids(See Chapter: **The Sun Food Connection: Omega Fatty Acids**) will dramatically boost and maintain ones equilibrium and mental focus. Saturated fat from coconut oil may lead the list in brain protecting foods as well as helping to body naturally form the cholesterol required for healthy hormone production.

The top mental problems in society are increasing the more deficient our food supply becomes, such afflictions include Autism, ADD/ADHD, Depression, Bipolar, Anxiety, Insomnia, Schizophrenia, and multiple Neurodegenerative disorders such as MS and Parkinson's disease. As these issues grow so does the rate of pharmaceutical prescriptions being distributed. Children are being labeled with certain afflictions without in depth testing or nutritional advising leading to early child hood drug addictions, "medication" addictions to be exact. According to Dr. Hyla Cass pharmaceutical medications tend to disrupt our brain chemistry by depleting the nutrients that are needed to create neurotransmitters. The production of these brain transmitters allows for the proper chemical signals to take place in the brain through the transferring of information. This information(neurotransmitters) is carried through the brain by what is known as VMAT(Vesicular Monoamine Transporter) in order to reach the receptor site that informs our synaptic connections(thought patterns). The long term use of synthetic medications such as antidepressants to correct irregular Neurotransmitter health can actually lead into serious side effects such as lack of libido, cardiovascular issues, and chemical depression(suicide). Once our serotonin or our dopamine(See Chapter: **Leaving Behind Excess: The Adrenals)** is depleted the initial burst received from these drugs(or any others) lose their effect. The tolerance to any substance will increase the use of it in an effort to recreate the initial stimulation experienced from the drug.

The big cause for excessive medication is a lack of a conceptual understanding for how nutrition and the chemical balance of our overall being relate. It has been suggested by many leading health educators that the number one reason for depression is lack of sun light, not a pharmaceutical deficiency(See Chapter: **The Sun Food Connection: Vitamin D**). The triple combination of adequate sun exposure, electrical sufficiency through a skin to earth connection, and the highest quality water for proper hydration could be the most successful package you ever subscribe too(See Chapter: **The Triangle of Life**). The PH level in our body helps determine many personality tendencies regarding acidic or alkaline behavior. I suggest you study the chapter **Alkalinity** very carefully, as the pendulum swings from either alkaline dominant or acid dominant our brain chemistry changes. The exploration into raw living foods can radically shift someones balance due to the flush of alkaline minerals and as a result positively alter the way someone interacts in the world.

An attribute of especial interest should be in the quality of protein we consume or more specifically the amino acid profile we require. What is not always understood is how the quality of protein actually determines how our body utilizes nutrients. As you may realize after studying this information amino acids are the building blocks that help the formation and performance of our entire body. Neurotransmitters are made of amino acids which go into activating the chemical response based on the intelligence of high grade nutrition. The acidic nature of most forms of protein (meat, dairy, cooked, processed) produce adverse reactions in the body and contribute to the deactivation of our higher intellectual powers. (See Chapter: **The Raw Naked Truth: Meat**). Two foods come to mind that have been receiving great interest in alternative nutritional strategies, Cacao and Blue Green Algae. These two super foods contain compounds that do great service in assisting the neurotransmitter production for long term brain health. Blue Green Algae contains many unique characteristics but the one of interest is what is known as 'The Love Chemical" otherwise known as Phenylethylamine. Cacao is the only other food in the world that we know of that contains the exact same chemical constituent but also does work from many different points of entry. For Serotonin to be effectively secreted a conversion must take place, the start of this transition begins with the amino acid Tryptophan(heavily present in cacao) which converts into 5-HTP and then serotonin. Cacao also contains large amounts of magnesium as well as the metabolic stabilizing mineral chromium. A big part of neurological disorders and addictive habits are related to blood sugar imbalances, Chromium is known as a regulator for blood sugar. One more thing to point out about cacao is that it most likely contains MAOI's(Monoamine Oxidase Inhibitors) or something extremely similar to it. These compounds allow the extension of our neurotransmitter production through inhibiting the recycling process in our brain keeping us in a feel good state longer.

Co-factors that improve the uptake of these unique nutrients found in certain foods and everything that has been mentioned are B Vitamins. B Vitamins are depleted when we experience stress which is what these vitamins help to alleviate. The adequate storage in the body of b vitamins are said to be co factors in neurotransmitter production, B2, B3, B6, & B12 seem to be the most important for this.(See Chapter: **The Sun Food Connection: B Vitamins**)

(Recommended Books: Natural Highs: Dr. Hyla Cass)

I have found in my own life and many others that the one factor that could outweigh all others in comparison was being fully intact with their purpose in life. If I had to pinpoint what the master switch was that could change the course from drug addiction to sobriety and focus it would be finding ones true calling, their mission in life. The nutritional and chemical components of addictive behaviors are absolutely important, otherwise I would not have gone to great depths to search them out, but understand these are merely tools to assist us over the hill we are looking to climb.

There is a saying in business which is "its who you know that gets you in the door but its what you know that determines how long you stay there". The choice to align with the proper lifestyle habits will get you in the door of where you are going but in order to get there you must find out why, like Anthony Robbins said, "*You need to turn your should's into musts*". Goals or a strong purpose in life can replace the dependency to use drugs, most of the time people participate in destructive behavior out of pure boredom, the down time in life is not appropriately used therefore it must filled with distractions, with noise in order to deflect that nagging voice that is calling you for something much higher. (See Chapter: **Integration**)

Overview of Drug Addiction Prevention and Healing Protocols:

Habits to Avoid:

- Remove all processed foods from the diet.
- Remove all conventional dairy and meat consumption from the diet.
- Remove artificial stimulants (coffee, cigarettes, marijuana, street drugs, pharmaceuticals, etc.)
- Remove all unsaturated fats used for cooking, (vegetable oil, olive oil, canola oil) replace with coconut oil.
- Remove tap water from your life (make sure you get a quality filter on your sink and shower!)
- Remove plastics from food or drink products (make sure to only purchase water in glass!)
- Remove all negative associations from your core circle.
- Remove all activities that drain your energy and attract negative behaviors from arising.

Habits to Increase:

- Increase the consumption of green leafy vegetables, fresh fruits, nuts, and seeds.
- Increase the green vegetable juices(at least one a day).
- Increase the healthy fats(coconut oil, flax oil, hemp oil, sacha inchi oil, krill oil, cacao butter)
- Increase the "soaked" raw nuts and seeds in place for standard snack food.
- Increase the consumption of fresh organic berries.
- Increase protein rich super foods(spirulina, goji berries, marine phytoplankton, chlorella, hemp seeds, chia seeds, maca).
- Increase the cacao consumption in place of standard chocolate bars. Add a serving or two of raw chocolate to your daily diet.
- Increase the amount of water you drink. Drink 2 liters a day with at least 1/2 tea spoon of celtic sea salt.
- Increase activities that bring out the best in you.
- Increase positive and supportive people in your life.

Orthorexia

Orthorexia is the clinical or psychiatric term for obsessive eating disorder or someone who is entirely focused on eating "health" foods. This condition is considered by the medical community to be a mental disorder where the individual will avoid all food perceived as toxic in order to purify their body, so to speak. This sort of situation has been most heavily related to raw foodism as seen by the general public as being far too restrictive and alienating from society. I strongly feel this type of situation is a by product of the abusive enforcement of our artificial marketing culture, the need for perfection is coupled with the desire to be different. There are those (myself included at one point) that feel the pull to disassociate from the negativity and flimsy moral foundation in which our fast food nation stands. This is an example of the neurosis of our society, where there is rarely a middle ground for balance and one will swing much too far into one extreme or another.

What we know of today as the modern day raw food movement was started largely in the early 1900's with what is referred to as Natural Hygiene. This way of life was predicated on the idea that self healing is achieved through cleansing, cleanliness, caloric restriction and self maintenance. These ideas are part and parcel to vitality and natural living which in those days, strangely enough, were radical approaches to what is now known as "disease care". The major push through the early and mid 1900's of this movement was by Herbert Shelton, who was a medical doctor and alternative health advocate. Dr. Shelton experienced a long list of legal troubles yet persisted to promote his message that fasting vs medical intervention towards disease was the most appropriate path to follow for healing. The natural hygiene approach has been shown to be very effective in alleviating dietary illness's and therefore was a powerful option for short term healing. The philosophy of this movement was very strict and relied heavily on certain views I would personally describe as dogmatic excluding foods or alternatives that have shown to bring balance for many people. I have found that this central philosophy has found it's way into the modern day health culture creating conflict, confusion, and a false sense of identity in many cases. When one becomes too ingrained in a single idea or philosophical imposition they will inevitable break down either due to physical needs or psychological unrest. Dr. Herbert Shelton spent 13 years battling a degenerative neuromuscular condition we may now call Parkinson's Disease that eventually took his life. The ideas he once implemented to heal others became unsuccessful to heal himself over the course of his later years. I believe this could have been avoided if he had adjusted to the times and explored other options that were available, not necessarily medical approaches, but alternative routes that were available outside of his personal comfort zone.

If someone has become far too invested into their diet to the point it becomes harmful to their overall life this is a clear definition of orthorexia. The need for balance has different meaning for different people, for vegans or vegetarians it will most likely operate within their own ethical beliefs. However you can bring harmony into your life do yourself a favor and explore those options, the end result of putting all your "eggs into one basket" so to speak will most likely lead to disappointment and sometimes much worse.When people become aggressive, rude, or irrational about food choices this is no longer about health, it becomes more of a false agenda.

Alkalinity

The choices we make through our day may be leading us in one of two states of living, an acidic state or alkaline state. The way in which we experience life is massively filtered through the internal terrain of our physical make up. Those that wish to experience more clarity, relaxation of the mind, muscular ease, improved cardiovascular strength, and overall richness in life will want to stack their chips on the side of alkalinity. When we are alkaline our electrical conductivity or capacity is greatly enhanced, when we are more acidic we become more dense which ultimately slows us down and enhances the aging process. We are seeing the greatest epidemic of age related illnesses at younger and younger ages through the scope of modern medicine. On the other side we are also seeing a great revival of youth related vitality in more accelerated ages as the power of a positive lifestyle becomes more popular.

In order to better understand the importance of maintaining a healthy lifestyle its good to know about the acid-alkaline-balance. In general terms its 80% alkaline to 20% acid ratio to keep in proper biological balance, of course this will fluctuate through different lifestyle changes and the simple nature of life. Imagine a sea saw with acid and alkalinity on each side, we want most of the weight on alkalinity while a small portion rests along the acidic end. We want to have both sides of the coin present, the only time we want to focus almost entirely on alkalinity is when we are cleansing from too much acidic foods and/or other negative contributors such as heavy metals, plastics, calcium deposits, chemicals, etc. Another time it is appropriate to completely alkalize your body is when your soul searching, the reduction of acidic food and calorically dense foods periodically can open up energetic pathways allowing for greater insights and focus.

A startling realization that came to me along my raw food journey was that almost 100% of food in western civilization was acidic and very few people even understand what this meant. The primary factor that makes food alkaline or acid is in its mineral composition. All foods contain dominantly alkaline minerals, acidic minerals, both or absolutely none in between which mostly deems those foods obsolete. All cooked food is acidic which reinforces my original statement regarding the popular western diet which has traveled worldwide. Alkaline minerals such as magnesium, silica, calcium, potassium, manganese, and iron are all found in organic vegetables. Acidic minerals such as phosphorus(found in nuts, seeds), and Sulfur(hemp seeds, MSM) are essential for aiding in bone, skin, hair, and muscle/tendon elasticity health.

The basis for the standard diet of society is centered around the root, seed, and muscle program which constitutes a fast food menu. The root would be the french fries(potatoes), the seed would be the bun, and the muscle is the piece of meat. If you take a close look at almost every commercial restaurant it is exactly the same formula in a slightly different form such as a bigger portion of fries or a baked potato, a bigger burger or a steak, and all the familiar sides of soda(chemical soup), milk or milk shake(Dairy). If this line up looks even remotely familiar then its definitely time to start stacking the chips on the other side of the sea saw. The easiest way to alkalize your body right away is by drinking as many green juices as you feel like through the day. The alkaline minerals & chlorophyl content will help replenish the blood helping to release the overgrowth of acidity and restore the body into natural balance. When eating acidic based foods combine it with green vegetables as much as possible as the chlorophyl helps create more oxygen in the blood cells improving digestion & nutrient absorption.

In his book **The Ph Miracle**, *Dr. Robert Young* firmly says the ideal Ph(Potential Hydrogen) level is at 7.365. Dr. Gabrielle Cousens believes a PH of 7.46 is ideal, Dr. David Jubb believes the perfect PH point 7.3 is perfect. I personally believe you will be just fine in this general range given the extremely alkaline nature of a well balanced life style of incorporating fresh organic vegetables, water rich fruits, super foods for increased nutrition, specific herbs(herbs are very alkaline), and the best quality water you have available. The blood requires high levels of oxygen(hydrogen) to send out information through the body signaling different responses needed for basic and advanced functions alike, these foods have the magic!

In the 1950's a biochemical researcher and professor named Dr. George Watson came to discover the role the dominant PH levels of our blood had to do with psychological and personality imbalances. Dr. Watson's research was focused on metabolic individuality and helping to get people back into balance using what was appropriate for their own constitutional type. He found people fell into three groups which are fast oxidizers, slow oxidizers, and sub oxidizers which determines the rate in which one metabolizes food into energy. Because many people are eating foods that do not agree with their unique needs it can swing them dramatically out of balance leading into personality disturbances. Dr. Watson found that when most people stray too far from the optimum PH of 7.46, which is slightly alkaline, the susceptibility of disease increases as well as psychological disorders such as paranoia, depression, anxiety, and a variety of other neurological conditions. He found when he brought the ideal PH back into balance the brain became much more effective in resolving these previous conditions.

Vegetables are extremely calming, eating a big salad at night is effective to calm our nervous system and reduce stress built up from the day. The normal inclination for a late night snack is something other than the best food for you. I believe one of the worst ways to prepare for a new day is to increase the level of acidity before sleeping, this will most certainly disrupt brain wave formations, constrict blood vessels, hinder cellular intelligence and ultimately promote inflammatory responses through out the body. If this pattern is continued for too long what eventually happens is the acceptance within the mind of mankind that getting sick for any reason is a natural facet of life. I propose that being sick is the furthest thing from nature and is entirely attached to an acid lifestyle. In nature animals who consume wild plants seem to beam with energy and never become struck down by civilized illness. Animals domesticated within concrete cities that adopt a processed or cooked diet also adopt city related disabilities.

According to Dr. Robert Young at around 2 pm in the afternoon your alkalinity should be at its highest and around 2 am it should be at its most acidic which is why many people find themselves getting up in the middle of the night to eliminate, the acidity has become so great the body needs to release toxins.

Lifestyle Factors:

There are other lifestyle considerations we should look at besides just food alone, its good to remember food is merely a tool that can open the doors to a higher quality of enjoyment in all areas of life. It was Bruce Lipton(**Biology of belief, Spontaneous Evolution**) the famous cellular biologist that taught me that each one of our trillions of cells is a mirror reflection of the entire human being. If we are out of balance in any way then so are our cells as they form the microscopic community that is built into our every experience in our lives. An easy way to grasp this concept is to consider the emotional response that is created from everyday occurrences and activities. Every thing we do from the words we speak, to the words we write, to the conversations we engage in have what I would describe as a cellular flooding effect through out our physiology.

Deepok Chopra brought to our attention that our body recreates itself every seven years or so. That means that we are constantly given the opportunity to turn back time on the repercussions of past mistakes or harmful actions. According to Dr. Gabriel Cousens in his book **There is A Cure for Diabetes**, "*Muscles get replaced every 6 months to 3 years. The pancreas replaces every 5-12 months. The liver replaces every 3 months. Our bones replace every 8 months to 4 years. Red blood cells replace every 90-120 days. The intestinal lining replaces every 5-30 days*". Everyday is truly the first day of the rest of our lives, all setbacks become a set up for personal reinvention. Every choice we make has negative or positive response on the biological nature of our body or perhaps we could say an alkaline or acidic effect. The concept of the alkaline battery is exactly the same as when we connect barefoot to the negatively charged grid of the earth. We automatically become alkaline because we are being "electrically charged" with clean energy opposed to the dirty energy of electro magnetic pollution.

The way we feel about ourselves from moment to moment is leading us in an alkaline state or acidic state much like the long term effects of what we put into our body. When we smile we release tension, yet when we are upset we induce constriction, whether it be food or emotions they have the same effect on the body. The beauty of following the live-it lifestyle approach is that it is all about self empowerment and choosing the best option at any given time. If you had no food, water, or money available what would be the most opportune thing to take action on. In my opinion it would be tapping into the power of laughter, the effort it takes to smile is the same as it does to frown, but the benefits are far different. In India there has been a movement going on called the Laughter Yoga started by *Dr. Madan Kateria* who believes this simple tool can be the best medicine. Laughter is one of the main reasons for social gatherings, the anticipation of positive interactions with others is what stimulates certain endorphins which attract us to one another. In Dr. Kateria's program groups of people get together to laugh hysterically at each other and themselves with great results. This idea came from the scientific research indicating the benefits of laughter and overall positive emotions on the body. Laughing helps release serotonin, and seems to allow for our immune system to work more efficiently, smiling also has a youthening effect on our appearance. Those who are happier in life tend to not only outlive negative individuals but also age more gracefully regardless of alternative lifestyle factors.

The great example of using laughter and positive emotion as a viable avenue for self healing is of the holistic health and peace activist, Norman Cousins. Cousins had been diagnosed with heart disease, told he did not have very much time to live he decided to take his life into his own hands and create a personal self revival strategy based on his beliefs towards healing. He began locking himself in a room watching old Marx Brothers comedy movies. He focused his attention on creating an environment of positivity, love, joy, and laughter. He believed that at least 10 minutes of genuine laughter would provide him with at least two hours of pain-free-sleep. He stated that, "When the pain-killing effect of the laughter wore off, we would switch on the motion picture projector again and not infrequently, it would lead to another pain-free interval".

Music is the great medium in which we experience the different sensations of life. The symphony of natures orchestra is continuously playing its tune, influencing the very vibration we are living our lives at. We have all grown up listening to different forms and genres of music which unknowing to most of us have either raised our awareness or dampened it depending on the tune in which it resonates. A perfect example can be shown from someone playing with the different tunes of a piano. If you play further to the left side of the keyboard the tone is uplifting and light on the ear, the further to the right it is more dense and heavy. Music in all of its forms has a powerful effect on the way we perceive reality and the feeling state in which we are interacting with the world. The levels of alkalinity in the body are increased by the amount of light we take in, the food that has absorbed the most light provides a more alkaline and fluid terrain. The tune in which we transmute sound has the same response because when we are more at ease, stress free and generally enjoying our own company everything operates better. When we listen to music that is heavier such as heavy metal or watch a horror movie our adrenaline is kicked on instigating more of a defensive and "stressed" state. When we watch a comedy, love story or indulge in music such as jazz, Rhythm & Blues, or orchestra our stimuli is no longer aggressive but moves into a place of restful inspiration.

The more inspired you can become each and everyday you will influence your physiology in a profound way. Remember happy joyful people generally live longer and more fulfilled lives than anal retentive health fanatics. Something to keep at the forefront of your conscious awareness. Flexibility in all areas of life is highly encouraged!

Inflammation

The chronic and debilitating conditions that the mass population are struggling with are a result of nothing more than an inflammatory lifestyle. When we consume too much highly acidic foods it has a heating effect on us, almost like spraying acid rain on our cells which then causes a defensive response in the body thus creating inflammation. The swelling that occurs from a cut, bruise, infection, burn or injury are white blood cells rushing to that area to ward of dangerous pathogens and invoke a healing response. Inflammation is the bodies natural response to an infection or injury and without it our wounds would never heal but when we have chronic inflammation that is a clear sign our body needs to cool down. Imagine a house on fire blazing out of control, that is what is happening on the inside of every human being eating a standard diet and living a standard lifestyle. When we eat a diet primarily of cooked or processed foods our body activates a white blood cell response(See Chapter: **The Raw Naked Truth, Cooked Foods**) stimulating inflammation in the stomach and digestive system.

When I worked in the emergency room I saw some very disturbing situations involving patients that had been treated for every kind of ailment one can think of. I worked with a lot of Hiv patients who most likely came in with alternative problems which were being blamed as a symptom of a weakened immune system due to the Hiv or AIDS Virus. Looking back on those years what I realize is that the lifestyle those individuals had committed themselves to had completely collapsed their immune system leaving them in an everyday state of acidity. It was not just those individuals but almost everyone involved in the hospital, whether patients or employees, who were deconstructing their own immunology and opening themselves up to colds, illness's, injuries, and all kinds of infections. The food selections in the cafeteria for friends and family of patients were likely to cause them to become patients very soon, the food being served to ER patients was much worse. Every single person exposing themselves to that type of "treatment" is not only putting a bandaid on the real problem, they are constantly inflamed from the inside out.

One of the main reasons for consistent inflammation in the body can be traced back to food allergies or food sensitivities. Everyone who has healed themselves of some kind of condition by changing what they ate knows exactly what this feels like. We can grow up most of our lives eating foods that do not agree with us, are causing us to have any number of road blocks in our health and never even make the connection that our problem may have something to do with what we are eating. Just as we have talked about before when we eat something that does not agree with our biological preference(hybridized/cooked food) our body immediately goes into an inflammatory state as a defensive mechanism. If we do not get the clues early on and continue to eat food that is not good for us our cells will swell up thus creating an environment more suited for parasitic organisms, and harmful bacteria. Most of us are coming from a situation where we have become easily addicted to foods we are really allergic too such as contaminated meat, and dairy products, every kind of fried oily food, an over abundance of sugar coming from soda, artificial fruit juices, high fructose corn syrup and every kind of junk food candy bar we can recount. The kind of stress these foods have placed on us has actually collapsed the immune system of most westerners making it difficult to consciously tell what food is good or bad for us anymore. It is imperative to make changes right away to reroute the direction of ones health, there is no time to wait to be as vibrant and free of illness as you can be.

The majority of our health problems are coming from what is going on inside of us, not necessarily what is going on around us. The key to getting our health back in many situations is not entirely dependent on what we put into our body but what we leave out of it.

Excessive alcohol and smoking have a very negative effect on our blood causing thickening to the stream, clogging our cells and reducing the cellular transportation of oxygen. The blood flow to our brain gets interrupted and that is what causes the light headed effect of smoking or the intoxicated feeling of drinking, its actually a suppression of oxygen being sent to the brain. All these things hinder our ability to become all we can be and therefore should be considered as extremely important factors to look into.

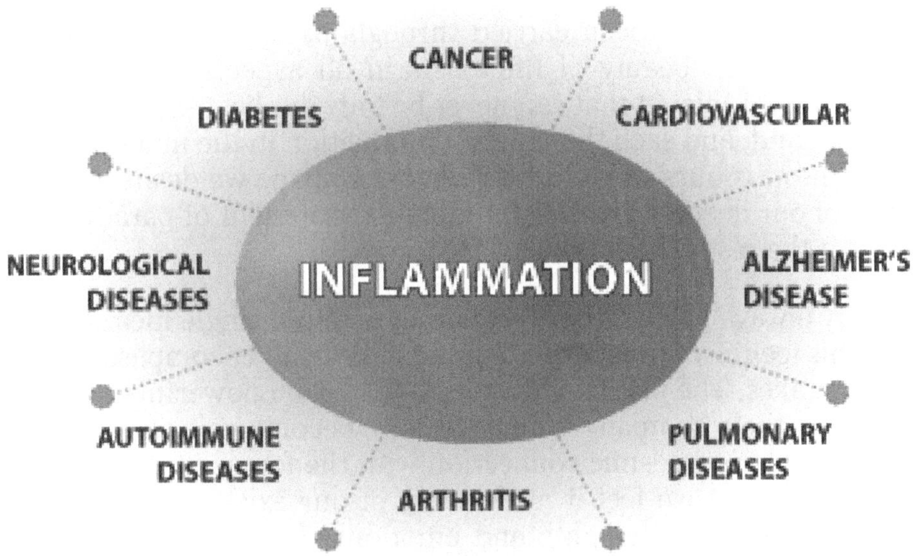

True Beauty

"Beauty awakens the soul to act"
Dante Alighieri

"Beauty is a manifestation of secret natural laws, which otherwise would have been hidden from us forever"
Johann Wolfgang Von Goethe

"The human body is the best picture of the human soul"
Ludwig Wittgenstein

The idea of beauty has been carried throughout the pages of time before pages were even available. The beauty of life exists in all aspects of creation, creating an everlasting mark on this planet that can never be fully duplicated. Each breath is special, each smile is profound, and each thought is a production in the making. The life we have right here, right now, is ours to mold into whatever shape we desire. We can be guided by the pleasure of our deepest dreams, building a monument of paradise that will stand as a testament for the rest of history to aspire towards.

True beauty always begins from resonating within a single idea. It can be any idea that transmits this feeling of prosperity. For me, it is an all encompassing passion for life in all the forms it takes. The plants of this earth hold such powerful energy that all those that spend time in their company will eventually become one with all of nature. The pure essence of beauty is a cosmic connection with the forces of the universe we do not rationally understand yet we feel it at the core of our existence. We mirror the exact reflection of our innermost thoughts and emotions. If our character is one of noble intentions it will become apparent on the surface. Those who focus on lack and disharmonious intentions will become burdened with the outer afflictions those energies attract.

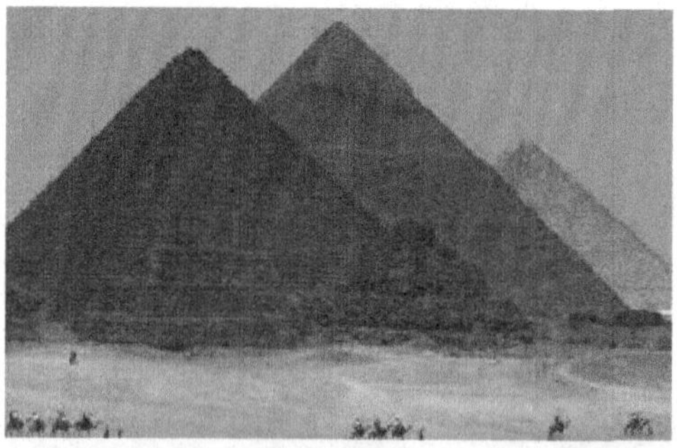

I believe in our exciting time of transparent transition. We must redefine the popular conception of beauty. In general terms, our socially accepted take on what beauty means is in complete opposition to the true nature of such a gracious word. Beauty never needs to be covered up with synthetic substitutes; it never needs to be air brushed because it holds no flaws or imperfections. The very idea that we have imperfections is our own insecurity that has been ingrained in our consciousness by a system that fears the result of inward thinkers. Beauty is expressed in the confidence of a person who has captured their heart's desire. They exude charisma and smile contagiously because life's brilliance is shown in every moment.

As we dive deeper into our own genius we come to find what has been missing all along- the search all human beings do for that one thing that will finally complete our soul. When we open the pathways to our heart, spilling out imagination that has the power to alter the tint of the world, we no longer need anything else. We must re-learn what beauty means by living in a way that promotes such an ideal. We must communicate with beauty, we must do business with beauty, we must eat for beauty, and, above all else, we must live with beauty.

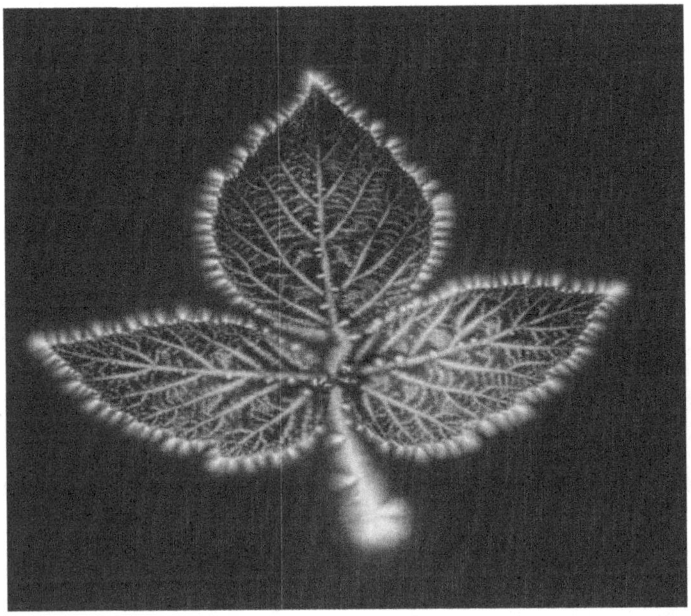

The beautiful energetics surrounding a leaf displayed through Kirlian Photography

Beauty Nutrition

The essence of our nutritional program should be held within the idea of beautifying our entire life. It should not only sustain our life, but should emphatically express our life force to the world. The energy we absorb through our food will translate to the world through our pores, the clarity in our eyes, the confidence in our speech, and the stride in our walk.

In many cases, what you put onto your skin is far more important than what you put into your mouth. It is always a good idea to consider that the cells of the body require nourishment before any other area of the body does but, on average, the meat of the body is being fed while the cells starve. The cells create the genetic blueprint for our entire body and the health of our cells will further translate to the outer coating of our skin. The skin is nourished by transdermal absorption from the substances that we put onto it as well as into it.

The cosmetic and skin care industry have for years been marketing products that claim to be beneficial for our outer glow but, in reality, the chemical additives and inorganic compounds found in these materials are not only detrimental for our skin, hair, nails, eyes, but also to our lives. Food has always been the most helpful aid for our skin health and outer appearance.

In order to achieve natural radiant beauty that is associated with soft subtle skin, clear of wrinkles, and unnecessary acne, we must choose a lifestyle centered around beauty. The thoughts we think should be positive in nature as our thoughts have cellular responses proportionate to the energetic resonance behind it. The intentions of our choices lead us to make additional choices that will either guide us towards beauty or its direct opposite. Everything we partake in has a corresponding effect on our exterior health. You can tell when someone has had a rough life because it shows up in their skin quality.

Foods that are high in antioxidants are especially important since many of the obstructions in our world such as pollution, calcification, pesticide exposure, rancid fats, radiation, and chlorine contribute to the destruction of all areas of health by showing up first in the skin. Oxidation occurs when there is damage to an atom or cell coming from a loss of electron transfers in the body, basically meaning damaged oxygen molecules getting in the way. This can happen from various injuries, toxicity in the body, or an open wound which is freely exposed to air. The same effect happens when you cut open a fruit and it soon changes colors. The fruit is being oxidized at this stage and eventually is beyond the point of healing. The same thing can happen in the body. That is why it is crucial to clean it up from the inside and introduce foods high in antioxidants. These foods can include all kinds of multi-colored berries, whole cacao beans, fresh fruits in season such as peaches, apricots, apples, kiwi, watermelons (with seeds), cherries, and especially seed-bearing grapes. Specifically the seed and skin of grapes contain a compound called *Resveratrol* which has been noted extensively for its antioxidant effects being linked to reducing inflammation, lowering blood sugar, and also aiding in cardiovascular health. The herb called japanese knot weed (polygonum cuspidatum) has been said to be the best source of resveratrol of any food source known.

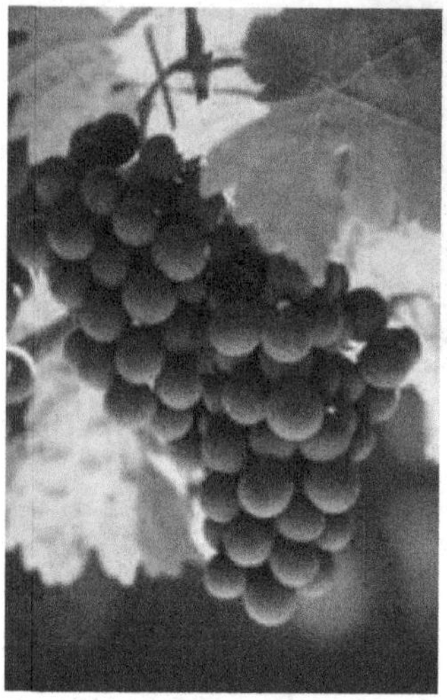

The best foods to eat in addition to those high in antioxidants are those with high quality oils, fatty acids, mineral rich, raw sources of protein, and generally alkaline in nature. Maintaining a lifestyle high in alkalinity is very important which is why we want to color our palate with fresh vegetation as we have talked about in the section on **Chlorophyll**. The wide assortment of natures rainbow mixed with herbs is possibly the best tactic for beautifying the body, mind, and spirit. This will aid in keeping the body well hydrated, limber (reducing the inflammatory issues that can cause skin break outs), and provide the right kinds of beauty minerals the body requires such as magnesium, sulfur, zinc, manganese, boron, and silicon. Foods such as celery, cucumbers, arugula, bell peppers, heirloom tomatoes, beats, figs, pumpkin seeds, hemp seeds, radishes and cold-pressed extra virgin olive oil are fantastic to make a salad with.

The skin is developed from collagen which is a type of protein integral for a flourishing display. In his book, **Eating for Beauty**, *David Wolfe* explains how collagen is subject to free radical damage caused by unstable oxygen (oxidation) and can be turned around by applying healing oils on the skin such as hemp oil, coconut oil, and stone crushed olive oil. It has been my personal experience that this is accurate as I have improved my skin quality by doing this, most specifically with coconut oil and consuming hemp and olive oil in my salads. He also states that the skin condition Eczema is often caused by the organs being filled up with unbearable amounts of toxicity that the body is forced to push excess toxins into the blood stream, making it necessary to get rid of them through the pores of the skin. In the chapter **The Triangle of Life,** specifically the section on The Sun, I explain how the sun contributes to our skin health and how toxic products are working against us in relation to the sun and actually how the sun increases our natural vibrance.

I would highly recommend you read **Eating for Beauty** along with all of David Wolfe's other works. I believe this book in particular to be the most complete and honest look at how our interaction with food and life affects our beauty not only on the outside but on the inside as well.

(Recommended Book: Eating for Beauty, David Wolfe)

The Law of Attraction

The spiritual laws of the universe are truly what governs our existence; not the artificially imposed laws of man. The law of attraction has been imprinted into our consciousness before we were enlisted into these physical bodies. Somewhere inside we all know that what we think about comes about. What we focus on manifests itself in our world one way or another. The moment we are able to accept this magnificent law of attraction we grant ourselves permission to become the beautiful artists who craft our dreams from the template of the stars.

In order to attract health we must become health conscious. In order to attract wealth we must become wealth conscious. This is the dynamic of creating what we want in our lives. We must become conscious as to what we are attempting to pull into our lives. It is important to open ourselves to the beauty that surrounds us at all times. Even when things seem bleak there is a pocket of light that can lead our way to a truly abundant reality. We never attract what we are unable to handle at any given time. Every situation that presents itself is a possibility to grow and move to a new level. If we wish to have more we must first become more and that usually means we must learn more. The road to beauty is sometimes taken through passages of contrast to deepen our appreciation for what we already have. A beautiful soul is one who has witnessed both light and dark, now able to decide which is most appealing.

I was turned on to an idea that has shifted the frame of how I view life: all of life plays out exactly the way a movie does. The world is not based in a linear straight and narrow way; it is lucid, expansive and always developing like a good story. The story of our lives play out moment to moment, and the more you can get yourself into the flow of your day the more you will pick up on the subtle coincidences that show up, leading you to where your thoughts are dictating. As soon as I adopted this attitude I adopted goal setting. I had been goal setting previous but I decided to do it in a completely new way. I learned from David Wolfe that when you spell something out you are actually casting a spell into the universe. It is key to write down your goals with a pen and paper. Do not do goal setting on the computer because as you use your hands to write you are activating your neural pathways in the brain to condition the mind in a way that lines up with what you want. Recall *Maxwell Maltz's* work **Pyscho-Cybernetics**- the brain is like a heat seeking missile aiming to find its target. You must condition your mind in such a way.

When you do write down your goals, do it in such a way that it becomes less about black and white statements and more about creating a story. Design your intentions in a way that it plays out exactly the way you wish for it to happen. Get creative and flood this experience with positive emotions as if you were living it already. When our thoughts are aligned with our emotions the our lives becomes ever more magical. The story begins to unfold in ways we could never predict because the surprise becomes the intention.

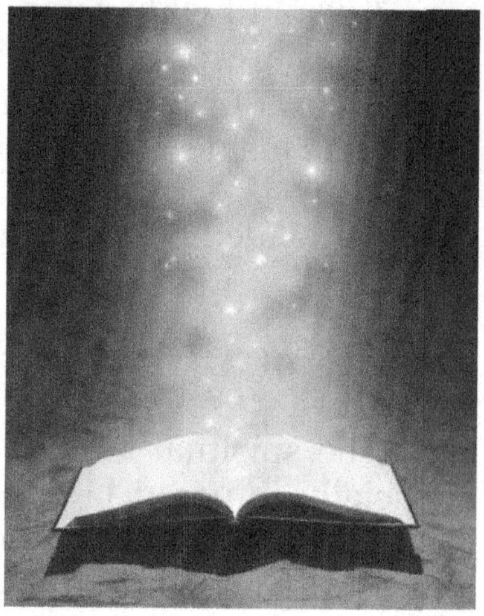

The best way to attract what we want in life is to develop the character of someone who is most deserving of that reality. If we wish for more paradise on earth we must synchronize our thoughts and actions towards its realization. We pull together the events that are in the nearest field of attraction as we are at each moment in time. As we change our thoughts we begin to attract different circumstances, and as we change our actions we attract different results. If we have not yet received what we passionately desire perhaps it is because we are not able to hold that idea in our current space, and perhaps we are blocking the entrance and must first clean out the closet, so to speak. The universe is intelligent. There is a higher mind at work which knows exactly what we need and when we need it. If we are merely bringing things into our life without letting outdated things go then all we do is create clutter. This can not serve our greatest good and that is exactly what the higher mind is aiming for.

Abstinence

One definition for abstinence is a voluntary restraint from indulging in bodily activities that are widely experienced as giving pleasure. The more you wish to increase your vitality, clarity, spiritual identification, and overall life force then giving consideration to the stripping of non-essentials is important. In the media-driven culture, consumerism is among the core values: to pile as much as we can in efforts to avoid the thought of lacking what others around us have. This idea has given birth to psychological turmoil in many and has nothing to do with health, wealth, happiness, or beauty. When we move away from a highly processed cooked food diet we come to terms with the beauty of achieving more by consuming less. As we strip the blockers from our lives we can see how each choice we make has an impact on the environment, the wild life, our economics, our food supply, and most definitely each other. It's very hard to receive abundance in your world when one is holding two catchers mitts focused on what they can get rather than what they can release.

In many cultures and religions the art of abstinence is practiced in different ways. Muslim tradition teaches fasting from dusk until dawn for an entire month on Ramadan which is the ninth month on the Islamic calendar. The Buddhists completely abstain from eating meat of any kind for health and spiritual purposes. In order to obtain true beauty that is supported by not only clean food but clean energy, we should involve ourselves in periodic abstentions of different kinds. The release of flesh foods and conventional diary from the diet is crucial for our times of great health challenges and spiritual evolution. At the very least it should be cycled in and out if one is not ready to completely let go. The goal is to produce the highest quality energy possible and to abstain from acts that place barriers to this process if done in excess.

The act of sex is the most common idea when anyone mentions abstinence. One's power comes directly from their reproductive organs. When one is sexually stimulated, all other functions of the body are up taken. A sure fire way to see if you are in good health is to look at your sex drive. I do not mean entirely your drive for sex, but the ambitious drive you have in your goal-orientated world. *Napoleon Hill* wrote a brilliant chapter in the book **Think and Grow Rich** which is titled **The Mystery of Sex Transmutation**. The word transmute means to literally transfer one form of energy into another, to condition the constraints of a specific desire to serve a more appropriate purpose. The desire for sex is by far the most powerful channel that motivates one's actions. Many will risk careers, reputations, relationships, and even personal values for the obtainment of it. The desire for sex is completely natural and is a sign of a hormonally healthy individual. Studies of the most successful men show they generally have high testosterone levels, indicating high sex drive. Those that have learned to focus their passion into creative outlets outside that of purely physical needs can create wonders this world can hardly explain.

Destroy the sex glands, whether in man or beast, and you have removed the major source of action. For proof of this, observe what happens to any animal after it has been castrated. A bull becomes as docile as a cow after it has been altered sexually. Sex alteration takes out of the male, whether man or beast, all the FIGHT that was in him. Sex alteration of the female has the same effect.

Napoleon Hill

Knowing that our power lies in our sexual glands we should take extra care of the direction of our lifestyle. We can literally modulate the increase or decrease of sexually driven energy by diet and living conditions. If ones desire for sex is too strong then it will cloud the mind, hindering his or her ability to make well thought out decisions. If the desire becomes too low it can lead to complacent or passive behavior. This can be the result of a hormonal imbalance and adrenal fatigue. The majority of foods being eaten from restaurants, fast food joints, and grocery stores are causing premature aging, resulting in lack of libido and motivation in life. There is an epidemic of over stimulation, hormonal disruptions, depression, and infertility. The long list of preservatives, fried fatty foods, chemicals, contaminated materials in the water supply, and processed animal products are creating a docile generation. When someone has lost there zest for life they have lost touch with their desire to live on purpose. Living foods can snap them back unlike anything I have ever seen.

The results are nothing short of amazing by introducing organic fruits, vegetable juices, mineralized super foods, and time tested herbs into the picture. By adding in more of these foods you are unconsciously abstaining from the lesser options of the commercial menu. It is not about reduction as much as it is about giving yourself a better option in place of the lesser one.

It is important to abstain from certain raw foods at pivotal points in our life for maximum results. I find in times of growth or confusion eating less opens up gateways to more creative outlets. When someone moves more into raw foods they can become very stimulated in many different ways. The unseen factors encoded in the foods actually transfers to the mind of whoever eats it. I have seen floods of artistic ideas come to fruition as ordinary folks make lifestyle changes. I believe in order to take full advantage of the increased desire for expression we should arrange our eating habits in a way that enhances that. There are many living foods that can increase libido and sexual drive, causing us to make physical desires the focal point of our attention. Abstaining from sexual activity of all kinds for a selected period of time can prove beneficial in many ways. The mind can transmute that powerful focus into any direction of your choosing. You can become much more in tune with your spiritual quest by cleansing sexual energy, especially if you have abused this aspect in the past. The body benefits tremendously because every time we ejaculate we lose important trace minerals that must be replenished through our nutrition. This time of abstaining from all sexual activity should be focused on cultivating power within oneself which will reflect on the outside as a confident, charismatic, and centered human being.

Foods that increase sexual potency are nuts of all kinds, raw seeds, cacao, maca root, coconuts and coconut oil, durian fruit, avocados, olives and olive oil, all bee products such as raw honey, bee pollen, and royal jelly. Fruits of all kinds such as figs, berries, watermelons (with seeds), and kiwi can be very effective for sexual boosting.

The act of sex is very important for a healthy lifestyle and brings two people together if done correctly. The act of making love has been left out of the bedroom in many cases, and replaced with a more Neanderthal-like activity where the spirit is not present. By taking time to do a sexual cleanse physically and nutritionally a new source of energy will come through you in all that you do. Sex helps clear the mind and as a raw foodist it is an experience that is completely unlike its cooked counterpart. When two people are spiritually connected the physical senses explode and the emotions run high, and when both participants are laying next to one another the energy is sustained.

(Recommended Books: Think and Grow Rich: Napoleon Hill)

Cultivating Love

Love is the driving force that creates and sustains all things. The deeper our love the more beauty we will experience on a daily basis. The flow of life literally moves in proportion to the current our river of love is moving. If we are moving with ease so will the events in our life, and they will generally be filled with joyful outcomes. Love is the center piece of all religious and spiritual practices. Beyond the superficial differences, it all ties back together through the act and cultivation of loving oneself, loving others, and loving our planet. The Garden of Eden and how that looks like in our world is the result of transferring the seeds that have been planted in our hearts to the fertile soil of the earth. The idea of heaven and hell being some far off locations is a bit farfetched. We are living those experiences right now. We are creating those experiences on earth based on the energies we are flooding our brain and heart with. If they are fear driven then hell will be an unavoidable outcome. But if they are filled with gratitude and love, heaven shows up every time.

Love moves through the atmosphere with the grace of a seasoned dancer, open your arms wide with a smile knowing in each moment you are the greatest expression of the Creator's brilliance.

I believe the most beautiful people in the world are those who have made a life path out of happiness and being in love with life. All the designer cosmetics will never cover up the ugliness of someone who has let their soul degrade and rot. No matter how much teeth whitener one uses, eventually they lose their teeth from committing too much time in destructive practices. When you eat foods that carry the energy of the earth you become deeply effected by it. In some way your mind becomes the mind of the earth. You gain insights and ideas that begin to lead your life in a much different direction than you could have imagined while eating dead foods. The cell wall of living foods still holds a consciousness; it has the ability to relay information to anyone who consumes it. Once you cook, broil, fry, or bake food then that information is lost forever, just as a library of knowledge is lost once a human life exits this planet unfulfilled.

Prepare your food with a conscious intention focused on peace and love. The field of energy we produce has powerful influences on all that are engulfed in it, especially the food and drink we will be putting into our temple. When you chop up your vegetables to make your salad do it with care, speak to your food if it feels right, communicate the message of loving appreciation at all times. As Mother Teresa once said, "*Love is a fruit in season at all times, and within reach of every hand*". It is always a good time to show someone you love them, it is always an appropriate moment to stop and smell the roses, and it is always a good time to dig just a little bit deeper on a rough day and draw out the seeds of love that have been there all along. Love is never ending; it is all enduring, and will outlast every negative event you could come across. It is time to develop your love mentality and to activate your abundance gene. As the great author Og Mandino has said time and time again: "*DO IT NOW, whens a good time, Now!*"

Remember to always do It with Love!

Integration

"It's lack of faith that makes people afraid of meeting challenges, and I believed in myself."
Muhammad Ali

"Ever since I was a child I have had this instinctive urge for expansion and growth. To me, the function and duty of a quality human being is the sincere and honest development of one's potential."
Bruce Lee

The true beauty in life is the step by step integration of our greatest skillsets and passions. Only we have the capability to share our gifts in the profound way we were born to. I am convinced beyond a shadow of a doubt that each human being was placed into this world to help shape the direction of our planet. The bottomless depth of the human experience up to this point has been unexplored. The true potential you have as you read this is available. It is urging your acceptance at this critical time in our world. By opening yourself up to the power of your own talents and abilities you unconsciously give others the permission to do so without enforcement or preaching.

The world right now is craving for people to wake up to their inner truth. The illusions of a surface-based reality where many are striving for material rewards while losing sight of the spiritual lessons is wearing thin. Many are taking up truly noble causes that resonate in their heart and promote a deep healing for all those that share this mission. As long as we are all moving towards our strengths and using our lives as vehicles for growth we are in direct accordance with the massive healing of not only our world but the universe that governs the great network of all life.

The children of our world are special beyond words. We must nurture their lives with all of our energies, and we must encourage all of their interests and focus much less on enforcing out dated theories. Each child that incarnates on this planet carries with them new strands of evolutionary DNA that will eventually birth new insights, new progressive ideas and potentialities we never considered but will one day grasp immediately. The future will one day rely on the decisions of the youth. We must have the foresight to be shining examples so that they may evolve their gifts and create a perpetual cycle of inspiration.

The most consistent quality of the super successful entrepreneurs, actors, artists, musicians, and all those embarking on their journey is the ability to be easily inspired. To inspire literally means to be in spirit; to be in the frequent frequency of your heart center or simply to move towards what excites you as much as possible. The feeling of inspiration is like the motion of strokes from an artist's brush. What the colors create from an empty canvas are similar to the rainbow that emerges from a rainy day. No matter how hard things seem at the moment or have been up to this point right now you can experience your greatest excitement. To see yourself as a gift to this world is what it feels to be inspired or to be in spirit. After discovering my gifts not a day passes that I am not inspired to reach as far as my imagination will take me.

It has become my experience that our nutrition should be up to par with what our personal mission is in life. When many get involved in new health ideas and approaches the great mistake is that there is no definitive goal associated with it. With every choice we make it should be taking us somewhere. Actually, it is taking us in one direction- we just have to make sure it is the one we wish to go. Every time we choose something to eat it is pulling us in a certain direction. It may seem faint but over time the destination we find ourselves in can be traced back to the seemingly insignificant choices we have made in the past.

Your own mission in life is completely personal to you and cannot be dictated by others. Everywhere in the world people are running around, focusing their energy on telling others what they need. In reality, only we know what we actually need. The best way to find your passion in life is to line up with what brings you the greatest joy. This feeling has been locked in a treasure chest for most people which is why many are trapped in a reality that causes stress, inflammation, poor relationships, and drives these individuals to make self-destructive choices. Nothing influences us more than the food we take into our body. The closer you get to nature the closer you get to your heart. The more you eat harshly processed foods the more you have to process your reality, making it nearly impossible to authentically express your gifts to the world.

Living foods over time will begin to change the way one thinks in the normal constructs of society. Your goals become something completely different because your values become something completely different. Instead of placing value on false beliefs and material symbolisms we are taken inside to discover the true value of who we are, the recognition of our soul which is the surest and quickest route to finding our true mission on this planet. When we ingest the negative energies of the world through false foods that do not agree with our life direction we are lured off the path of prosperity which the Essenes spoke of so long ago.

In order to gain full access to your magical powers you must learn the sacred art of integration. The ability to apply good information consistently like an intuitive scientist is paramount in importance. You must learn to filter out the non-essentials and allow the essential building blocks to form the solid foundation in which you walk your path. The true benefits of a raw plant-focused lifestyle only take shape when we integrate our highest thought patterns with our most authentic spiritual nature. To achieve success in all of these categories we need to apply the foundational principles every pillar of success is built upon. Incorporate more raw plant foods into your lifestyle as a step by step approach while focusing on the grand unfolding of your most pristine visions. This is not a short term solution that promises instant results in hopes of showing off your body for the summer and revert into old habits. This is a lifestyle design where you take ahold of the wheel. With every positive addition you make a negative subtraction takes place and, before you realize it, your entire reality becomes a masterpiece that all those around you now aspire to emulate.

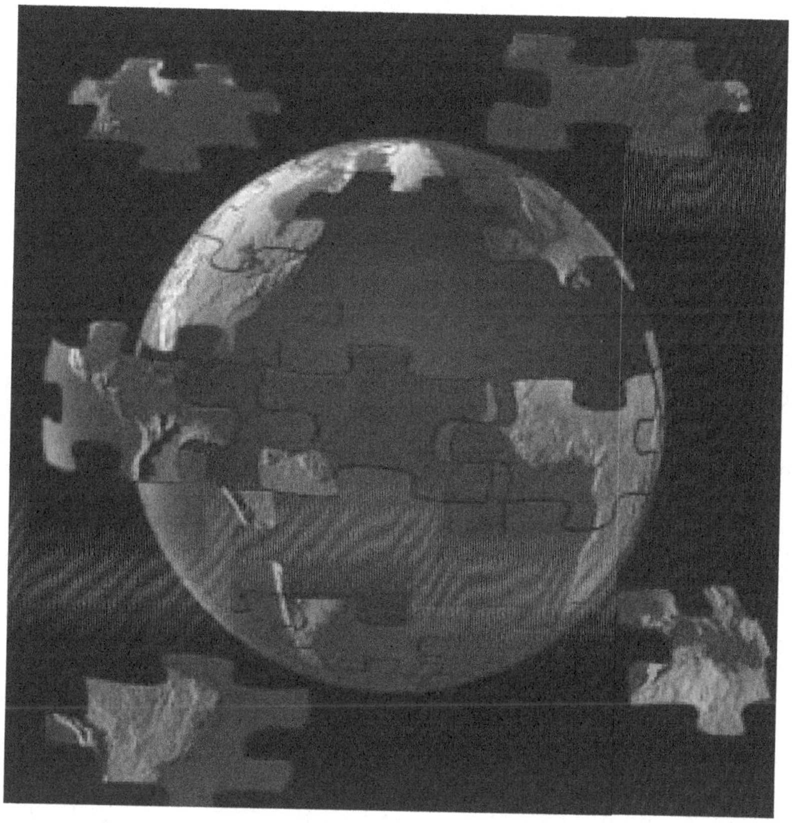

Global integration begins by integrating our individual efforts into the bigger picture

Message to the Reader: The Need for Soul Searching

I know well what I am fleeing from but not what I am in search of.
Michel de Montaigne

Trying to define yourself is like trying to bite your own teeth.
Alan Watts

This is a sincere message to all living food advocates, freedom of choice activists, and progressive individuals. You have made it to the final lesson sealed within these pages and an important lesson it is. We find ourselves in the strangest of times where each day is either a gift or a curse. The choice of how we approach any situation rests entirely on our shoulders. The responsibility of our lives is ours to bear with grace and courage. Every tool you need is already in your capable hands even though it may seem contrary to the fact. As you step out on your mission in life the secrets will begin to reveal themselves in the most mysterious ways, some a bit more obvious and some much more hidden. Therefore it is critical to pay attention to each intention that is sent out into the world like a rocket of desire cracking through every excuse and barrier of resistance left over from years of preconditioning.

We all begin with an equal start in life but the first 6 years of influences begin to shape the way we see ourselves and the world. We can use this fact as a crutch to rest on the hinges of mediocrity or we can use it as a launching pad to explore the untold stories that exist as the movie of your life unfolds. Whichever route you decide to take know that you are the director of your own fairy tale and the next chapter begins as soon as you wake up. We all get 24 hours in each day. The only difference between us is what we choose to do with those hours.

I have spent my teenage years and entire adult life studying the patterns of life and those who seem to be the most successful at it. The quotes in this book were carefully selected to invoke ideas and insights that you may use to deepen your understanding. The references used were delivered from searching out the most cutting edge, inspirational, and thought provoking pioneers in the fields of health, nutrition, personal development, and liberating leadership. I highly suggest you take what resonates with you and study some of these teachings from the past in order to create a solid foundation for the future. One day not far from now we will either be the long forgotten relics of time or unshakable monuments of what our children aspire to become.

This is a truly beautiful and artistic way to live which promotes exuberant health, a shining personality, radiant skin, ethically sound practices, and genuine relationships. As you progress in your living foods lifestyle the need for soul searching has never been more important than it is right now. The world is at a turning point in its history, leaving many in a state of fear and uncertainty. It is up to each one of us to be those light towers that serve to guide our brothers and sisters out from the darkness. This does not mean we impose ourselves or force feed our own belief systems onto others. We must express our message with hope and compassion because that is what the world needs at this time. The absolute most effective way to attract anyone to your way of thinking is to be the best version of that which you speak day in and day out. This is much easier said than done; it requires a daily one on one session with yourself. It can be easy to wrap ourselves up in some theory when talking to the public but it is very difficult to lie ourselves to sleep. I find that as I open myself to the magic of the universe and get out of my own preconditioning I change my mind about something constantly. What was once concrete has become softened in order to allow new ideas to take shape.

Remember the true purpose of this book is to provide new options for all who seek them. I am merely a dedicated voice for the most important message of our time. You are what you eat exists at the forefront of every natural law in which this world operates; there are no exceptions. What we eat influences our relationships, it determines our genetic expression, our food contains information that educates our cells in how we wish to experience our own reality. The greater our health the better we feel, translating into improved ways of treating all living beings around us. We become one with nature, no longer fearing its pure love. All those around us benefit as we center our lives on promoting this idea of a live-it mentality. The preservation of a single animal can create magnificent leaps in our consciousness. If we focus on nature's path to health we will get there naturally. When one human heals then a portion of this planet becomes healed instantly as the natural disasters we see are the result of all human life being thrown off balance. We are all one, connected to an infinite source of love and everlasting health.

Share this book with everyone you know as it contains insights that were literally downloaded from somewhere outside of my own understanding. However this work's true origins came to be, it has worked to heal my life in ways that still remain a mystery. I am in deep gratitude for finding the raw living food lifestyle for it has given me that edge in life that was missing. We are truly embarking on new and exciting times where the ways of the past can no longer sustain a future of progress. Take what makes sense to you and can be easily applied from where you stand. Do not worry about what is not useful for you but do not disregard it completely until you have experienced it first hand. We only know what we know at this very moment and that is an ever evolving reality.

I wish you the greatest experience your life has to offer and as always encourage you to take on all challenges as they serve to assist and propel you to new heights!

About the Author

I want to first share my deep appreciation for your interest in not only this particular book, but the field of study in which it lies. We are all students of life. As students, it is critically important we open ourselves to the possibilities that lie before us, and the ones we can not see visually but know by faith is just around the horizon. This work is the result of my own journey of searching for what it meant to feel alive; not just in the obvious sense, but that deep yearning for more than what I knew was available.

Early on, I was exposed to many different cultures and people that had their own traditions, beliefs, and philosophies that were different from what those around me were comfortable with. As I grew older, and took even greater interest in personal pursuits, I learned to take what was specifically important to me, and leave what remained for another to investigate. I also learned the importance of hard work and the subtle rewards such values would bestow on my life. The immortal words of one of my late mentors, Jim Rohn, have rung true through the years in which he advised "*Work harder on yourself than you do on your job!*" I have taken these words to heart and have never looked back.

I have spent the majority of my life involved as a dedicated martial artist and athlete. This is what has driven me for so long in working diligently towards increasing my abilities to one day become a professional athlete and Olympic champion. When I was nineteen I had encountered my first major knee injury and my first surgery followed. This event devastated me because I had relied on my athletic endeavors as a sign of self worth and identity. This would become my greatest catalyst for personal liberation. I had already worked years to correct the previous injury by the time my next surgery took place on the opposite knee. These were experiences that I did not realize at the time that would be the launching pads for the work I am doing now.

I spent the following 6 years after the surgeries working to heal my body as I moved towards my dream of playing professional basketball as well as becoming a world-class peak performance coach. I would be the first in the gym at 5:00 AM to do my first workout, and be one of the last to leave after the second, or sometimes third, training session in the day. My drive to become a professional athlete was the energy that fueled my life but obstacles in the form of injuries would keep popping up. These signs in the road would lead me to take my head out of the sand and eventually explore the world around me. You never know when the seeds of transformation will sprout, and that is what I always think about when looking back on this story. A close friend of mine told me when I had my first injury: "Ronnie you have trained your body your entire life, now it is time to train your mind". I would never forget those words.

I remember the day my first awakening happened. I was getting ready to do a training session but was so irritated with an ankle injury that I had I decided to investigate it further. I had spent years studying physical therapy, nutrition and the human body, but somehow the most obvious truth was still eluding me. I was introduced to a book by *Christopher McDougal,* titled **Born To Run**, which talks about barefoot running and the dangers of conventional shoes. As I played with this information, I began to witness instant results that drove my curiosity further. My further curiosity lead me to an online video about barefoot healing by David Avocado Wolfe, a health lecturer and raw food pioneer. This began my journey into what would become my life mission: to become one of the biggest voices for raw foods and generational sustainability in the world!

In the beginning, I slowly integrated this information by playing with it, and seeing where it would take me day by day. I had been studying nutrition and health-related modalities for years prior to this new direction, but much of it was within the confines of mainstream education and the misinformed fitness world. I now see why I am healing quicker, recovering from workouts instantly, and even performing better after moving away from the advice of mainstream "professionals"- something was very wrong with the system which health and nutrition is taught. This is what has initially led me to become a live food and health advocate. Eventually, I was able to move into a completely vegetarian lifestyle; leaving meat and conventional dairy products alone. This was such an eye opening experience for me because it truly allowed me to see the world with different lenses. I was now fully aware of the problems that most people face and don't even realize.

The defining moment came in the summer of 2010 when all the hard work on my health was paying off, and my first professional basketball tryout was coming up. This was the pivotal time in my life where I was going one direction and went completely another direction literally one week before the tryouts. I decided to not go through with the tryouts as I knew in my heart something had changed. I had learned too much, and I knew I had to use this opportunity to share what I had learned with others. I completely dedicated myself to the study and application of raw food nutrition, super foods, accelerated learning, and every bit of information I could get my hands on. I have been exposed to self development material since the age of 15, and have been applying it to business ventures and sports. Now I have a new purpose, and knew I could take these key principles to the next level: world wide healing.

The experiences I have had since day one have all been crucially valuable in my own development. I urge everyone reading this to value your own experiences and see the gifts in the struggle at all times. I have been a life-long athlete. I have been a full-time martial arts instructor who taught children, teenagers, and adults of all ages, and even managed and ran the martial arts studio at one point. I have been a basketball coach, and have spent a considerable amount of time around many other great coaches, athletes, and highly successful individuals in their own respective areas of expertise. I have spent up to three years working in the ER of a medical hospital in Oakland, seeing the absolute lowest levels of disease and despair which had greatly shaped my perspective in this field. I have also been around those who exude the heights of glowing enthusiasm. I have learned that true health and appreciation is a choice we make, and it is not dependent on just circumstances. We decide the lives we are to live, every step of the way; that is what this book is all about. Make the choices that will eventually lead you to the dreams you harbor deep inside because your dreams are waiting for you!

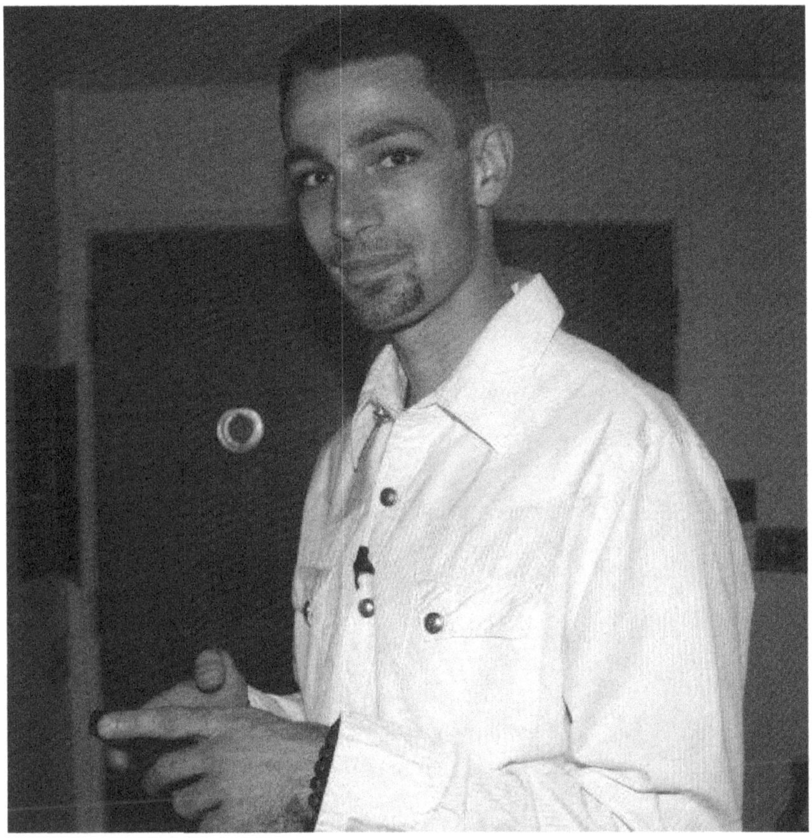

Raw Food Resources

Healing Clinics :

- The Hippocrates Health Institute (West Palm Beach, Florida)
- The Tree of Life Healing Center (Patagonia, Az)
- Hallelujah Acres (North Carolina & Ontario)
- Happy Oasis (Prescott, Az)
- Living Foods Institute (Atlanta, Georgia)
- Optimum Health Institute (San Diego, Ca)

Raw Food Resturaunts:

- Euphoria Loves Rawvolution: 2301 Main Street, Santa Monica, CA (310) 392-9501
- Au Lac Humanese Cuisine: 16563 Brookhurst St Fountain Valley, CA
- Life Food Organic: 1507 North Cahuenga Boulevard, Los Angeles
- (323) 466-0927
- Sun Cafe: 3711 Cahuenga Boulevard, Studio City, CA (818) 308-7420
- Real Raw Live: 5913 Franklin Avenue, Hollywood, CA (323) 461-4545
- Organic Avenue: 216 8th Ave (at 21st St.) New York, NY 10011
- Pure Food & Wine: 54 Irvining Place, New York, NY 10003
- Planet Raw: 609 Broadway Street, Santa Monica, CA (310) 587-1552
- Cru: 1521 Griffith Park Boulevard, Los Angeles, CA (323) 667-1551

Raw Food Recipe Books:

- Rawvolution- Matt Amsden
- Raw Food for Real People- Rod Rotondi
- I Am Grateful- Terces Engelhart & Orchid
- The Raw Food Detox Diet- Natalie Rose
- Everyday Raw Express- Mathew Kenney
- Raw Food Real World- Mathew Kenney & Sarma Melngailis
- Live Raw: Raw Food Recipes for Good Health and Timeless Beauty- Mimi Kirk
- Easy Sexy Raw- Carol Alt
- Ani's Raw Food Kitchen: Easy, Delectable Living Foods Recipes- Ani Phyo
- Bethanne Wanamaker: Super Food Beauty Elixirs
- Get Naked Fast! A Guide to Stripping Away the Foods That Weigh You Down- Diana Stobo
- Naked Bliss, Naughty and Nutritious Dairy Free Milkshakes that Make You Feel So Good!- Diana Stobo
- Chef Belive: Going Going Gone Raw
- Raw: The Uncook Book: New Vegetarian Food for Life- Juliano Brotman

The best efforts were made in reaching out to all published works for permission to use information. If anyone connected to any information or images that was used specifically for this book feels they did not receive the appropriate credit or reference for their influence please feel free to contact us and we will make all efforts to do so. The resources used for the informational content of this work have been recorded below within our best intentions and capabilities, some references may have slipped out due to the pace in which I have put this information together. All works were used for the best interest and health concerns of the reader and I ask that the reader use these resources as a way to further educate themselves!

Resources

Book used for Resources:

- The Answer is in your Blood Type: Steven M. Weissberg, Joseph Christiano
- Earthing: Clint Ober, Stephan Sinatra
- The Sunfood Diet Success System: David Wolfe
- The Longevity Now Program: David Wolfe
- Blatant Raw Foodist Propaganda: Joe Alexander
- Super Foods: David Wolfe
- Naked Chocolate: David Wolfe
- Eating for Beauty: David Wolfe
- Fats that heal, Fats that Kill: Udo Erasmus
- The 6 Week Cure for the Middle- Aged Man: The Simple Plan to Flatten your Belly Fat: Michael R. Eades, Mary Dan Fades
- Adaptogens: David Winston, Steven Maimes
- Water & Salt: The Essence of Life: Dr. Barbara Hendel, Peter Ferreria
- World without Cancer: Edward Griffin
- The Zone Diet: Barry Sears
- Biochemical Individuality: Roger J. Williams
- Natural Highs: Dr. Hyla Cass
- The Calcium Bomb:Douglas Mulhall & Katja Hansen
- Biology of Belief: Bruce Lipton
- Charlie & the Chocolate Factory: Roald Dalh
- The Structure of Scientific Revolutions- Thomas Khun
- Left in the Dark- Tony Wright
- Synthesis in Healing: Judy Jacka
- As a Man Thinkth: James Allen
- Think and Grow Rich: Napoleon Hill
- The Miracle of MSM:Stanley W. Jacob M.D., Ronald M. Lawrence M.D., Martin Zucker
- The Alchemist: Poelo Choehlo
- Enzyme Nutrition: Dr. Edward Howell
- The Veganist: Kathy Freston
- The Essene Gospel of Peace: Edmond Bordeaux Szekely

- ParasiteREX: Carl Zimmer
- Dr. Bernards Program for Reversing Diabetes: Dr. Neal Bernard
- There is a cure for diabetes: Dr. Gabriel Cousins
- Psycho Cybernetics: Maxwell Maltz
- Adrenal Fatigue: Dr. James Wilson
- Spiritual Nutrition: Dr. Gabriel Cousins
- The Evolution of the Brain & Intelligence: Harry Jerison
- The Ego & its Own: Max Stirner
- The Secret Life of Water: Dr. Masaru Emoto
- Your Bodies many Cries for Water: Fereydoon Batmanghelidj
- The Detox Miracle Diet: Dr. Robert Morse
- The Coconut Oil Miracle: Bruce Fife
- Cleaning Up! The Ultimate Body Cleanse- Kim Evans
- How to Eat, Move, and Be Healthy- Paul Chek
- The Origins of Human Diet and Medicine- Timothy Johns
- Secrets of an Alkaline Body- Dr. David and Annie Jubb
- Silica The Forgotten Nutrient- Klaus Kaufman
- Wellness Secrets For Life: A. True Ott, Ph.d
- 2012 The Return of Quetzalcoatl: Daniel Pinchback
- The Evolution of the Brain and Intelligence: Henry Jerison

Film/Documentary Resources:

- Discover the Gift-Producer Damien Lichtenstein, Co-Producer Shajen Joy Aziz
- Food Matters-Enzo Tedeschi
- Simply Raw: Reversing Diabetes in 30 Days- Nick Ortner, Mark Perlmutter, Keith Lyons, Scott Mader, Michael Bedar and co.
- Food Inc.- Elise Pearlstein, Robert Kenner
- Forks Over Knives- John Corry
- The Secret- Rhonda Byrne
- What the bleep do we know- William Arntz, Mark Vicente, Betsy Chasse

Scientific Research Studies & Valuable Articles:

Calcification

- http://articles.mercola.com/sites/articles/archive/2003/05/14/vitamin-k-part-one.aspx
- http://en.wikipedia.org/wiki/Hydroxylapatite
- http://en.wikipedia.org/wiki/Calcium
- http://www.thatsfit.ca/2010/08/06/calcium-supplements-can-cause-heart-attacks-and-do-little-for-bo/
- http://articles.latimes.com/2010/jul/29/news/la-heb-calcium-supplements-20100729

Aloe Vera

- http://www.internethealthlibrary.com/Plant-Remedies/AloeVera-research.htm

Maca

- http://www.ncbi.nlm.nih.gov/pubmed/19260845
- Subjective effects of Lepidium meyenii (Maca) extract on well-being and sexual performances in patients with mild erectile dysfunction: a randomised, double-blind clinical trial.

Vitamin D

- http://www.grassrootshealth.net/media/download/garland-gorham-mohr_sip_vit_d_prevent_2009.pdf
- http://www.grassrootshealth.net/media/download/johnson_sip_vit_d_breastcancer_2009.pdf
- http://www.grassrootshealth.net/media/download/grant-
- mohr_sip_eco_ultra_b_vit_d_cancer_2009.pdf
- http://www.vitamindcouncil.org/health-conditions/neurological-conditions/autism/
- http://www.ncbi.nlm.nih.gov/pmc/articles/PMC2913107/
- http://en.wikipedia.org/wiki/Vitamin_d
- http://www.psychologytoday.com/blog/evolutionary-psychiatry/201104/autism-and-vitamin-d

Dairy

- http://notmilk.com/deb/jd.html
- http://notmilk.com/j.html
- http://www.nutritionmd.org/nutrition_tips/nutrition_tips_understand_foods/dairy.html
- http://www.vibrancyuk.com/dairy.html

Diabetes

- http://www.effectsofdiabetes.org/
- http://www.immortalhumans.com/tissue-glycation/
- http://www.treehugger.com/culture/dr-gabriel-cousens-on-curing-diabetes-with-raw-food-and-on-why-going-vegan-makes-sense.html
- http://www.naturalnews.com/023012_diabetes_food_toxins.html
- http://www.naturalnews.com/028341_diabetes_living_foods.html
- http://www.gabrielcousens.com/PROGRAMS/REVERSINGDIABETESPROGRAM/tabid/1923/language/en-US/Default.aspx

- http://www.thelivinlowcarbshow.com/shownotes/2909/dr-neal-barnard-on-vegetarian-and-vegan-diabetes-control-episode-415/
- http://www.NaturalNews.com/032141_soy_products_diabetes.html

Genetics/Epigenetics

- http://www.phschool.com/science/science_news/articles/invasive_genes.html
- http://www.time.com/time/magazine/article/0,9171,1952313-2,00.html-Epigenetics
- http://www.anapsid.org/aboutmk/biochem.html- Biochemical Individuality
- http://www.ronsblogworld.com/?s=epigenetics&x=0&y=0- two epigenetic articles

Enzymes

- http://www.living-foods.com/articles/enzymes.html
- http://www.qualityenzymes.com/html%20pages/researchmiracle.htm
- http://www.enzymeessentials.com/HTML/enzyme_research.html

Cooking

- http://www.towardsfreedom.com/CookedFoodEffects.html
- http://www.ncbi.nlm.nih.gov/pubmed/18430446
- The effects of subchronic acrylamide exposure on gene expression, neurochemistry, hormones, and histopathology in the hypothalamus-pituitary-thyroid axis of male Fischer 344 rats.
- http://www.ncbi.nlm.nih.gov/pubmed/22459607
- Effects of acrylamide exposure on serum hormones, gene expression, cell proliferation, and histopathology in male reproductive tissues of Fischer 344 rats.
- http://www.ncbi.nlm.nih.gov/pubmed/21721575
- Acrylamide formation in almonds (Prunus dulcis): influences of roasting time and temperature, precursors, varietal selection, and storage.
- http://www.ncbi.nlm.nih.gov/pubmed/22992282
- Steam-cooking rapidly destroys and reverses onion-induced antiplatelet activity.

Meat

- http://www.forbes.com/sites/michellemaisto/2012/04/28/eating-less-meat-is-worlds-best-chance-for-timely-climate-change-say-experts/

Genetically Modified Food

- http://localnourishment.com/2011/05/13/genetically-modified-pesticide-found-in-umbilical-cord-blood/

Water

- http://www.cleanwater.com/types-of-water-contaminants.php

Environmental Pollutants

- http://www.chem.unep.ch/gpa_trial/14ddt.htm -DDT in Meat
- http://www.guardian.co.uk/environment/2008/mar/24/climatechange.fossilfuels
- http://en.wikipedia.org/wiki/Soot
- http://www.stoveaid.org/index.php?p=1_5_Environment
- http://www.foodispower.org/factory_farm_workers.htm
- http://www.savatree.com/whytrees.html

Detoxification

- http://www.gorhams.dk/html/the_lymphatic_system.html
- http://www.narryecaldwell.com/2010/07/the-truth-about-salt-and-your-digestion/

Brain Health

- http://www.thedoctorweighsin.com/obesity-is-also-in-your-head/
- http://www.pheromonetalk.com/studies-abstracts/second-brain-stomach-113.html
- http://www.huffingtonpost.com/daniel-amen-md/weight-brain_b_1182078.html
- http://leftinthedark.org.uk/node/4- Left in the Dark-Tony Wright
- http://en.wikipedia.org/wiki/Tony_Wright_(sleep_deprivation)

Grounding/Earthing

- http://earthing.com/index.php

Youtube Resources:

- Are Food Allergies Making you fat?- Ultra Wellness
- Gabrielle Cousins speaks about Reversing Diabetes 1-10- FreshandAlive
- Holistic Living with Gabrielle Cousins-Supreme Masters TV
- There is a Cure for Diabetes 1–2 - Conference of Life
- 20- Fruitarianism, Fructose, and Sugar- Drgabrielecousinsmd
- Dr. Neal Barnard program for reversing diabetes-sistsang
- Reversal of Diabetes???-naturalhealthrevival

- A cure for Diabetes through veganism: In-Depth with Drs. Neal Barnard & Gabriel Cousens- Part 1-2- Supreme Master TV
- Dr. Fuhrman- Value of High Fat Foods-headveg
- Is a 100% Fruit Diet Healthy ?- Dr. Gabriel Cousens-TheCoolVegetarian
- David Wolfe - Part 1-5-rawfor30
- Milk Causes Type 1 Diabetes & Autoimmune Diseases-headveg
- Effects of Diabetes-David Wolfe- naturalhealthrevival
- David Wolfe University Lecture Part one-Eight- Thebestdayever37
- Dr. Udo Erasmus: Healthy Fats & Oils for Vegans & vegetarians-Morealivede
- Let Food Be your Medicine and Medicine be your food- With David Wolfe- Longevitydvds
- David Wolfe on Calcium Part 1-6- TempleoftheRaw
- Why Soy is not a health food-Mercola
- Dairy & Diabetes- upcycle
- Essential Information about Vitamin D Pt.1-7- Mercola
- Roger J. Williams and the Science of Individuality] By Jeff Riggenbach

Additional Internet Websites:

- http://www.bewellbuzz.com
- http://www.thebestdayever.com
- http://www.naturalnews.com
- http://www.sacredchocolate.com
- http://www.mercola.com
- http://www.notmilk.com

Product Resources:

- http://www.longevityreview.com

Photo Credits:

- Many of the images used were found online and the direct source of these images were not found.

Made in United States
North Haven, CT
05 November 2026

21766164R00174